AF324323

Environmental CNS Stimulation in **Aging, Health** and **Disease**

Environmental CNS Stimulation in Aging, Health and Disease

Lei Cao

The Ohio State University, USA

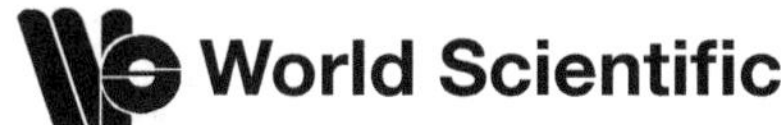

World Scientific

NEW JERSEY · LONDON · SINGAPORE · BEIJING · SHANGHAI · HONG KONG · TAIPEI · CHENNAI · TOKYO

Published by

World Scientific Publishing Co. Pte. Ltd.

5 Toh Tuck Link, Singapore 596224

USA office: 27 Warren Street, Suite 401-402, Hackensack, NJ 07601

UK office: 57 Shelton Street, Covent Garden, London WC2H 9HE

British Library Cataloguing-in-Publication Data
A catalogue record for this book is available from the British Library.

ENVIRONMENTAL CNS STIMULATION IN AGING, HEALTH AND DISEASE

ISBN 978-981-125-033-0 (hardcover)
ISBN 978-981-125-034-7 (ebook for institutions)
ISBN 978-981-125-035-4 (ebook for individuals)

For any available supplementary material, please visit
https://www.worldscientific.com/worldscibooks/10.1142/12667#t=suppl

Typeset by Stallion Press
Email: enquiries@stallionpress.com

Preface

Social and environmental factors have profound impacts on health and diseases across the life span. Yet many experimental studies utilize animals in laboratory conditions without adequate social interactions. The goal of our research is to understand how environmental stimuli to the central nervous system (CNS) shape biological processes and disease pathology, and how this knowledge can be harnessed to improve health and treat diseases. Our recent findings provide insights on how one's living condition, social contact, and lifestyle can efficiently influence brain activity (cognition, stress, mood, *etc.*) and how these changes in brain interact with other systems (fat, endocrine, immune systems, *etc.*) both at the molecular level and at the systemic level to influence the metabolism and various diseases including obesity, diabetes, autoimmune disease, and cancer. Specifically, we demonstrate that environments that are more complex and challenging, but not stressful *per se*, have robust effects on body composition, energy balance, immunity, peripheral cancer progression, and healthy aging. One underlying mechanism is the activation of a specific neuroendocrine brain-adipocyte axis with brain-derived neurotrophic factor (BDNF) as the key brain mediator. This book summarizes this work and discusses how environmental enrichment (EE) can serve as a valuable animal model of an active lifestyle. Moreover, the book integrates our discoveries into the body of literature regarding the environment, health, and disease, and discusses its translational potential.

Acknowledgments

I am grateful to all past and present lab members, coauthors of research papers, and collaborators for their data and discussions that make the book possible. Cao lab is funded by grants from the National Institutes of Health and The Ohio State University Comprehensive Cancer Center.

Contents

Chapter 1

Environmental Enrichment: A Model of an Active Lifestyle

Introduction

Large majority of basic biology research and preclinical studies are conducted in laboratory animals, mostly in mice. Unfortunately, many promising results from preclinical animal studies often fail to translate to the humans. The cost is undoubtedly huge given the waste of efforts, time, and funds. The underpinnings of the failure are not fully understood but certainly multifactorial. Differences in genetics and physiology between species are obvious reasons whereas living conditions are much less and inadequately appreciated as an important variable. As long as animal studies remain necessary to elucidate mechanisms and to assess the efficacy and safety of therapeutic interventions, it is utterly important to employ proper animal models and understand their limitations. It is impossible to recapitulate real-world human life in rodents, not even in nonhuman primates. Nevertheless, humans and rodents are both social animals. A variety of behavioral traits and emotional states can be modeled in laboratory mice and rats. These animal models have greatly facilitated the progress of neuroscience. Hence, providing housing for laboratory animals resembling their natural habitat may improve animal modeling for human physiological and pathological research.

We have long-term interest in understanding how an individual interact with one's physical and social environments, and the impacts on health, well-being, and disease risk. For such research, we have been using environmental enrichment (EE) as a model of an active lifestyle in the past 15 years. In this book, lifestyle is loosely defined as one's living condition but not necessarily self-option, habit, or natural instinct.

What Is Environmental Enrichment?

EE refers to a laboratory animal housing condition that provides complex physical, social, cognitive, motor, and sensory stimuli to improve health and well-being.[1,2] EE was described firstly by Hebb in 1947. Hebb reported that the rats being allowed to move freely in his house performed better on cognitive tasks compared to those housed in standard cage.[3] In the early 1960s, Rosenzweig and colleagues placed mazes and toys in the rat cages and frequently reconfigured these objects. They found that the sensory cortex, the brain region processing all of the senses (sight, smell, sound, touch, and taste), was larger in rats living in EE than in their counterparts living in standard housing.[4] Bennett and colleagues demonstrated that rats in EE housing developed heavier and thicker cerebral cortices compared to standard housing cohorts,[5] and the cortical thickening was attributed to an increase in the number and length of glial cells.[6] The 1990s saw a boom of interest in EE as Gage and colleagues revealed that EE enhanced neurogenesis, a process of generating new neurons, in adult brain.[7]

In the past six decades, neuroscientists have investigated a wide range of EE effects on behaviors, cognitions, brain structure, and functions. Generally speaking, EE exerts beneficial effects on the central nervous system (CNS) including enhancing learning/memory, stimulating neurogenesis, promoting recovery from brain insults, and increasing resistance to drug addiction. Moreover, EE has been shown to lessen neurological symptoms and behavioral deficits in animal models of a wide range of neurological disorders.[1,2] Numerous research papers have documented EE as a positive behavioral intervention for neurological diseases including Alzheimer's disease,[8] Parkinson's disease,[9] Huntington's disease,[10] autism,[11] depression,[12] schizophrenia,[13] amyotrophic lateral sclerosis,[14] traumatic brain injury,[15] stroke,[16] epilepsy,[17] among others.

Key Components of Environmental Enrichment

Standard housing environment (SE) for laboratory mice commonly constitute cages of the size of a shoebox (30.5 cm × 19 cm × 14 cm) with bedding, and single-sex housing in groups (typically three to five mice per cage). Mice have *ad libitum* access to food and water, and living in air-conditioned rooms. Although life in SE is comfortable and safe from predators, it is artificial and "boring" in the sense of being deprived of rich real-world experiences.

EE housing protocols vary between laboratories and there is still no consensus on which EE settings are ideal to achieve optimal benefits on behavior and the nervous system. The lack of standardization of EE protocol sometimes hinders the direct comparison of EE studies conducted by different labs, which underscores the importance of reading the fine-print of the EE protocol. On the other hand, numerous studies have shown various EE protocols achieve similar results, demonstrating reliability and reproducibility of core components of an EE. Common EE housing typically includes larger surface area, increased levels of bedding, more companions, and supplementation of objects to interact with (toys, running wheels, tunnels, and shelters). The essence is to offer animals opportunities to engage physically, socially, and cognitively. Animals are not forced to do anything but free to choose engagement versus retreat.

Which components are important for eliciting specific effects of EE? This frequently asked question has been addressed previously. Studies have compared the individual impacts of physical enrichment,[18–21] social enrichment,[22,23] and cognitive/sensory enrichment[24–26] to the impact of combined EE. The overall consensus is that a single contributing factor of EE is unlikely to be isolated for most of benefits associated with EE.[20,21,27,28] Instead, the "whole package" in which components of EE work together holistically to exert overlapping, unified, or emergent effects on animals living within EE housing. Any one of these components cannot account for all of the effects of a typical EE, which supports the description of EE as "a combination of complex inanimate and social stimulation".[22]

Another question is the dose of EE, in other words, is there a threshold of EE? This might depend on particular effects.[29] What is clear is that the duration of an EE exposure can greatly impact the observed outcomes. The durations for EE exposure used in mouse studies are mostly from one week to a couple of months. The phenotypes of EE do not occur at the same time (examples in Chapters 2, 3, 6, and 7). EE can be delivered either continuously (living in EE housing continuously), or at interval exposures, such as daily for a few hours.

Our Environmental Enrichment Settings

We have been using two EE settings in our studies on cancer, obesity, and aging. Figure 1.1 shows the EE housing in a large container of 120 cm × 90 cm × 76 cm supplemented with running wheels, tunnels, igloos, huts, retreats, wood toys, a maze, nesting material. Two regular mouse cages with holes at the side are placed in the EE container allowing mice to access food and water *ad libitum*.

Environmental complexity is a key aspect of EE which is usually achieved by objects providing a variety of opportunities for visual, somatosensory, and olfactory stimulation (e.g. toys and mazes). Environmental novelty is another key aspect that is achieved by exchanging or reconfiguring the objects, and rearranging the locations of the objects weekly.[2] The larger space and the running wheels encourage freely roaming and physical activities. Larger number of animals living in the EE housing increases social contact (10–20 mice per cage). Hiding places are also important because they allow animals to retreat to safe havens and thereby enhancing the sense of self-control.

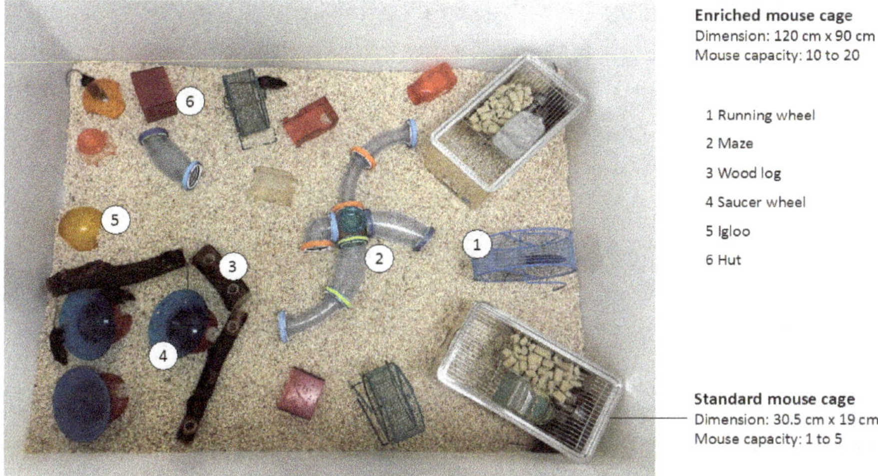

Fig. 1.1 An enriched environment for laboratory mice. The enriched environment has larger space with two modified standard mouse cages for free access to food and water. Running wheels and saucer wheels provide opportunity of exercise. Mazes and other toys stimulate cognition. Wood logs may give mice a sense of nature. Igloos and huts provide a safe haven to boost feeling of safety and self-control.

Mice are nocturnal, we therefore videorecorded the activities of mice living in SE and EE using a night-view camera at night.[30] In SE, mice had little to do except eating and sniffing around. In EE, different activities of individual mouse were observed: free-roaming around the cage, retreating in the huts, eating or drinking, playing with toys, exploring the mazes, running on the wheels, *etc.* I was particularly captivated by an episode. One mouse (Mouse A) was running on a wheel when two mice approached to the wheel. The two latecomers (Mouse B and C) circled the wheel a few times. Then Mouse B pushed the wheel but Mouse A refused to vacate the wheel. Next, Mouse B jumped on to the wheel. Mouse C watched Mouse A and B occupied the wheel simultaneously and the wheel stopped. Mouse C turned away to play something else. Mouse A eventually got off the wheel so that Mouse B could run.

This moment illuminated the rich social contact in this complex environment. Individuals achieve their goals by negotiation, taking turns, or sometimes by force — a different context compared to physical exercise of voluntary running, for example, one mouse in a cage with a running wheel.

In our later studies in which large number of mice are difficult to obtain, for example transgenic mice or aged mice, we have been using an EE protocol consisting a container (63 cm × 49 cm × 44 cm) in which five mice are housed. In general, this EE setting using midsize EE bin results in similar effects of EE as the large bin with more mice.

Numerous research work has characterized a breath of adaptive changes in the CNS and behavior induced by EE. Several excellent articles have reviewed comprehensively these robust and powerful influences of EE on brain function and the underlying mechanisms.[2,31–33] This book focuses on work showing the impact of EE on energy balance, cancer, immunity, and aging.

References

1. Cao L, During MJ. (2012) What is the brain-cancer connection? *Ann Rev Neurosci* **35**:331–345.
2. Nithianantharajah J, Hannan AJ. (2006) Enriched environments, experience-dependent plasticity and disorders of the nervous system. *Nat Rev Neurosci* **7**:697–709.
3. Hebb D. (1947) The effects of early experience on problem-solving at maturity. *Am Psychol* **2**:306–307.
4. Rosenzweig MR, Krech D, Bennett EL, Diamond MC. (1962) Effects of environmental complexity and training on brain chemistry and anatomy: A replication and extension. *J Comp Physiol Psychol* **55**: 429–437.
5. Bennett EL, Diamond MC, Krech D, Rosenzweig MR. (1964) Chemical and anatomical plasticity Brain. *Science* **146**:610–619.
6. Diamond MC, Law F, Rhodes H, *et al.* (1966) Increases in cortical depth and glia numbers in rats subjected to enriched environment. *J Comp Neurol* **128**:117–126.

7. Kempermann G, Kuhn HG, Gage FH. (1997) More hippocampal neurons in adult mice living in an enriched environment. *Nature* **386**: 493–495.

8. Merceron-Martinez D, Ibaceta-González C, Salazar C, *et al.* (2021) Alzheimer's disease, neural plasticity, and functional recovery. *J Alzheimers Dis* **82**:S37–S50.

9. Aumann TD. (2016) Environment- and activity-dependent dopamine neurotransmitter plasticity in the adult substantia nigra. *J Chem Neuroanat* **73**:21–32.

10. Mo C, Hannan AJ, Renoir T. (2015) Environmental factors as modulators of neurodegeneration: insights from gene-environment interactions in Huntington's disease. *Neurosci Biobehav Rev* **52**:178–192.

11. Gubert C, Hannan AJ. (2019) Environmental enrichment as an experience-dependent modulator of social plasticity and cognition. *Brain Res* **1717**:1–14.

12. Lee MM, Reif A, Schmitt AG. (2013) Major depression: A role for hippocampal neurogenesis? *Curr Top Behav Neurosci* **14**:153–179.

13. Burrows EL, Hannan AJ. (2016) Cognitive endophenotypes, gene-environment interactions and experience-dependent plasticity in animal models of schizophrenia. *Biol Psychol* **116**:82–89.

14. Sorrells AD, Corcoran-Gomez K, Eckert KA, *et al.* (2009) Effects of environmental enrichment on the amyotrophic lateral sclerosis mouse model. *Lab Anim* **43**:182–190.

15. de la Tremblaye PB, Cheng JP, Bondi CO, Kline AE. (2019) Environmental enrichment, alone or in combination with various pharmacotherapies, confers marked benefits after traumatic brain injury. *Neuropharmacology* **145**:13–24.

16. McDonald MW, Hayward KS, Rosbergen ICM, *et al.* (2018) Is environmental enrichment ready for clinical application in human post-stroke rehabilitation? *Front Behav Neurosci* **12**:135.

17. Akyuz E, Eroglu E. (2021) Envisioning the crosstalk between environmental enrichment and epilepsy: A novel perspective. *Epilepsy Behav* **115**:107660.

18. Suzuki K, Tagami K. (2005) Voluntary wheel-running exercise enhances antigen-specific antibody-producing splenic B cell response and prolongs IgG half-life in the blood. *Eur J Appl Physiol* **94**:514–519.

19. Lu Y-P, Lou Y-P, Nolan B, *et al.* (2006) Stimulatory effect of voluntary exercise or fat removal (partial lipectomy) on apoptosis in the skin of UVB light-irradiated mice. *Proc Natl Acad Sci* U S A **103**: 16301–16306.

20. McMurphy T, Huang W, Queen NJ, *et al.* (2018) Implementation of environmental enrichment after middle age promotes healthy aging. *Aging (Albany NY)* **10**:1698–1721.

21. Cao L, Liu X, Lin E-JD, *et al.* (2010) Environmental and genetic activation of a brain-adipocyte BDNF/leptin axis causes cancer remission and inhibition. *Cell* **142**:52–64.

22. Rosenzweig MR, Bennett EL, Hebert M, Morimoto H. (1978) Social grouping cannot account for cerebral effects of enriched environments. *Brain Res* **153**:563–576.

23. Van Praag H, Kempermann G, Gage FH. (2000) Neural consequences of enviromental enrichment. *Nat Rev Neurosci* **1**:191–198.

24. Jankowsky JL, Melnikova T, Fadale DJ, *et al.* (2005) Environmental enrichment mitigates cognitive deficits in a mouse model of Alzheimer's disease. *J Neurosci* **25**:5217–5224.

25. Stuart KE, King AE, Fernandez-Martos CM, *et al.* (2017) Environmental novelty exacerbates stress hormones and Aβ pathology in an Alzheimer's model. *Sci Rep* **7**:1–7.

26. Ferchmin P, Bennett EL, Rosenzweig MR. (1975) Direct contact with enriched environment is required to alter cerebral weights in rats. *J Comp Physiol Psychol* **88**:360.

27. Li G, Gan Y, Fan Y, *et al.* (2015) Enriched environment inhibits mouse pancreatic cancer growth and down-regulates the expression of mitochondria-related genes in cancer cells. *Sci Rep* **5**:7856–7856.

28. Cao L, Choi EY, Liu X, *et al.* (2011) White to brown fat phenotypic switch induced by genetic and environmental activation of a hypothalamic-adipocyte axis. *Cell Metab* **14**:324–338.

29. Mazarakis NK, Mo C, Renoir T, *et al.* (2014) 'Super-enrichment' reveals dose-dependent therapeutic effects of environmental stimulation in a transgenic mouse model of Huntington's disease. *J Huntingtons Dis* **3**:299–309.

30. Slater AM, Cao L. (2015) A protocol for housing mice in an enriched environment. *J Vis Exp.* 8:e52874.

31. Kempermann G. (2019) Environmental enrichment, new neurons and the neurobiology of individuality. *Nat Rev Neurosci* **20**:235–245.

32. Hannan AJ. (2014) Environmental enrichment and brain repair: harnessing the therapeutic effects of cognitive stimulation and physical activity to enhance experience-dependent plasticity. *Neuropathol Appl Neurobiol* **40**:13–25.

33. van Praag H, Kempermann G, Gage FH. (2000) Neural consequences of environmental enrichment. *Nat Rev Neurosci* **1**:191–198.

2 Cancer and Macroenvironment: What Is the Brain–Cancer Connection?

Hallmarks of Cancer

There are over 100 distinct types of cancer, and moreover subtypes can be found within a specific organ. Accumulating evidence suggests a small number of molecular, biochemical, and cellular traits are shared by most and possibly all types of cancer.[1] In 2000, Hanahan and Weinberg published a seminal paper "The Hallmarks of Cancer" proposing a logical framework for understanding the incredible diversity of cancer.[1] They synthesized decades of research on neoplastic diseases to six hallmarks of cancer — six biological capabilities acquired along the multistep development of human tumors. These six essential alterations in cell physiology collectively drive the progressive transformation of normal human cells into malignant cells and dictate malignant growth. The six cancer hallmark capabilities include sustaining proliferative signaling, evading growth suppressors, resisting cell death, enabling replicative immortality, inducing angiogenesis, and activating invasion and metastasis.[1,2]

The concept of cancer hallmarks is well received and seminal in our understanding of the common traits of cancer although not free of critique. A decade later, Hanahan and Weinberg summarized conceptual progress and updated the concept in another influential paper "Hallmarks of Cancer: The Next Generation."[2] They added two emerging hallmarks — reprogramming of energy metabolism and evading immune destruction. The genetic and epigenetic alterations underlying these hallmarks are incredibly complex, and continue to be heavily investigated.

Tumor Microenvironment

Another dimension of complexity is the tumor microenvironment. Tumors are not clusters of endlessly proliferating cancer cells, but instead complex tissues composed of multiple distinct types of cells including pericytes, cancer-associated fibroblasts, endothelial cells, local and bone-marrow-derived stromal stem and progenitor cells, and immune cells.[3,4] Cancer cells must create a tumor microenvironment enabling the full malignancy. In the case of solid tumors, the microenvironment provides a tumor ecosystem for bidirectional communications between cancer cells and the tumor-associated stroma to support tumorigenesis[1,4] (**Fig. 2.1**).

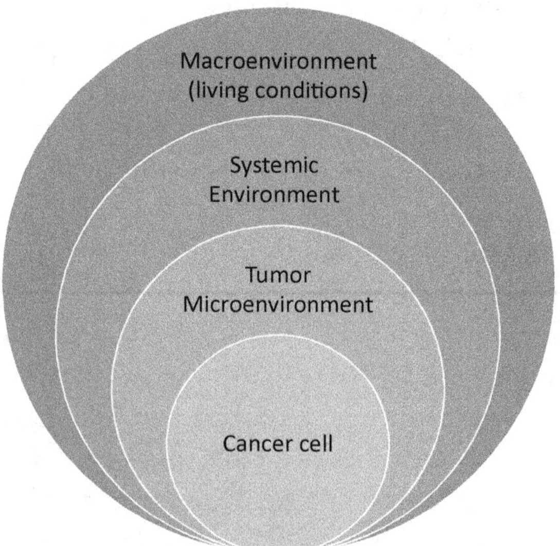

Fig. 2.1. The natural course of cancer is influenced by complex interactions between cancer and its environments.

Systemic Environment

This tumor microenvironment is influenced by systemic factors such as hormones, growth factors, cytokines, metabolites, to name a few. And the cancer itself induces both local and distant changes through paracrine signaling and interactions with the immune and nervous systems.[5,6] Cancer invasion and metastasis are serial events through which a locally growing tumor develops into a systemic, metastatic, and eventually morbid disease. The local invasion is initiated by signaling pathways that control cytoskeletal dynamics in cancer cells and the turnover of cell–cell junctions, followed by cancer cell migration into the adjacent tissue. Then metastasis occurs when invading cancer cells engage with blood and lymph vessels, disseminating through the vessel lumen to colonize distant organs. Cancer invasion is now thought to be a heterogeneous and adaptive process in which both tumor cells and the surrounding tissues experience reprogramming reciprocally.[7] Tumor metastasis is influenced by signals from destination tissues. An analogy is to view a cancer, although a part of self, as a parasite hijacking the body of host for its own survival and growth (**Fig. 2.1**).

Macroenvironment (Living Conditions)

Macroenvironment brings the complexity of cancer to the next level. Numerous evidences indicate that environmental factors and lifestyle exert profound effects in the initiation, promotion, and progression of cancer.[8,9] The past decade has seen increasing appreciation of the macro-physiological milieus shaping individual variability in the natural course of cancer and responsiveness to therapies[4,10] (**Fig. 2.1**). Social economic status, education, family and community support, accessibility and quality of healthcare are all important variables for an individual's risk of developing cancer and the prognosis. However, the impacts and mechanisms of the macroenvironment on systemic cancer, specifically an individual's interaction with its physical living and social environment, are poorly defined.

Environmental Enrichment Suppresses Cancer Progression

Our long-term interest is to understand how environmental stimuli to the central nervous system (CNS) shape biological processes and disease pathology; and how this knowledge can be harnessed to improve health and treat diseases. Decades of neuroscience research has demonstrated that environmental enrichment (EE) is a remarkable environmental model exerting profound impacts on brain structure and function. In 1991, my mentor Dr. Matthew During and colleagues published that EE reduces spontaneous apoptotic cell death in the hippocampus, a brain region critical for learning and memory, and protects rats against kainic acid–induced seizure and neural injury. These neuroprotective effects are associated with induction of glial-derived neurotrophic factor (GDNF) and brain-derived neurotrophic factor (BDNF).[11] I also started EE research focusing on hippocampus-dependent learning and memory. We published that EE improves spatial memory and increases hippocampal neurogenesis together with an upregulation of vascular endothelial growth factor (VEGF) expression in the hippocampus. Our mechanistic studies elucidate a mechanism in which VEGF, acting through kinase insert domain protein receptor (KDR), mediating EE effects on neurogenesis and cognition.[12,13]

It is well known that EE has considerable impacts, mostly positive, on the phenotypes of a variety of toxin- and genetically induced models of human neurological diseases.[14] That intrigued us to ask the question, whether an environment, like EE, that improves brain function and resiliency to brain insults, can also affect the body's overall state of health and the progression of a peripheral disease. Dr. During and I both lost family members to cancer. We were also fascinated by the large individual variability in the natural course of cancer. Thus, we decided to tackle the abovementioned question using the EE and peripheral cancer models in mice. The results were nothing short of remarkable.

B16 Melanoma

First, we assessed whether simply placing animals in EE could result in effects powerful enough to significantly alter the growth of a highly malignant cancer using syngeneic tumor implantation models in which cancer cells proliferate following implantation and develop to highly reproducible solid tumors. We housed mice in EE (similar setting as shown in **Fig. 1.1**) for 3 weeks and implanted B16 melanoma cells, 1×10^5 per mouse, subcutaneously to the flank. At 19 days post tumor inoculation, the mean volume of tumor in EE mice was 43% smaller than those in the standard environment (SE) housing **(Fig. 2.2(a))**. Extending EE exposure to 6 weeks prior to tumor inoculation further enhanced the anticancer effect — a remarkable 80% decrease in tumor mass **(Fig. 2.2(b))**. Furthermore, the rate of tumor growth over time was more linear in EE mice without the exponential growth curve found in SE mice **(Fig. 2.3(a))**. Notably, ~17% mice in EE displayed no palpable tumor at the end of the experiment 17 days post inoculation, whereas all mice in SE developed visible tumors[15] **(Figs. 2.2(c), 2.3(b))**.

Histological analysis revealed reduced cell proliferation and increased apoptosis in tumors collected from EE mice compared to those from SE mice. Melanoma cells have been associated with activation of a number of signaling transduction enzymes critically involved in the tumor growth. The tumors from EE mice displayed robust decreases in multiple signal transduction pathways including phospho-AKT, phospho-ERK1/ERK2, and phospho-p38α, consistent with inhibition of tumor growth. In addition, the levels of factors promoting angiogenesis were decreased in tumors from EE mice consistent with reduced staining of vascular marker **(Fig. 2.3(c))**. We were astonished by these remarkable results because B16 melanoma is an aggressive murine tumor model. Thus, we repeated the experiment a few times and the results were reproducible.

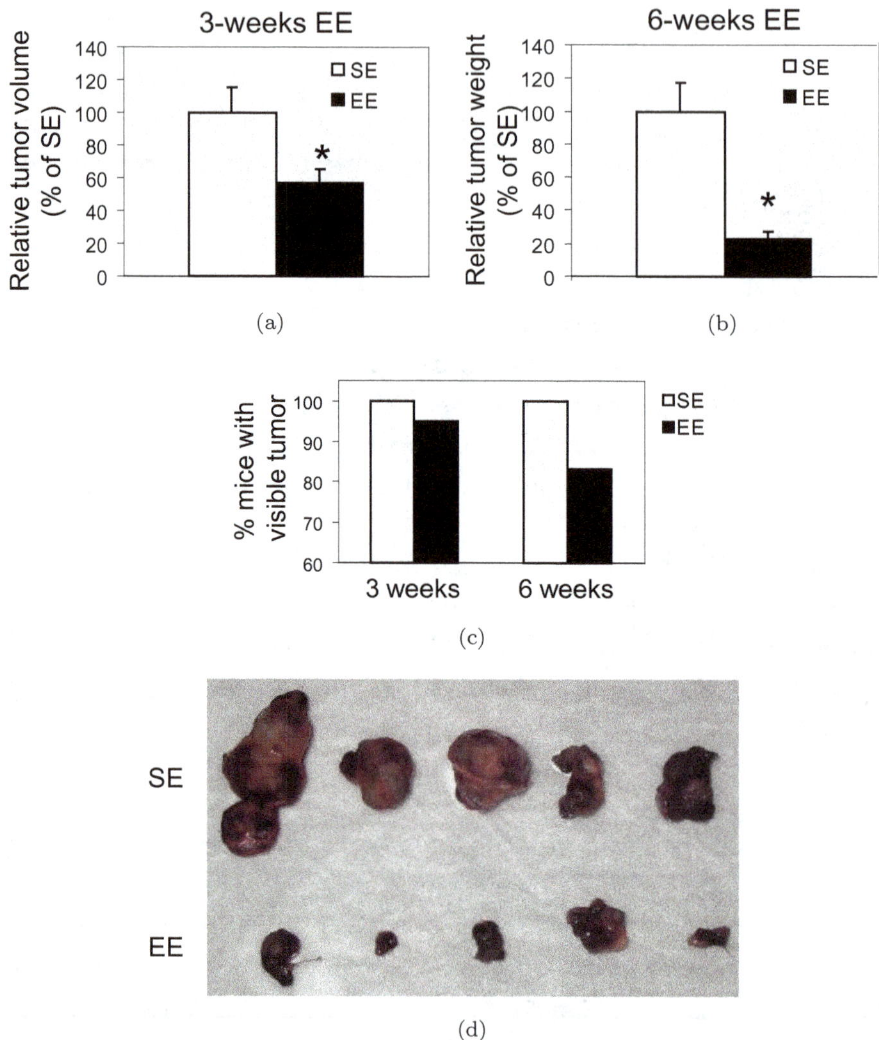

Fig. 2.2.   EE suppresses B16 melanoma growth. (a) EE housing for 3 weeks prior to tumor implantation reduced tumor volume day 19 after inoculation, $n = 20$ per group. (b) EE housing for 6 weeks prior to tumor implantation further decreased tumor weight day 17 after inoculation, $n = 18$ per group. (c) EE induced complete tumor resistance in a subset of mice at sacrifice for respective experiment. All SE mice showed visible tumors. (d) Representative B16 melanoma dissected from the 6-week EE experiment. Data are mean ± SEM. * $P < 0.05$. Reprinted from *Cell* Vol 142, Cao *et al.* Environmental and genetic activation of a brain-adipocyte BDNF/ leptin axis causes cancer remission and inhibition, 52–64, Copyright (2010), with permission from Elsevier.

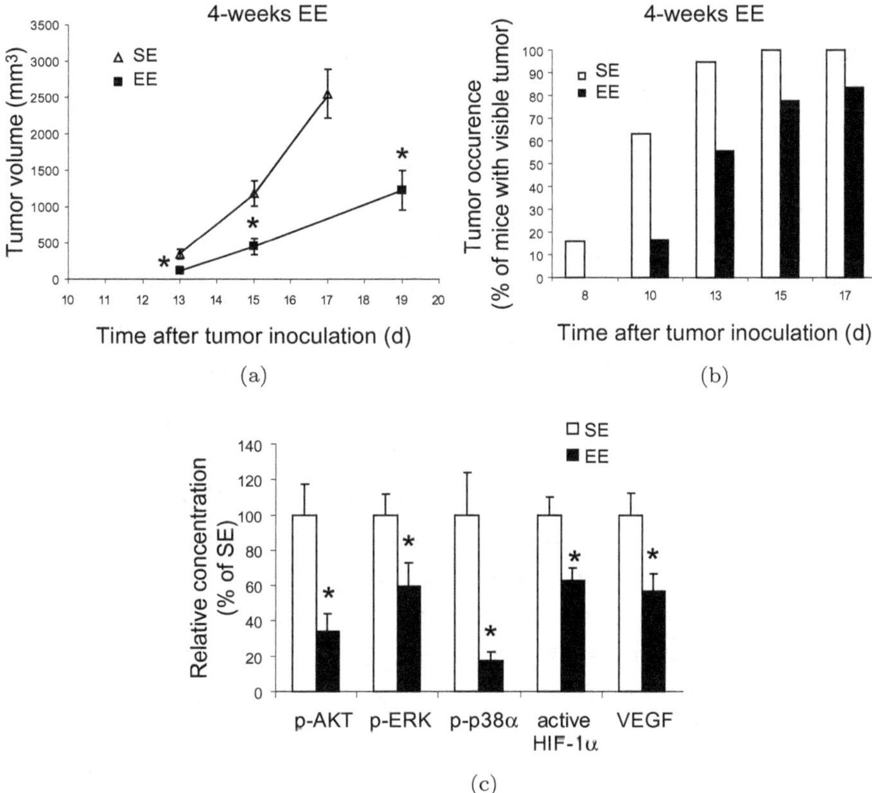

Fig. 2.3. EE slows B16 melanoma growth rate and affects signaling pathways in the tumor. (a) EE housing for 4 weeks prior to tumor implantation decreased tumor growth rate, $n = 20$ per group. (b) Four weeks of EE delayed the occurrence of tumor. (c) Phospho-AKT1 (*S473*), Phospho-ERK1 (T202/Y204)/ERK2 (T185/Y187), Phospho-p38α (T180/Y182), active HIF-1α activity, and VEGF concentration in tumors, $n = 7$ per group. Data are mean ± SEM. * $P < 0.05$. Reprinted from *Cell* Vol 142, Cao *et al.* Environmental and genetic activation of a brain-adipocyte BDNF/leptin axis causes cancer remission and inhibition, 52–64, copyright (2010), with permission form Elsevier.

MC38 Colon Cancer

To determine whether the anticancer effect of EE could be generalized, we studied mouse models of colon cancer. Colorectal cancer is the second leading cause of cancer death in women and the third in men worldwide.[16] Risk factors associated with colorectal cancer include advanced age, deficiencies in mismatch repair proteins and adenomatous polyposis coli (APC), inflammation, smoking, poor diet, lack of physical activities, alcohol consumption, and imbalance of intestinal microbiota.[17]

To examine whether EE is effective when the tumor is already established, we used two models: first, a minimal disease model in which EE was implemented 4 days after the implantation of the MC38 colon cancer cells but prior to the occurrence of any visible tumors (**Fig. 2.4(a)**); second, an established tumor model in which EE was delayed until the MC38 colon cancer became visible (**Fig. 2.4(c)**). In the minimal disease model, tumor mass was significantly reduced in EE mice by 40%, with 10% of EE mice bearing a barely palpable tumor when large tumors were observed in SE mice (**Fig. 2.4(b)**). In the established model, all mice received equal number of MC38 cells and lived in identical housing for 6 days until visible tumors were found, and then randomized to either EE or SE. Delayed EE still markedly slowed the growth rate of established colon cancer and reduced the tumor mass by 55% at 18 days post implementing EE (**Fig. 2.4(d, e)**).[15]

Genetic Tumorigenesis Model APC$^{min/+}$ Mice

Next, we examined the effect of EE in APC$^{min/+}$ mice, a spontaneous tumor model with a germline mutation in APC similar to humans with familial adenomatous polyposis, and a gene in which somatic mutations occur in 80% of human colon cancer. The mutation makes APC$^{min/+}$ mice highly susceptible to spontaneous intestinal adenoma formation.[18] Therefore, APC$^{min/+}$ mice have been extensively used in studies on colon cancer biology and evaluation of therapeutic interventions. EE was initiated at 7 weeks of age. One mouse from SE housing died at 11 weeks of age, whereas all mice in EE survived to the end of the experiment at 13 weeks of age. The entire intestine was examined blindly and all visible polyps larger than 1 mm in

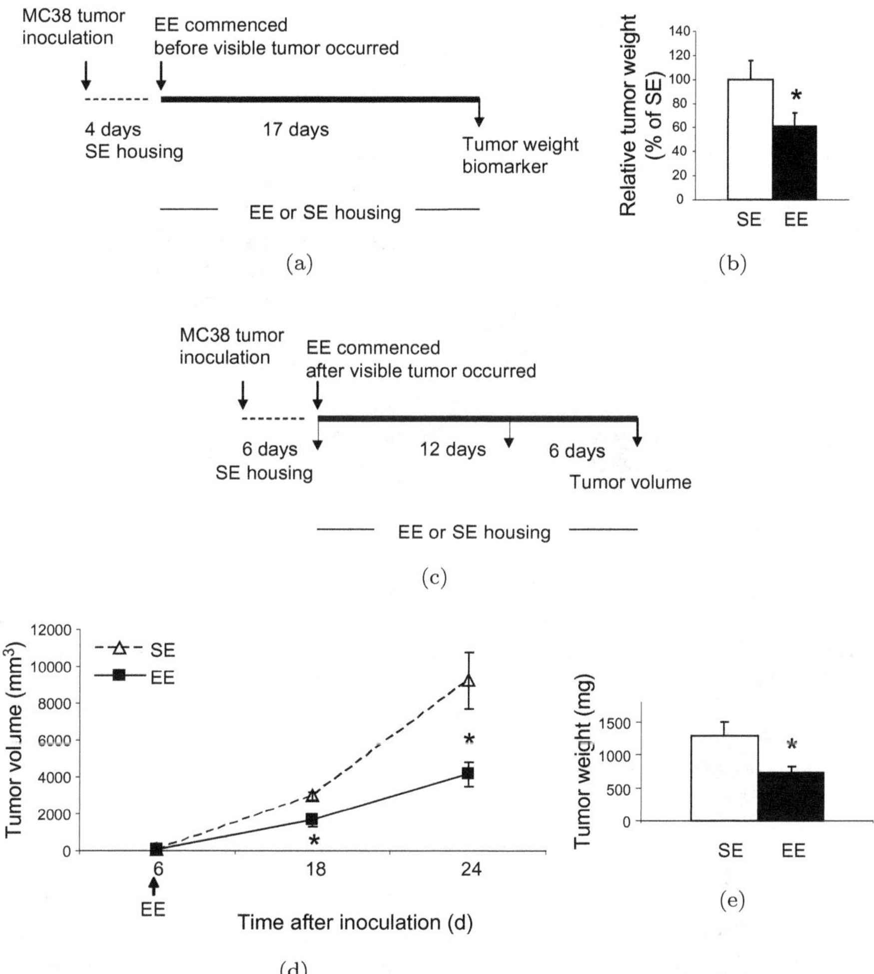

Fig. 2.4. EE inhibits colon cancer growth when commenced after implantation of MC38 colon cancer. (a) Study design of the minimal disease model. (b) EE reduced tumor mass in minimal disease model, $n = 20$ per group. (c) Study design of the established cancer model. (d) EE initiated after visible tumor occurred decreased tumor growth rate, $n = 6$ per group. (e) EE reduced tumor weight day 24 after tumor implantation in the established disease model, $n = 6$ per group. Data are mean ± SEM. *$P < 0.05$. Reprinted from *Cell* Vol 142. Cao *et al.* Environmental and genetic activation of a brain-adipocyte BDNF/leptin axis causes cancer remission and inhibition, 52–64, Copyright (2010) with permission from Elsevier.

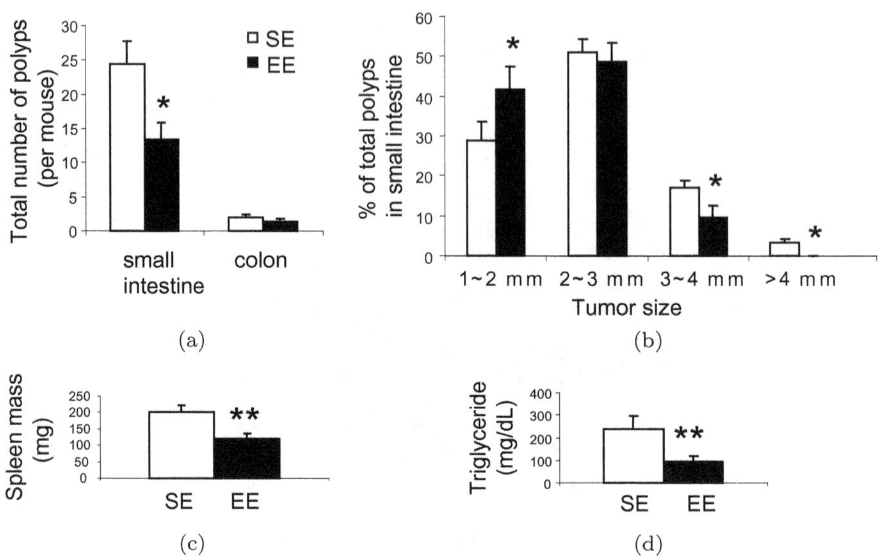

Fig. 2.5. EE inhibits intestinal tumorigenesis in Apc$^{Min/+}$ mice. EE was initiated at the age of 7 weeks for a 6-week EE housing. (a) Total number of visible polyps larger than 1 mm in diameter. (b) EE reduced the size of polyps in small intestine. (c) EE reduced splenomegaly. (d) EE reduced serum triglyceride level. N = 15 for EE, n = 14 for SE. Data are mean ± SEM. *P < 0.05, ** P < 0.01. Reprinted from *Cell* Vol 142, Cao *et al.* Environmental and genetic activation of a brain-adipocyte BDNF/leptin axis causes cancer remission and inhibition, 52–64, Copyright (2010), with permission form Elsevier.

diameter were scored. EE decreased the total number of polyps in the small intestine by approximately 50% and substantially reduced the size of polyps by ~50% in all polys larger than 3 mm, with no polyps greater than 4 mm in diameter. Alleviation of splenomegaly and hyperlipidemia were observed in EE mice consistent with the reduction of polyp burden[15] (**Fig. 2.5**).

In Search of the Underlying Mechanisms

We were convinced that EE exerted significant anticancer effects in multiple mouse models of cancer. As this finding was completely novel at the time, we started the search for underlying mechanisms by screening factors known to be implicated in tumor growth.

Systemic Metabolic Changes

Because a slight alteration in body weight was observed in EE mice, we examined the systemic metabolic changes in EE prior to tumor implantation. Insulin-like growth factor-1 (IGF-1) levels have been associated with cancer risk and progression.[19,20] EE significantly reduced serum IGF-1 level by ~30% while its major binding protein, IGFBP3, did not change (**Fig. 2.6**).

Adipose tissues secrete hundreds of adipokines and cytokines that potentially affect tumor progression. We measured two major adipokines in EE. The serum level of adiponectin, an adipocyte hormone, was higher in EE mice than that in SE mice (**Fig. 2.6**). This abundant protein is associated with insulin sensitivity but it has also been shown to have pleiotropic properties including suppressing carcinogenesis and inhibiting angiogenesis in cancer models.[21,22] In contrast, EE sharply reduced the serum level of leptin to 13% of SE mice (**Fig. 2.6**). Leptin is a major adipocyte hormone often trending opposite direction to adiponectin in obesity. Leptin plays

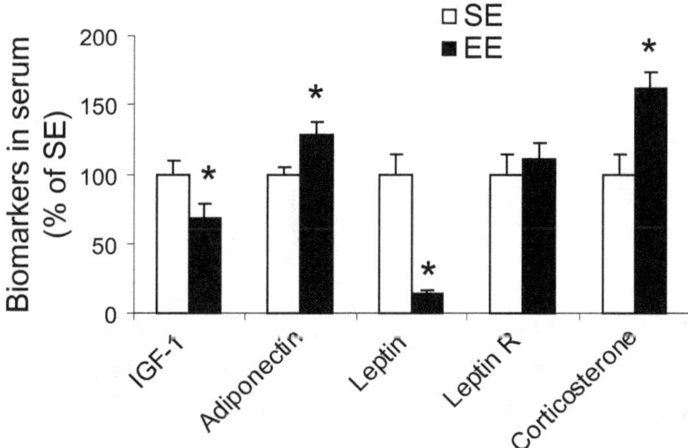

Fig. 2.6. EE effects on biomarkers in serum. Serum samples were collected after 6-week EE exposure prior to melanoma implantation. n = 20 per group. Data are mean ± SEM. * P < 0.05. Reprinted from *Cell* Vol 142, Cao *et al.* Environmental and genetic activation of a brain-adipocyte BDNF/leptin axis causes cancer remission n and inhibition, 52–64, Copyright (2010), with permission from Elsevier.

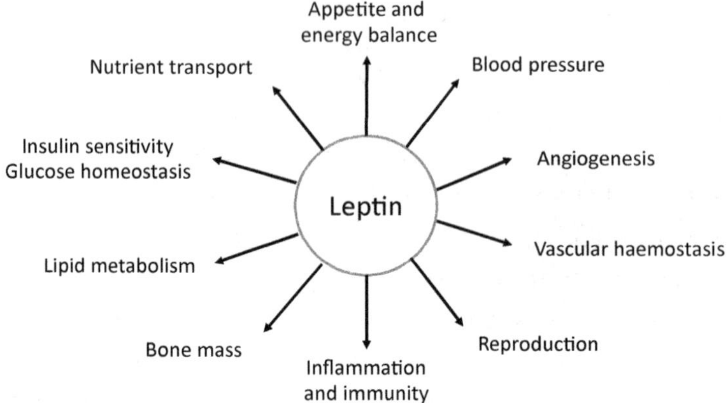

Fig. 2.7.   Leptin is an adipocyte hormone with pleiotropic functions.

a critical role in regulation of appetite and energy expenditure by conveying metabolic information to the brain.[23,24] Leptin is also a pleiotropic hormone[25] that involved in multiple pathways affecting many peripheral organs as a mitogen, metabolic regulator, survival or angiogenic factor, depending on the tissue type.[26,27] Some clinical reports and animal data have linked elevated serum leptin levels with an increased risk of certain types of cancer including prostate,[28,29] breast cancer,[30,31] endometrial cancer,[32] colon cancer,[33] and melanoma[34] (**Fig. 2.7**).

Immune Changes

Antitumor immunity is an obvious target to examine. Compared to SE mice, spleens from EE mice were significantly enlarged after B16 melanoma cells were implanted. The splenic lymphocytes from EE mice showed ~2-fold higher cell proliferation in response to the T cell mitogen Concanavalin A before (day 0) as well as several time-points (days 9, 13, and 17) following tumor inoculation. Moreover, natural killer (NK) cell cytotoxicity was enhanced by EE before tumor inoculation. In addition, CD8[+] T cell cytotoxicity was also increased in EE mice bearing tumors.[15] Both NK cells and CD8[+] T cells function as an important defense against cancer. How EE regulates immunity and its contribution to anticancer effects are discussed in Chapter 6.

Leptin as Peripheral Effector

One of the most drastic changes observed in EE mice was a sharp drop of leptin level in circulation. We examined whether the serum samples obtained from mice living in EE versus SE could influence B16 melanoma cell growth in culture. Indeed, sera from EE mice significantly slowed melanoma cell proliferation. A leptin-neutralizing antibody also inhibited tumor cell growth suggesting leptin as a mitogen for B16 melanoma (**Fig. 2.8**).

We investigated the relevance of leptin using both pharmacological and genetic approaches. First, we implanted mice with leptin-releasing liposomes before assigning them to the EE. The leptin-encapsuled liposome vesicles continued to release exogenous leptin and thereby attenuating the drop of circulating leptin

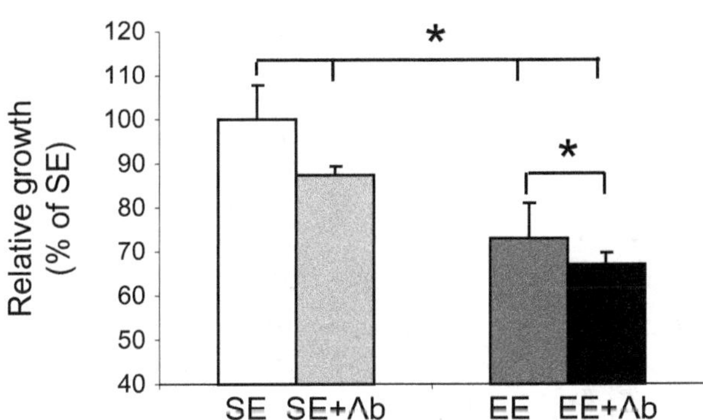

Fig. 2.8. Serum from EE mice slows B16 melanoma growth in culture compare to serum from SE mice. Pretreatment with leptin-neutralizing antibody inhibited the effect of serum on B16 melanoma cell growth. $n = 4$ per group. Data are mean ± SEM. *$P < 0.05$ between groups indicated. Ab, leptin-neutralizing antibody. Reprinted from *Cell* Vol 142, Cao *et al.* Environmental and genetic activation of a brain-adipocyte BDN/leptin axis causes cancer remission and inhibition, 52–64, Copyright (2010), with permission form Elsevier.

induced by EE. Accordingly, the tumor-inhibiting effect of EE was blocked as well (**Fig. 2.9**).

Second, we used a genetic model of leptin deficiency. *ob/ob* mice lack functional leptin and therefore manifest obesity and metabolic syndromes.[35] *ob/ob* mice were randomly assigned to live in SE or EE housing for 3 weeks, and were implanted with B16 melanoma cells. Tumors were larger in *ob/ob* mice than in wild type mice, likely due to the general effects of obesity.[36] Of note, in contrast to wild type mice, EE failed to inhibit tumor growth in leptin-deficient *ob/ob* mice although substantially lowered body weight (**Fig. 2.10**).

To further define the specific role of leptin on tumor growth from general effects associated with obesity, we conducted a leptin replacement experiment in *ob/ob* mice using osmotic minipumps to deliver leptin constantly for 14 days followed by melanoma implantation (**Fig. 2.11**). The leptin replacement reconstituted physiological levels of leptin and reduced food intake by ~50% compared to *ob/ob* mice receiving saline. The third group of mice receiving saline but pair-fed to the leptin replacement mice, meaning eating the same amount of food as the leptin replacement mice. The leptin-infused mice had similar body weight and fat mass as the pair-fed saline-infused mice. However, the tumor weight was 140% greater in leptin-infused mice than pair-fed saline mice, further supporting leptin's role in melanoma growth.

Taken together, these results demonstrated a consistent inverse relationship between circulating leptin and B16 melanoma mass, independent of body weight. Moreover, the presence of a decrease in leptin was required for EE-induced tumor inhibition, indicating leptin as a major peripheral effector linking EE to tumor progression.[15]

Molecular Signature in the Hypothalamus

When we found systemic metabolic and immune alterations in EE, we reasoned that the brain region crucial for the regulation of both was likely to play a critical role in mediating the anticancer effect of EE. Thus, we chose to target the hypothalamus, an area of the

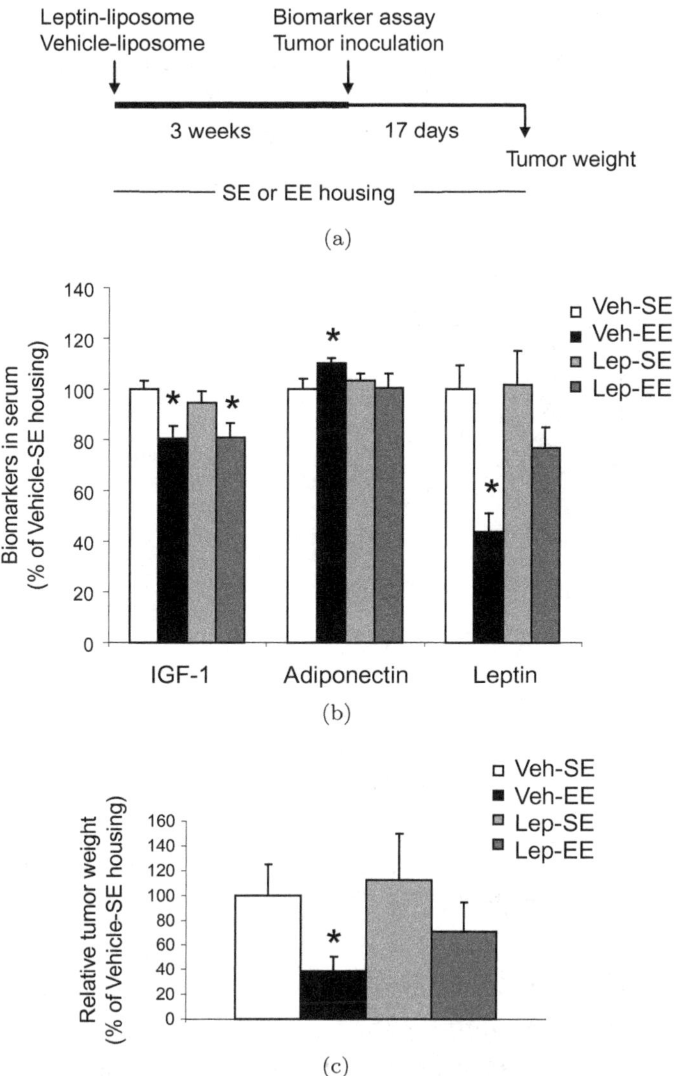

Fig. 2.9. Administration of leptin-releasing liposomes attenuates the EE-induced drop of circulating leptin and inhibits the anticancer effect of EE. (a) Study design. (b) Serum biomarkers after 3-week EE housing prior to B16 melanoma implantation. (c) B16 melanoma weight. n =10 per group. Data are mean ±SEM. * $P <$ 0.05 compared to mice receiving vehicle-lip some and living in SE. Reprinted from *Cell* Vol 142, Cao *et al*. Environmental and genetic activation of a brain-adipocyte BDNF/leptin axis causes cancer remission and inhibition, 52-64, Copyright (2010), with permission from Elsevier.

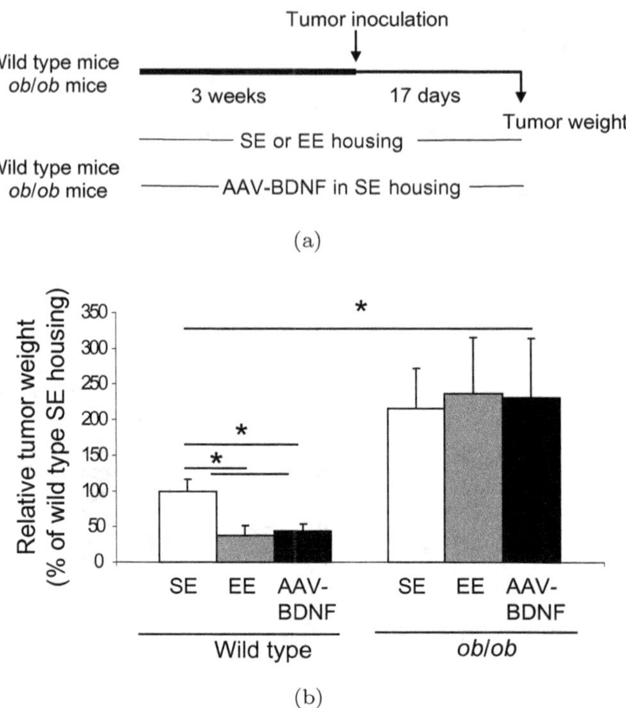

Fig. 2.10.   EE and hypothalamic overexpression of BDNF fail suppress B16 melanoma growth in leptin-deficient *ob/ob* mice. (a) Study design. (b) B16 melanoma weight. *n* = 10 per group. Data are mean ± SEM. *P < 0.05 between groups as indicated. Reprinted from *Cell* Vol 142, Cao *et al.* Environmental and genetic activation of a brain-adipocyte BDNF/leptin axis causes cancer remission and inhibition, 52–64, Copyright (2010), with permission from Elsevier.

brain that is critical in the regulation of both energy balance and neuroendocrine–immune interaction.[37,38]

As the CNS neuroendocrine coordinator for the body, the hypothalamus regulates many critical physiological processes, including energy balance, circadian rhythms, social drives, reproduction, homeostasis, thermoregulation, and stress responses.[39] These physiological processes are coordinated across discrete neuronal nuclei within the hypothalamus. These hypothalamic nuclei are responsive to endocrine signals and are interconnected with the

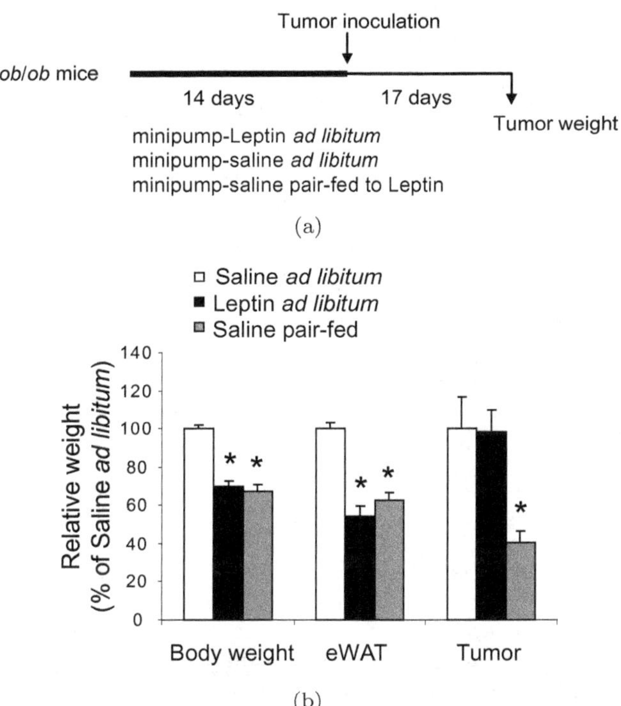

Fig. 2.11. Leptin replacement alleviates obesity but increases B16 melanoma growth in *ob/ob* mice. (a) Study design. (b) Body weight, epididymal white adipose tissue (eWAT) weight, and B16 melanoma weight. *n* = 10 per group. Data are mean ± SEM. *P < 0.05 compared to saline-infused mice and *libitum*. Reprinted from *Cell* Vol 142, Cao et al. Environmental and genetic activation of a brain-adipocyte BDNF/leptin axis causes cancer remission and inhibition, 52–64, Copyright (2010), with permission from Elsevier.

autonomic nervous system. The feeding and satiety circuitry of the hypothalamus plays a critical role in energy homeostasis and the development of obesity as well as related metabolic syndromes, and is located across the medial basal hypothalamus, including the arcuate nucleus of hypothalamus (ARC), paraventricular nucleus of hypothalamus (PVN), ventromedial hypothalamus (VMH), dorso-medial hypothalamus (DMH), and lateral hypothalamic area (LHA) (**Fig. 2.12**). The ARC is thought to receive information regarding metabolic status from peripheral circulating factors including leptin,

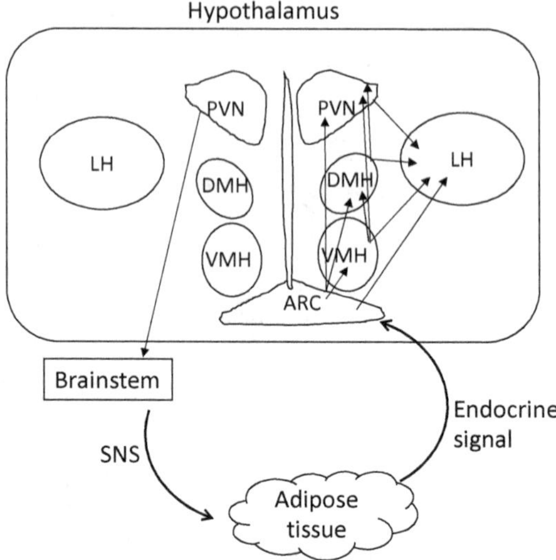

Fig. 2.12. Simplified schematic overview of the hypothalamus-adipose crosstalk regulating energy homeostasis. The arcuate nucleus (ARC) integrates peripheral endocrine signal (e.g. leptin). Leptin acts on its receptor in the ARC to modulate the expression and release of neuropeptides (e.g. NPY, POMC). The ARC drives other hypothalamic nuclei including ventromedial (VMH), dorsomedial (DMH), and paraventricular (PVN) nuclei (satiety centers) and the lateral hypothalamic area (LHA, hunger center). These neuronal populations communicate within the hypothalamus. Neuronal signaling, particularly from the PVN, modulates the activity of sympathetic nervous system (SNS) via the nucleus of the solitary tract located in the brainstem. The resulting change of SNS tone regulates energy expenditure such as lipolysis and/or thermogenesis in adipose tissue.

insulin, glucose, and the gut peptides like ghrelin.[38,40,41] The neuronal projections from the ARC to other brain areas mediate the effects of the ARC on energy balance. Anorexigenic pro-opiomelanocortin (POMC) neurons signal for satiety whereas orexigenic neuropeptide Y (NPY)/agouti-related peptide (AgRP) neurons drive feeding. Both neuronal populations express leptin receptor and are responsive to leptin. In light of leptin as the most drastic change among circulating growth factors and hormones examined, we zoomed in to the ARC that is the main action area of leptin.

At first, we used the candidate gene approach to screen a number of genes known to be involved in metabolic regulation and neuronal immune crosstalk at different durations of EE. The ARC was microdissected by laser capture and messenger RNA (mRNA) expression was examined by quantitative reverse transcription polymerase chain reaction (qRT-PCR) (**Fig. 2.13(a–c)**). At the early timepoint of 2 weeks of EE, among the 14 genes screened, the BDNF was the only gene showing a significant change, a 2-fold increase. The upregulation of *Bdnf* expression sustained at 4 weeks and 9 weeks of EE. In contrast, upregulation of *Npy* and *Agrp* expression occurred at 4 weeks of EE and increasing further by 9 weeks of EE. More genes regulating feeding and energy expenditure (serum/glucocorticoid-regulated kinase, *Sgk1*, and nerve growth factor inducible, *Vgf*) were stimulated only after 9 weeks of EE. These data revealed a dynamic gene expression pattern responding to EE. Those genes displaying changes after extended EE exposure may reflect a secondary response to the metabolic outcomes, but unlikely the key mediators in the CNS driving the peripheral phenotypes.[15]

Moreover, 2-week EE-stimulated *Bdnf* expression by 2-fold in the VMH and DMH, the hypothalamic nuclei crucial for the suppression of appetite[42,43] (**Fig. 2.13(d)**). Of note, *Bdnf* expression responded to EE in a pattern similar to neuronal activation markers *Junb* and *Fos*, consistent with BDNF as a plasticity-related and effector immediate early gene.[44,45]

Hypothalamic BDNF as the Key Brain Mediator

The gene expression profiling experiment drew our attention to BDNF as an attractive candidate gene mediating the peripheral phenotypes induced by EE. BDNF is one of the most intensively studied molecules with diverse functions in brain development and plasticity[46] (**Fig. 2.14**). BDNF null mice are embryonic lethal due to severe deficit in brain development. It is well known that BDNF expression is highly responsive to neural activity and environment[11] particularly in brain regions crucial for learning and memory.

BDNF transcription is controlled by calcium responsive elements and is significantly induced by calcium influx in neurons responding to

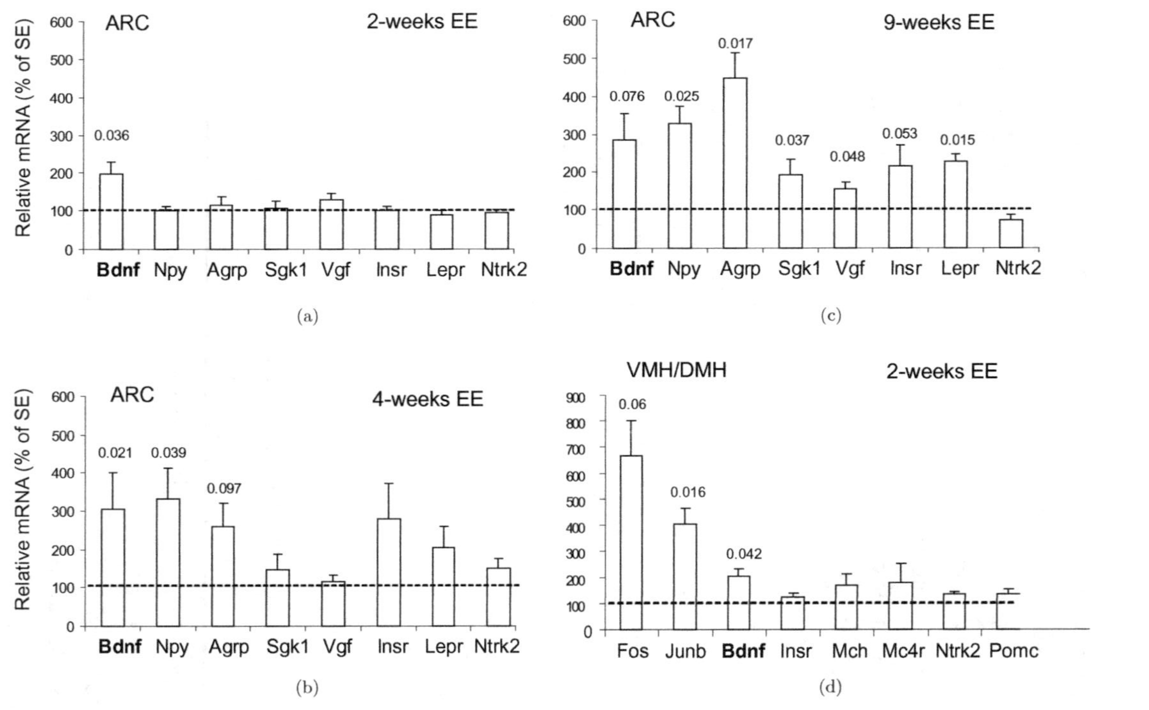

Fig. 2.13. EE induces gene expression changes in the arcuate nucleus of hypothalamus (a–c) and ventromedial (VMH)/dorsomedial (DMH) hypothalamus (d) at various duration of EE. $n = 5$ per group. Data are mean ± SEM. *P* values of significance or strong trends are shown above the bars. Reprinted from *Cell* Vol 142, Cao *et al.* Environmental and genetic activation of a brain-adipocyte BDNF/leptin axis causes cancer remission and inhibition, 52–64, Copyright (2010), with permission from Elsevier.

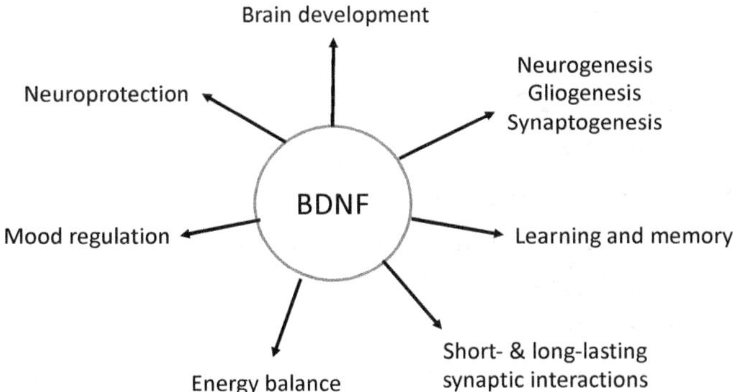

Fig. 2.14. BDNF is a neurotrophin with diverse functions.

neuronal activity.[47] The mouse *Bdnf* gene contains eight 5′ noncoding exons, each with distinct promoter regions, resulting in alternatively spliced mRNA isoforms. The exon IX contains the one coding region of the *Bdnf* gene.[48] Human BDNF gene shares a similar structure with 11 noncoding exons, splicing to a single coding exon.[49] BDNF is initially synthesized as precursor form — pro-BDNF, which is processed by proteases intracellularly to produce C-terminal mature form of BDNF.[50] Intracellular mature BDNF (m-BDNF) is generally trafficked via the activity-regulated synaptic packaging pathway to be stored both pre- and postsynaptic at dendrites for exocytosis.[51] In addition, BDNF can act via autocrine and paracrine release.[52] BDNF is present in almost all brain regions. Its functions vary depending on both the stage of brain development and the neuronal, glial, and vascular constituents of the brain.[53]

The BDNF isoforms bind to different types of receptors leading to a large variety of signaling cascades and functional consequences. The m-BDNF binds to the high-affinity neurotrophin receptor tropomyosin receptor kinase B (TrkB, also known as tyrosine receptor kinase B), leading to receptor dimerization and autophosphorylation. The m-BDNF/TrkB receptor complex triggers multiple downstream pathways including phospholipase C-γ (PLCγ), MAPK/ERK, PI3K/AKT, and guanosine triphosphate hydrolases (GTP-ases). Through these pathways, m-BDNF regulates cell function, growth, survival, and synaptic plasticity. TrkB receptor also has several isoforms adding more complexity to BDNF signaling. The full-length isoform (TrkB.FL) is predominantly expressed on neurons whereas a truncated isoform lacking receptor tyrosine kinase activity (TrkB.T1) is predominantly expressed on astrocytes.[54] These TrkB receptor isoforms have distinct or antagonizing actions.

Pro-BDNF can be released in some contexts to directly bind the p75 neurotrophin receptor (p75NTR) or to be processed extra-cellularly into m-BDNF.[50] Pro-BDNF is not an inactive precursor but rather a signaling protein-mediating diverse responses. Pro-BDNF preferentially interacts with p75NTR via its mature domain, and with the sortilin receptor via its pro-domain, thereby activating signaling pathways related with RhoA, JNK, and NF-κB. Pro-BDNF and m-BDNF have distinct or sometimes opposing effects on the regulation of neurophysiological processes. Hence, BDNF actions are regulated by the form of BDNF (mature or pro) secreted by cells, by extracellular proteolytic process, and by the presence of different types of receptors. This complexity allows proper control of signaling pathways critical for maintaining a dynamic balance between stimulating and inhibitory effects of BDNF that are exerted upon processes of brain development, synaptic plasticity, and brain regeneration after injury.[53,55]

Perhaps, more relevant to our study, BDNF is an important component of the hypothalamic pathway that controls energy homeostasis[56,57] (also see Chapter 3). Both peripheral and central administration of BDNF protein suppresses feeding, increases energy expenditure, and leads to weight loss.[58,59] Obesity is observed in mice with abnormal low BDNF levels such as BDNF heterozygous mice,[60] conditional knockout mice,[43] and selective deletion in VMH/DMH of adult mice.[61]

To elucidate the role of BDNF in the anticancer effect of EE, we genetically manipulated BDNF specifically in the hypothalamus of mice. First, we used a recombinant adeno-associated virus (rAAV) to deliver human BDNF gene to the hypothalamus of mice. A rAAV vector carrying the green fluorescent protein (GFP) was used as a control. rAAV vectors were injected to the hypothalamus via stereotaxic surgery, and all mice were housed in SE (**Fig. 2.15(a)**). Hypothalamic gene delivery of BDNF completely reproduced the metabolic (**Fig. 2.15(c)**) and immune changes (see Chapter 6) observed in EE, including a decrease in IGF-1 and leptin, an increase in adiponectin in the circulation, and enhanced immune responses. Importantly, rAAV-mediated overexpression of BDNF in hypothalamus resulted in remarkable suppression of tumor growth, a 75% reduction of B16 melanoma weight in BDNF-treated mice compared to GFP control mice (**Fig. 2.15(d)**).[15]

Next, we wanted to test whether the upregulation of hypothalamic BDNF expression was necessary for the EE-induced metabolic outcomes and anticancer phenotype using RNA interference (RNAi) approach. We generated a rAAV vector expressing a microRNA-targeting mouse *Bdnf* gene (miR-Bdnf). This miR-Bdnf could specifically suppress *Bdnf* mRNA and protein levels up to 80%.[15] A microRNA targeting a scrambled sequence (miR-scr.), interfering no known genes, served as a control. Mice were randomized to receive miR-Bdnf or miR-scr, and then split to live in EE versus SE (**Fig. 2.16(a)**). The miR-scr treatment did not interfere with the metabolic and anticancer effects of EE. In contrast, mice receiving miR-Bdnf in the hypothalamus were unable to respond to EE. In other words, preventing the EE-induced upregulation of *Bdnf* specifically in the hypothalamus completely blocked the anticancer effect of EE (**Fig. 2.16(b, c)**).

Furthermore, we investigated melanoma growth in BDNF heterozygous (BDNF+/-) mice whose BDNF protein levels in the hypothalamus is ~40% lower than wild type mice.[60] Both BDNF+/- mice and their wild type littermates were housed in SE. BDNF+/- mice were heavier with elevated serum leptin level, and their melanoma mass was increased almost 2-fold.[15]

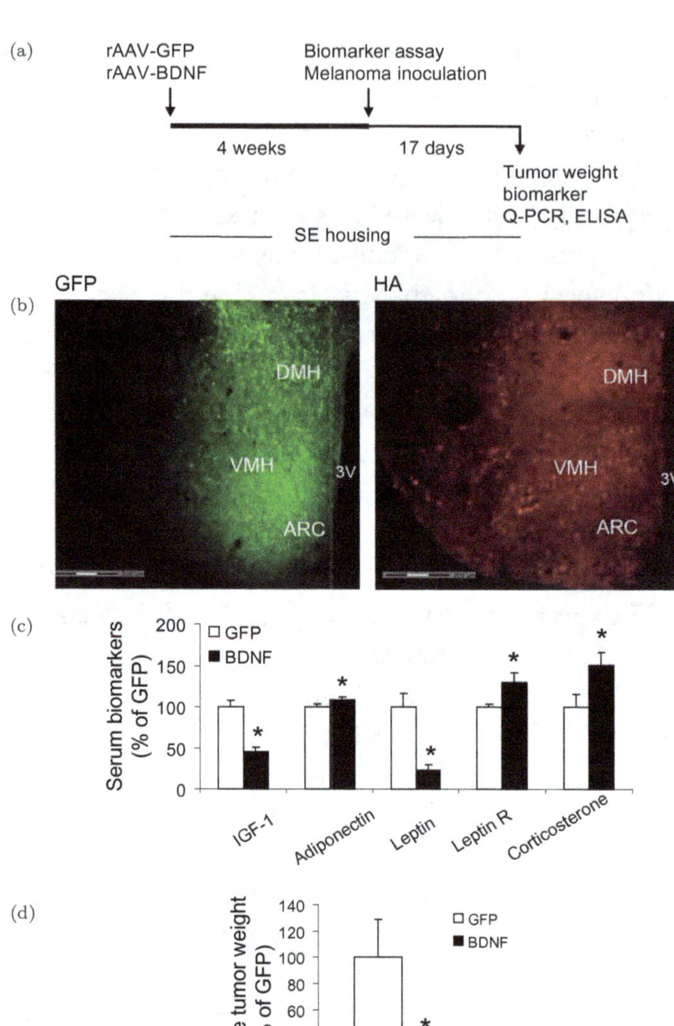

Fig. 2.15. Hypothalamic gene transfer of BDNF reproduces EE-induced metabolic changes and reduction of B16 melanoma growth (a) study design. AAV vectors were injected to the hypothalamus bilaterally. Mice were housed in SE. (b) Transgene expression in hypothalamus: GFP fluorescence; HA immunofluorescence (human BDNF has HA tag at 3′ terminal). (c) Biomarkers in serum. (d) Tumor mass. n = 10 for AAV-BDNF, n = 16 for AAV-GFP. Data are mean ± SEM. $P < 0.05$. Reprinted from *Cell* Vol 142, Cao *et al*. Environmental and genetic activation of a brain-adipocyte BDNF/leptin axis causes cancer remission and inhibition, 52–64, Copyright (2010), with permission from Elsevier.

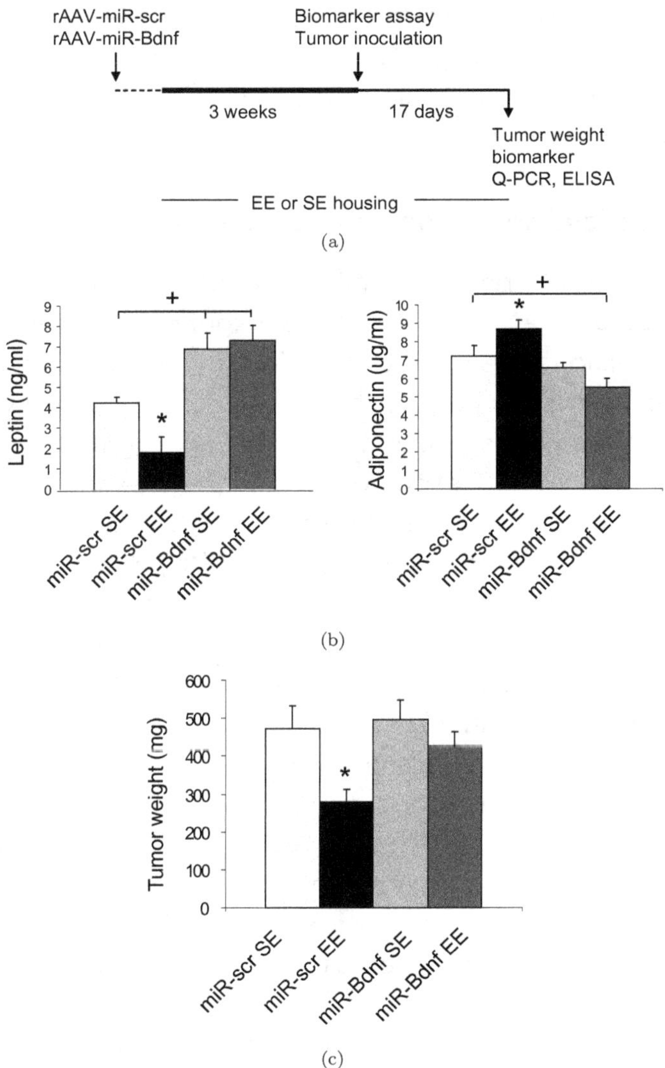

Fig. 2.16. Hypothalamic BDNF knockdown inhibits EE-induced metabolic changes and tumor resistance. (a) Study design of RNAi knockdown of hypothalamic Bdnf expression. (b) Biomarkers in serum 4-week post AAV injection and 3-week EE housing. $*P < 0.05$ miR-scr EE versus all other groups, $+ P < 0.05$ between groups as indicated. (c) B16 melanoma mass. $*P < 0.05$, miR-scr EE versus all other groups. $n = 7$–17 per group. Data are mean ±SEM. Reprinted from Cell Vol 142, Cao *et al.* Environmental and genetic activation of a brain-adipocyte BDNF/leptin axis causes cancer remission and inhibition, 52–64, Copyright (2010), with permission from Elsevier.

These data collectively have identified hypothalamic BDNF as a key brain mediator linking the environment to cancer growth in the periphery. The next question is how the hypothalamic information relays to the periphery.

Sympathetic Modulation of Adipose Tissue

Given leptin as key peripheral effector of EE, we hypothesized that the sympathetic nervous system (SNS) might connect hypothalamic BDNF signaling to the change of leptin in the adipose tissue. Leptin is secreted predominantly by the white adipose tissue (WAT), and circulating leptin levels reflect synthesis and secretion in WAT,[62] indicating that WAT is responsive to EE. Gene expression analysis showed leptin expression was decreased ~50% in EE mice consistent with the drop observed in serum (**Fig. 2.17(a)**).[15]

There is evidence that leptin expression is suppressed by sympathetic tone via β-adrenergic receptors (ARs).[62,63] All of the three β-AR genes, *Adrb1*, *Adrb2*, and *Adrb3*, were upregulated by approximately 3-fold in WAT of EE mice but not in skeletal muscle (**Fig. 2.17(a)**). Upon SNS activation, norepinephrine is released from nerve terminal to act on β-ARs. EE significantly elevated the norepinephrine level in WAT (**Fig. 2.17(b)**) but not in the circulation, indicating elevated sympathetic drive preferentially to WAT.[15] Hypothalamic overexpression of BDNF also led to an increase in the WAT norepinephrine levels similar to EE (**Fig. 2.17(c)**). On the contrary, norepinephrine level was significantly reduced in WAT of BDNF+/- mice supporting a role of BDNF in sympathetic modulation of WAT (**Fig. 2.17(d)**).

We then sought to test if SNS activation is required for EE's metabolic and anticancer effects. β-blocker propranolol abrogated EE-induced leptin drop and completely blocked the anticancer effect of EE suggesting an essential role of SNS (**Fig. 2.17(e, f)**).

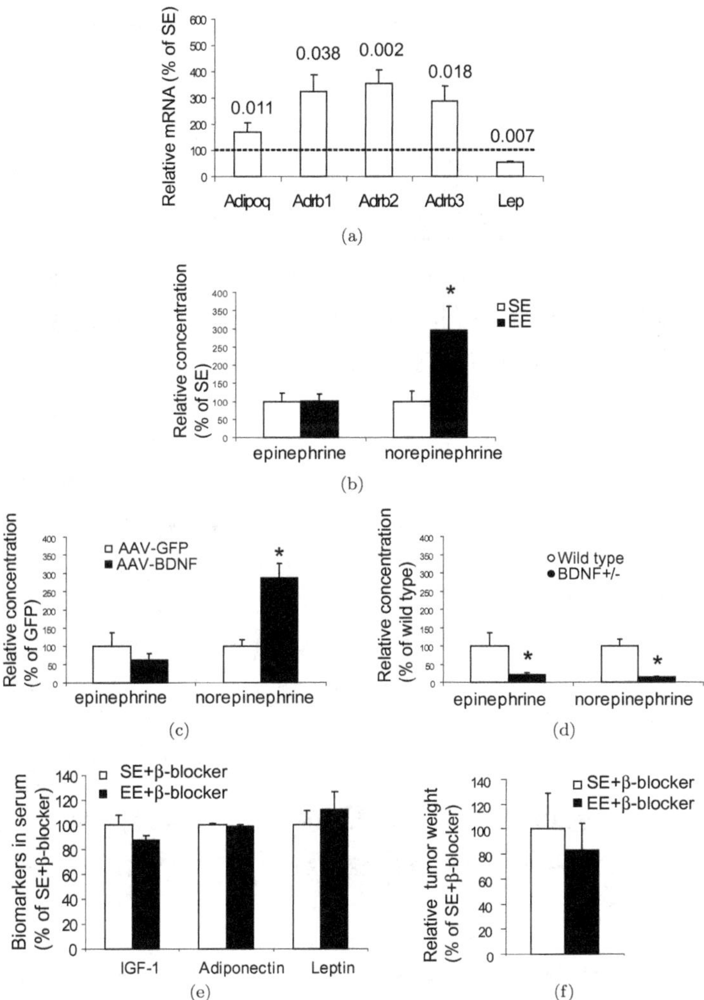

Fig. 2.17. Elevation of sympathetic tone to the white adipose tissue serves as a peripheral pathway mediating the EE-associated anticancer phenotype. (a) EE-induced gene expression changes in WAT after 9 weeks of EE. $n = 5$ per group. P values of significance are shown above bars. (b) WAT catecholamine levels after 9 weeks of EE. $n = 5$ per group. (c) WAT catecholamine levels in mice overexpressing BDNF in the hypothalamus compared to GFP-expressing mice. $n = 5$ per group. (d) WAT catecholamine levels in BDNF heterozygous mice compared to wild type littermates. $n = 4$ per group. (e and f) Propranolol completely blocked EE effects on serum biomarkers and melanoma growth. $n = 20$ per group. Data are mean ± SEM. * $P < 0.05$. Reprinted from *Cell* Vol 142, Cao *et al.* Environmental and genetic activation of a brain-adipocyte BDNF/leptin axis causes cancer remission and inhibition, 52–64, Copyright (2010), with permission from Elsevier.

Hypothalamic-Sympathoneural-Adipocyte Axis

In a comprehensive set of genetic and pharmacological experiments using somatic gene transfer, transgenic animals, controlled release liposomes, and osmotic minipump drug infusion, we teased out a key mechanism underlying the anticancer phenotype induced by EE. We coined the term "hypothalamic-sympathoneural-adipocyte" (HSA) axis to describe this brain–adipocyte axis — the specific neuroendocrine pathway linking the hypothalamus to WAT.[15] The hypothalamic component is mediated via BDNF. In response to the complex physical, social, and cognitive stimuli provided by EE, hypothalamic BDNF is induced as an effector immediate early gene and leads to activation of a component of the SNS, preferentially elevating the sympathoneural innervation of WAT. The activation of this axis therefore consists of an increase in hypothalamic BDNF, WAT norepinephrine, and via β-ARs on the adipocytes, and a suppression of leptin expression and release. The ensuring marked drop of leptin in circulation contributes critically to the suppression of tumor growth (**Fig. 2.18**).

Physical Exercise Alone Does not Account for the Anticancer Phenotype of Environmental Enrichment

One of the most frequently asked question is whether EE is just exercise. The answer is no at least in our models. To investigate whether physical exercise alone could mimic the EE-induced melanoma resistance, we housed mice in cages with free access to running wheels for 4 weeks followed by B16 melanoma implantation.[15] Mice love to run on wheels recording on average ~2 km per mouse per day. Wheel running resulted in several physiological alterations including lower body weight, reduced adiposity, and increased lean mass similar to that observed in the EE mice. However, runners displayed

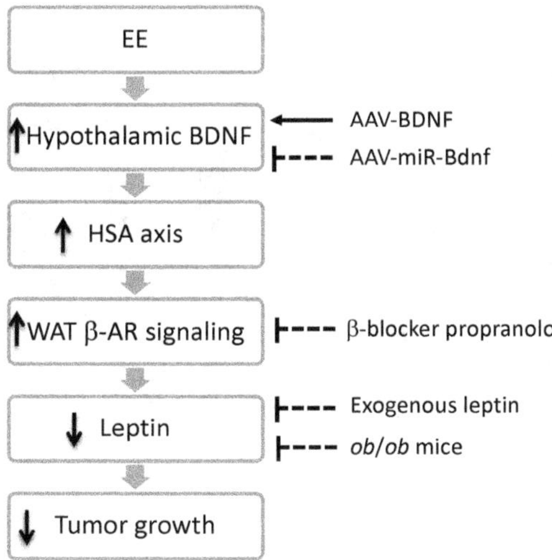

Fig. 2.18.   A specific brain–fat axis, the hypothalamic-sympathoneural-adipocyte (HSA) axis is one underlying mechanism of EE-induced inhibition of tumor growth. EE upregulates BDNF expression in the hypothalamus and subsequently elevates sympathetic tone to the adipose tissue. The resulting activation of β-adrenergic receptor signaling suppresses leptin expression and release, whereby decreasing tumor growth. Gain and loss of function studies identify each major component of the HSA axis.

altered biomarkers in serum with a pattern quite distinct to that of EE mice. In runners, IGF-1 was significantly reduced similar to that in the EE mice, but leptin was not changed in contrast to the drastic drop in the EE mice (**Fig. 2.19(a)**). Although an enhanced immune response was observed in runners, exercise alone did not significantly reduce melanoma weight (**Fig. 2.19(b)**). These data suggest that physical exercise alone is insufficient to account for EE-induced tumor resistance although it likely contributes.

EE consists of a much larger space, with various toys and objects to explore in addition to access to running wheels. We were aware that the total physical activities in EE were likely beyond the distance run on the wheels. To quantify the total physical activity, we video-recorded EE mice using a night-view camcorder throughout

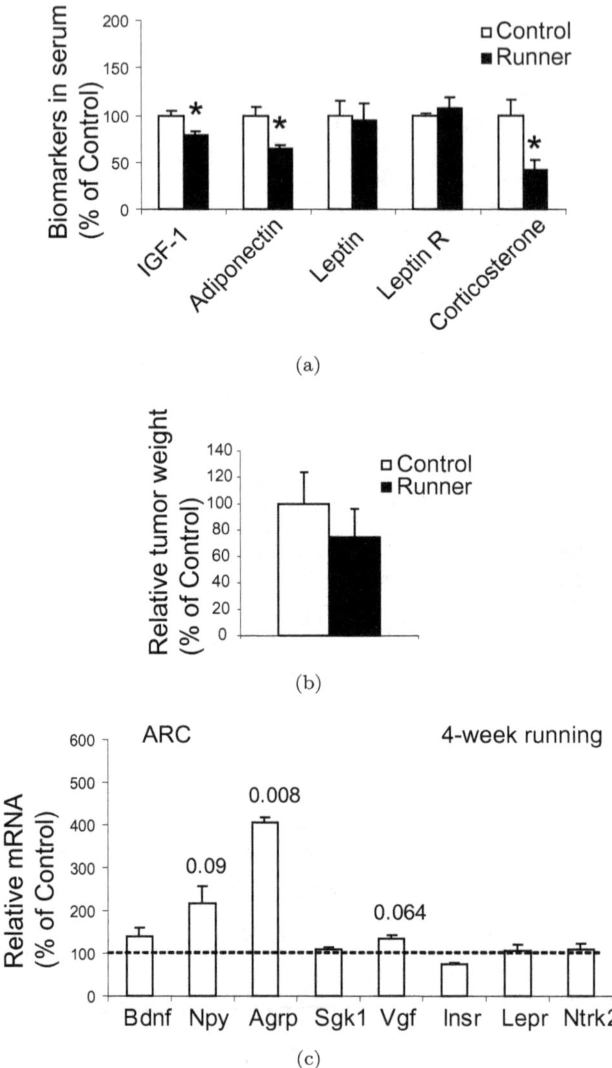

Fig. 2.19. Voluntary running does not account for the EE-associated anticancer phenotype. (a) Running led to some biomarker changes distinctive to those observed in EE. $n = 16$ for runners, $n = 13$ for control. $*P < 0.05$. (b) Running did not significantly reduce B16 melanoma mass. $n = 11$ for runner, $n = 10$ for control. (c) Running did not upregulate Bdnf expression in the arcuate nucleus as that observed in EE. $n = 5$ per group. P values with significance or strong trends are shown above bars. Data are mean ± SEM. Reprinted from *Cell* Vol 142, Cao *et al.* Environmental and genetic activation of a brain-adipocyte BDNF/leptin axis causes cancer remission and inhibition, 52–64, Copyright (2010), with permission from Elsevier.

the dark phase during which mice were active. We labeled the EE cage with grids visible in night-view recording, and marked the running wheel with a tape visible in night-view as well to facilitate counting rotation.[15] Our staff painstakingly watched hours of video recording and counted the total rotations of running wheel to calculate the distance of running. General motor activity was quantified by counting the total crosses of grids and calculated to the distance traveled. The total physical activity was represented as the sum of running distance on running wheels and distance traveled in the EE cage. The EE mice traveled on average a total distance of 0.64 km per day, ~66% less than the runners, further suggesting physical activity *per se* unlikely the major contributor to the EE-induced tumor inhibition.[15]

Noteworthy, wheel running led to a gene expression profile in the ARC qualitatively different compared to that in EE. In contrast to the EE mice whose *Bdnf* was upregulated 3-fold at 4-week timepoint, running for 4 weeks did not stimulate *Bdnf* significantly while the two orexigenic neuropeptides *Npy* and *Agrp* were increased (**Fig. 2.19(c)**).[15] Our later research has revealed additional differences between EE and wheel running alone which are discussed in Chapters 3 and 7.

These data by no means diminish the benefits of physical exercise. Large body of work has shown a wide range of beneficial effects associated with physical exercise on immune function,[64,65] metabolic homeostasis,[66,67] cognition and mental health,[68–71] and cancer.[72–74] Increased physical activity is an important and integral component of the complex EE. Accumulating evidence suggests that physical exercise alone unable to account for the phenotypic changes induced by EE including our studies.[15,75–77] In most cases, the whole package — commonly described EE providing physical, social, and cognitive stimuli, elicits optimal cerebral and physical benefits beyond each component alone (Chapter 1).

Imagine the physical activity in EE as team sports in contrast to running alone on a treadmill. Even if the physical activity is comparable, the mental impact certainly differs. Animal studies have revealed distinctive mechanisms underlying various outcomes of exercise and EE including those shared by both paradigms.[15,78] For example, both voluntary wheel-running and EE increase adult hippocampal neurogenesis, a process adding new neurons to the neural network, not just synapses and neurites. Voluntary running is thought to stimulate the proliferation and maintenance of the precursor cells from which adult neurogenesis originates. In contrast, EE primarily promotes the survival of newborn cells derived from the proliferating precursor cells. And these effects appear to be additive, which might be explained by their different cellular mechanisms.[79] Kempermann and colleagues propose that physical activity can "prime" the neurogenic region of hippocampus for increased neurogenesis when the animal is exposed to additional cognitive stimuli provided by EE.[80]

Publication and Impact

The journey to publishing the paper was long and ardent with several rounds of rejections from high impact journals. We understood from the beginning that the paper would not be immediately embraced by the reviewers, in part because emphasis of large majority of basic cancer research had been defining the disease at the molecular level. Indeed, some expressed disbelief that a simple change of housing could profoundly affect the growth of a highly malignant tumor. Others dismissed the significance of such research in animals on the ground that many clinical and epidemiology studies have shown influences of lifestyle on cancer. We persevered over a few years through several rounds of revisions. The paper was eventually published in *Cell* in 2010,[15] accompanied by a Leading-Edge Preview, featured on the cover of the issue (**Fig. 2.20**), and selected to show a PaperFlick on *Cell* website. This paper was at the top of the most downloaded papers by *Cell* in the month it was published. It was reported by *Nature, Science, Nature Reviews Cancer,* and

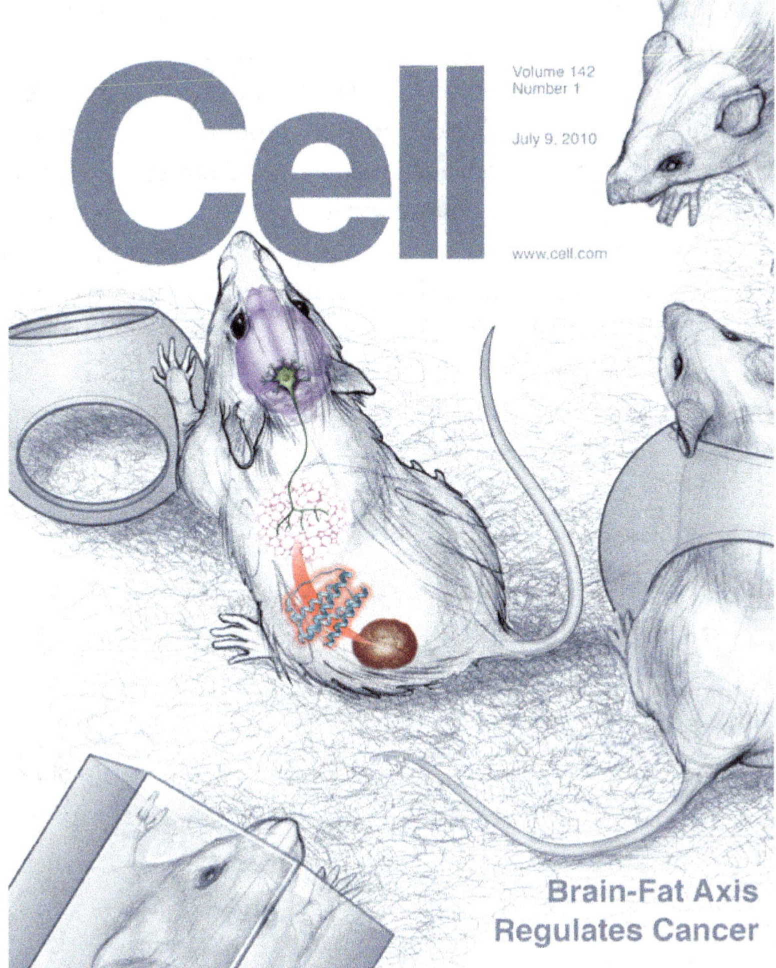

Fig. 2.20. Cover image. Reprinted from *Cell* Vol 142, Cao *et al*. Environmental and genetic activation of a brain–adipocyte BDNF/leptin axis causes cancer remission and inhibition, 52–64, Copyright (2010), with permission from Elsevier.

other scientific journals and also drew attentions from general media around the world.

Our work has brought some much-needed scientific rigor to a field that is of enormous public interest, but that has been considered soft, i.e., the "mind–body" connection, and the influence of the physical environment and mental state on physiological processes including cancer. This work is impactful because it not only demonstrates a highly consistent and rigorous effect of an environmental paradigm on cancer, where diet, exercise, and stress are not critical determinants, but also discovers a previously poorly defined neuroendocrine axis, the HSA axis. It is the first time that investigators have shown that the somatic manipulation of a single gene in the brain can influence systemic cancer, which may have broad implications in the field of stress biology (see Chapter 8) and public health.

Most satisfying to us is that our pioneering work has inspired others to investigate in this field, and the collective advance facilitates the shift to a more holistic view of cancer.

Generalization to Additional Cancer Types and Mechanisms

Since the first publication of the anticancer effect of EE, other investigators have generalized to additional types of cancer, demonstrating effectiveness of EE in pancreatic cancer,[81,82] glioma,[83] and lung cancer[81] models. These studies have explored mechanisms beyond the HSA axis.

Breast Cancer

Nachat-Kappes and colleagues investigated the effects of EE on normal mammary gland development and implanted mammary tumor growth.[84] Juvenile female C57BL/6 mice were housed in SE or EE for 9 weeks, followed by orthotopically transplantation of syngeneic EO771 mammary tumor cells into the right inguinal mammary fat pad. In non-tumor-bearing mice, EE influenced mammary gland development with enhanced side-branching and advanced development of alveolar structures of the mammary gland. In addition, EE led to a decrease of cells expressing cyclooxygenase-2 (COX-2) that has been implicated in breast cancer. Circulating level of adiponectin was significantly higher in non-tumor-bearing mice in EE compared to their counterparts in SE, but no difference in leptin, IL-6, TNF-α, PAI-1, MCP-1, PGF(2α), and F(2)-isoprostanes.

Mammary tumor volume and mass were smaller in EE mice. The decrease in tumor mass was associated with a reduction in COX-2 and Ki67 levels and an increase in caspase-3 level in the tumors. In the tumors collected from SE mice, COX-2 expression was positively correlated with leptin level. Both tumor-bearing groups showed increased levels of resistin, IL-6, TNF-α, PAI-1, and MCP-1 irrespective of housing environment suggesting higher inflammatory response due to the presence of mammary tumor. This study demonstrates EE effective in an implantation model of murine breast cancer associated with marked reduction in intra-tumoral COX-2 activity and an increase in the plasma level of adiponectin but short of mechanistic interrogation. The circulating leptin level was not changed in this study[84] inconsistent to our finding in male mice. The difference in EE setting and sex may cause this discrepancy.

We have investigated how EE influences breast cancer in obese conditions in female mice, which is described in Chapter 5.

Pancreatic Cancer

Li and colleagues extended EE to models of pancreatic cancer, among the most lethal cancers lacking effective treatment modalities.[82] The investigators adopted an EE protocol similar to our original report including the EE setting, the sex, age, and strain of mouse. They observed upregulation of *Bdnf* expression in the hypothalamus consistent with our report. Panc02 pancreatic cancer cells were implanted subcutaneously or orthotopically. EE significantly reduced the tumor burden in both models: subcutaneous — 53% reduction, and orthotopic — 41% reduction. They analyzed the tumor transcriptome and proteome and found a total of 129 genes showing differential expression at both the mRNA and protein levels in response to EE, 44 upregulated, and 85 downregulated. The majority of differentially expressed genes were localized to the mitochondria and enriched in the citrate cycle and oxidative phosphorylation pathways. Interestingly, nearly all of these mitochondria-related genes were downregulated in tumors from EE mice. This study provides evidence suggesting modulation of cancer metabolism by EE.

The investigators attempted to dissect essential component of EE in pancreatic cancer model. They evaluated single component of EE such as inanimate stimulation, social stimulation, and voluntary wheel running. None of the single component setting achieved comparative antitumor effect as the typical combined EE.

The Tu lab later investigated NK cell antitumor immunity using similar pancreatic cancer model and a lung cancer model, and described a SNS-dependent pathway enhancing NK cell activity in response to EE[81] (Chapter 6).

Glioma

In 2015, Garofalo and colleagues published a paper reporting a striking suppression of glioma growth induced by EE through immune and nonimmune mechanisms.[83] Malignant glioma is the most diffuse and aggressive neoplasm of the nervous system with a poor prognosis, characterized as high proliferation and invasiveness, diffuse apoptosis and/or necrosis, infiltration of astrocytes, and activation of microglia/microphage. This study has several intriguing findings but with some caveats.

The investigators randomized juvenile male C57BL/6 mice to live in SE or EE for 5 weeks followed by injection of syngeneic GL261 glioma cells to the right striatum. They monitored the tumor size at different times after brain transplantation of glioma. Starting 11 days post glioma implantation, the brains of EE mice showed smaller tumors and the difference became more remarkable by 17 days with a reduction in tumor volume by ~76% compared to that in SE mice. This robust inhibition of glioma growth was observed using different glioma cells such as the human U87MG (implanting to SCID [severe combined immunodeficient mice] mice) and the stem-like CD133$^+$ murine GL261 cells. EE profoundly improved survival of glioma-bearing mice by 3 folds. In addition, EE mice displayed an increased resistance to establish injected glioma. In SE, 3.5% of mice showed no visible tumor, while this value rose to 26.5% in EE. EE reduced tumor cell proliferation and astrogliosis but had no effect on microglia/macrophage infiltration of glioma.

The authors examined glioma cell invasiveness toward the healthy brain parenchyma and found EE mice having lower number of glioma cells protruding more than 150 μm from the main tumor mass, indicating reduced tendency to migrate and invade the surrounding tissue.

There is a caveat of this study regarding the controls. Control mice were housed in pair, in standard cage, which is atypical to most SE housing consisting one to five mice per cage. Housing two male mice in a cage could facilitate social hierarchy, one dominant, the other subordinate. The control setting in this study might make mice more vulnerable to glioma and therefore exaggerating the benefits of EE. Nevertheless, the authors examined the time dependency of EE exposure and conclude that EE is only effective when the brain is conditioned before glioma implantation and likely requiring longer periods (>3-week EE).

The investigators proposed two mechanisms of the glioma-inhibitory effects of EE. The immune mechanism is that EE increases IL-15 level in the brain of glioma-bearing mice and thereby promoting NK cell accumulation to the tumor site and enhancing NK cell activity. This immune modality is discussed in Chapter 6. The nonimmune mechanism is through BDNF actions. The brains of EE mice showed higher level of BDNF compared to SE mice. Two experiments were conducted to assess the effect of BDNF. First, SE mice were infused with BDNF protein 48 hr before and during glioma transplantation. BDNF treatment led to ~50% reduction in tumor volume by 17 days post glioma implantation. Second, BDNF was delivered 10 days after glioma injection to SE mice, and the infusion continued for 7 days. BDNF treatment resulted in significant reduction of glioma size, mimicking EE effect.

Furthermore, the authors examined the direct effect of BDNF on GL261 glioma cells and the signaling pathways involved. GL261 cells do not express the full-length form of BDNF receptor TrkB.FL. Instead, GL261 cells express the truncated forms TrkB.T1 and TrkB. T2. The *in vitro* studies revealed direct effects of BDNF on GL261 glioma cells, reducing the chemotactic activity of glioma cells through activation of TrkB.T1 and inhibition of the small G protein RhoA signaling. *In vivo*, BDNF infusion reduced microglia/macrophage infiltration in tumor mass. These are intriguing and novel findings. But there is a caveat in the authors' claim with regard to BDNF because the BDNF infusion experiments alone are insufficient to prove the role of BDNF in EE-induced glioma inhibition. Blockade of BDNF in the brain of EE mice is required for such investigations.

Colon Cancer

In 2017, Bice and colleagues reported a remarkable extension of life span induced by EE in a genetic model of colon cancer.[85] They previously developed a unique mouse model Tcf$^{Het/+}$ Apc$^{Min/+}$ mice in which heterozygous loss of a tumor suppressor, *Tcf4* gene (encoding T-cell factor 4), is combined with an initiating mutation in the *Apc* gene. This transgenic mouse line exhibits unregulated proliferation of colonic epithelial cells and significantly accelerated colon tumorigenesis. The investigators assessed whether long-term EE could affect the survival of Tcf$^{Het/+}$ Apc$^{Min/+}$ colon cancer mice and observed a drastic effect on both male and female mice. EE increased the median survival days by 32% in male $Tcf^{Het/+}$ $Apc^{Min/+}$ mice (173 days in SE versus 228 days in EE). EE had even more profound survival benefit in female $Tcf^{Het/+}$ $Apc^{Min/+}$ mice, extending median survival by 53% (156 days in SE versus 238 days in EE). Interestingly, tumor burden was reduced by EE only in female mice, which suggests survival benefit in males and females in response to EE may arise from different mechanisms.

The authors sought to characterize the systemic changes and alterations in tumor microenvironment in males because decrease of tumor number or size could not explain the striking extension of life span. Male $Tcf^{Het/+}$ $Apc^{Min/+}$ mice in SE lost more than 25% of body weight compared to wild type mice in SE, a sign of cachexia. EE mitigated this weight loss but did not alleviate anemia. Moreover, EE reduced serum levels of IL-6 by 45% and TNF-α by 70% indicating a strong anti-inflammatory effect. Because injection of IL-6 causes cancer cachexia in $Apc^{Min/+}$ mice, the authors conclude that EE improves the survival of male $Tcf^{Het/+}$ $Apc^{Min/+}$ mice, partially through reduction of IL-6- and TNF-α-dependent cachexia symptoms.

The investigators conducted RNA sequencing analysis of distal colon samples from male $Tcf^{Het/+}$ $Apc^{Min/+}$ mice. They found 205 upregulated genes and 105 downregulated genes in EE mice compared to SE mice. Of note, EE appeared to normalize the gene expression pattern of adenomas: reducing those genes that are upregulated in tumor while increasing those that are downregulated in tumor. EE also reduced the expression of many genes involved in Wnt/β-catenin-mediated tumor cell proliferation.

The comprehensive characterization of the tumor microenvironment revealed diverse effects of EE on wound repair processes.[85] The wound healing process is achieved through several different phases. Disruption of any phase causes chronic wounds that do not heal.[86] There is evidence that tumor microenvironment shares many features with defective wound healing. In other words, tumors can be seen as wounds that cannot heal. This study found that EE modulated multiple factors involved in different phases of wound repair process in $Tcf^{Het/+}$ $Apc^{Min/+}$ mice. EE activated several nuclear hormone receptors signaling including glucocorticoid receptor, thyroid hormone receptor, and oxysterol receptor. These nuclear hormone receptors play an important role in wound repair, and are often dysfunctional in colon cancer.[87]

Pericytes surround and stabilize blood vessels, and are important for wound repair. In $Tcf^{Het/+}$ $Apc^{Min/+}$ mice, EE recruited pericytes, reduced angiogenesis, and normalized tumor vasculature, resembling the later stages of revascularization in the wound repair process. This pericyte-mediated promotion of wound healing was associated with an increase in IgA level.

Disfunction of epithelial barrier in colon tumor tissue can result in microbial invasion and associated inflammation. EE was found to normalize gut microbiota composition in $Tcf^{Het/+}$ $Apc^{Min/+}$ tumor-bearing mice.

The authors propose a mechanistic model explaining the remarkable survival benefit of EE in $Tcf^{Het/+}$ $Apc^{Min/+}$ mice.[85] EE activates nuclear hormone receptors and thereby provoking tumor wound repair resolution through normalization of blood vessels, revascularization, plasma cell recruitment and IgA secretion, replacement of glandular tumor structures with pericytes ("scarring," or "seal the wound"), and restores biodiversity of microbiota. However, the phenotypic findings are associative, and the hypothesis of mechanism has not been tested due to lack of mechanistic interrogations. Nevertheless, this study provides exciting data and paves the way for future research.

Summary

Emerging evidence has shown that EE, a complex housing providing physical, social, and cognitive stimuli to laboratory animals, exerts remarkable anticancer effects in various murine models of cancer including melanoma, breast, colon, pancreatic, lung cancer, and glioma. The efficacy of EE as an intervention to combat tumor is considerably influenced by the type of tumor, the genetic defect of the cancer model, sex and age of the animals, and EE protocol. The underlying mechanisms are diverse and likely multimodal involving the nervous, immune, and endocrine systems. A specific brain–fat axis, the HSA axis, has been identified as one mechanism linking the brain activity to systemic cancer growth in response to EE. Although the past decade has seen significant progress, mechanistic studies remain scarce in the field of macroenvironmental impact on onco-genesis. This is a glaring gap in light of the vast amount of clinical and epidemiological data demonstrating the profound influence lifestyle and mental health on cancer risk and prognosis. As an experimental paradigm recapitulating certain aspects of an active or challenging lifestyle, EE can facilitate basic research bringing "hard science" to the traditionally soft "mind–body connection" in cancer research and beyond.

References

1. Hanahan D, Weinberg RA. (2000) The hallmarks of cancer. *Cell* **100**:57–70.
2. Hanahan D, Weinberg RA. (2011) Hallmarks of cancer: The next gen-eration. *Cell* **144**:646–674.
3. McAllister SS, Weinberg RA. (2010) Tumor-host interactions: A far-reaching relationship. *J Clin Oncol* **28**:4022–4028.
4. Green McDonald P, O'Connell M, Lutgendorf SK. (2013) Psychoneu-roimmunology and cancer: A decade of discovery, paradigm shifts, and methodological innovations. *Brain Behav Immun* **30 Suppl**: S1–9.
5. Aaronson SA. (1991) Growth factors and cancer. *Science* **254**:1146–1153.
6. Darnell RB, Posner JB. (2006) Paraneoplastic syndromes affecting the nervous system. *Semin Oncol* **33**:270–298.

7. Friedl P, Alexander S. (2011) Cancer invasion and the microenvironment: Plasticity and reciprocity. *Cell* **147**:992–1009.

8. Kolonel LN, Altshuler D, Henderson BE. (2004) The multiethnic cohort study: Exploring genes, lifestyle and cancer risk. *Nat Rev Cancer* **4**:519–527.

9. Baade PD, Youlden DR, Krnjacki LJ. (2009) International epidemiology of prostate cancer: Geographical distribution and secular trends. *Mol Nutr Food Res* **53**:171–184.

10. Castano Z, Tracy K, McAllister SS. (2011) The tumor macroenvironment and systemic regulation of breast cancer progression. *Int J Dev Biol* **55**:889–897.

11. Young D, Lawlor PA, Leone P, Dragunow M, During MJ. (1999) Environmental enrichment inhibits spontaneous apoptosis, prevents seizures and is neuroprotective. *Nat Med* **5**:448–453.

12. Cao L, Jiao X, Zuzga DS, *et al.* (2004) VEGF links hippocampal activity with neurogenesis, learning and memory. *Nat Genet* **36**:827–835.

13. During MJ, Cao L. (2006) VEGF, a mediator of the effect of experience on hippocampal neurogenesis. *Curr Alzheimer Res* **3**:29–33.

14. Nithianantharajah J, Hannan AJ. (2006) Enriched environments, experience-dependent plasticity and disorders of the nervous system. *Nat Rev Neurosci* **7**:697–709.

15. Cao L, Liu X, Lin E-JD, *et al.* (2010) Environmental and genetic activation of a brain-adipocyte BDNF/leptin axis causes cancer remission and inhibition. *Cell* **142**:52–64.

16. Ferlay J, Soerjomataram I, Dikshit R, *et al.* (2015) Cancer incidence and mortality worldwide: Sources, methods and major patterns in GLOBOCAN 2012. *Int J Cancer* **136**:E359–386.

17. Aran V, Victorino AP, Thuler LC, Ferreira CG. (2016) Colorectal cancer: Epidemiology, disease mechanisms and interventions to reduce onset and mortality. *Clin Colorectal Cancer* **15**:195–203.

18. Su LK, Kinzler KW, Vogelstein B, *et al.* (1992) Multiple intestinal neoplasia caused by a mutation in the murine homolog of the APC gene. *Science* **256**:668–670.

19. Jenkins PJ, Bustin SA. (2004) Evidence for a link between IGF-I and cancer. *Eur J Endocrinol* **151 Suppl 1**:S17–22.

20. Renehan AG, Zwahlen M, Minder C, *et al.* (2004) Insulin-like growth factor (IGF)-I, IGF binding protein-3, and cancer risk: Systematic review and meta-regression analysis. *Lancet* **363**:1346–1353.

21. Fujisawa T, Endo H, Tomimoto A, *et al.* (2008) Adiponectin suppresses colorectal carcinogenesis under the high-fat diet condition. *Gut* **57**:1531–1538.

22. Ando S, Naimo GD, Gelsomino L, *et al.* (2020) Novel insights into adiponectin action in breast cancer: Evidence of its mechanistic effects mediated by ERalpha expression. *Obes Rev* **21**:e13004.

23. Friedman J. (2016) The long road to leptin. *J Clin Invest* **126**:4727–4734.

24. Cui H, Lopez M, Rahmouni K. (2017) The cellular and molecular bases of leptin and ghrelin resistance in obesity. *Nat Rev Endocrinol* **13**:338–351.

25. Mantzoros CS, Magkos F, Brinkoetter M, *et al.* (2011) Leptin in human physiology and pathophysiology. *Am J Physiol Endocrinol Metab* **301**:E567–584.

26. Wauters M, Considine RV, Van Gaal LF. (2000) Human leptin: From an adipocyte hormone to an endocrine mediator. *Eur J Endocrinol* **143**:293–311.

27. Ray A, Cleary MP. (2017) The potential role of leptin in tumor invasion and metastasis. *Cytokine Growth Factor Rev* **38**:80–97.

28. Garofalo C, Surmacz E. (2006) Leptin and cancer. *J Cell Physiol* **207**:12–22.

29. Alshaker H, Sacco K, Alfraidi A, *et al.* (2015) Leptin signalling, obesity and prostate cancer: Molecular and clinical perspective on the old dilemma. *Oncotarget* **6**:35556–35563.

30. Cirillo D, Rachiglio AM, la Montagna R, *et al.* (2008) Leptin signaling in breast cancer: An overview. *J Cell Biochem* **105**:956–964.

31. Crean-Tate KK, Reizes O. (2018) Leptin regulation of cancer stem cells in breast and gynecologic cancer. *Endocrinology* **159**:3069–3080.

32. Ellis PE, Barron GA, Bermano G. (2020) Adipocytokines and their relationship to endometrial cancer risk: A systematic review and meta-analysis. *Gynecol Oncol* **158**:507–516.

33. Stattin P, Lukanova A, Biessy C, *et al.* (2004) Obesity and colon cancer: Does leptin provide a link? *Int J Cancer* **109**:149–152.

34. Gogas H, Trakatelli M, Dessypris N, *et al.* (2008) Melanoma risk in association with serum leptin levels and lifestyle parameters: A case-control study. *Ann Oncol* **19**:384–389.

35. Coleman DL, Hummel KP. (1973) The influence of genetic background on the expression of the obese (Ob) gene in the mouse. *Diabetologia* **9**:287–293.

36. Brandon EL, Gu J-W, Cantwell L, *et al.* (2009) Obesity promotes melanoma tumor growth: Role of leptin. *Cancer Biol Ther* **8**:1871–1879.

37. McEwen BS. (2007) Physiology and neurobiology of stress and adaptation: Central role of the brain. *Physiol Rev* **87**:873–904.

38. Dhillo WS. (2007) Appetite regulation: An overview. *Thyroid* **17**:433–445.

39. Burbridge S, Stewart I, Placzek M. (2016) Development of the neuroendocrine hypothalamus. *Compr Physiol* **6**:623–643.

40. Austin J, Marks D. (2009) Hormonal regulators of appetite. *Int J Pediatr Endocrinol* **2009**:141753.

41. Gaspar JM, Velloso LA. (2018) Hypoxia Inducible factor as a central regulator of metabolism - implications for the development of obesity. *Front Neurosci* **12**:813.

42. Rios M, Fan G, Fekete C, *et al.* (2001) Conditional deletion of brain-derived neurotrophic factor in the postnatal brain leads to obesity and hyperactivity. *Mol Endocrinol* **15**:1748–1757.

43. Xu B, Goulding EH, Zang K, *et al.* (2003) Brain-derived neurotrophic factor regulates energy balance downstream of melanocortin-4 receptor. *Nat Neurosci* **6**:736–742.

44. Nedivi E, Hevroni D, Naot D, *et al.* (1993) Numerous candidate plasticity-related genes revealed by differential cDNA cloning. *Nature* **363**:718–722.

45. Hughes P, Beilharz E, Gluckman P, Dragunow M. (1993) Brain-derived neurotrophic factor is induced as an immediate early gene following N-methyl-D-aspartate receptor activation. *Neuroscience* **57**:319–328.

46. Lu B, Pang PT, Woo NH. (2005) The yin and yang of neurotrophin action. *Nat Rev Neurosci* **6**:603–614.

47. Finkbeiner S. (2000) Calcium regulation of the brain-derived neuro-trophic factor gene. *Cell Mol Life Sci* **57**:394–401.

48. Liu QR, Lu L, Zhu X-G, *et al.* (2006) Rodent BDNF genes, novel promoters, novel splice variants, and regulation by cocaine. *Brain Res* **1067**:1–12.

49. Pruunsild P, Kazantseva A, Aid T, *et al.* (2007) Dissecting the human BDNF locus: Bidirectional transcription, complex splicing, and multiple promoters. *Genomics* **90**:397–406.

50. Lessmann V, Gottmann K, Malcangio M. (2003) Neurotrophin secretion: Current facts and future prospects. *Prog Neurobiol* **69**:341–374.

51. Leschik J, Eckenstaler R, Endres T, *et al.* (2019) Prominent postsynaptic and dendritic exocytosis of endogenous BDNF vesicles in BDNF-GFP knock-in mice. *Mol Neurobiol* **56**:6833–6855.

52. Mowla SJ, Farhadi HF, Pareek S, *et al.* (2001) Biosynthesis and post-translational processing of the precursor to brain-derived neurotrophic factor. *J Biol Chem* **276**:12660–12666.

53. Kowianski P, Lietzau G, Czuba E, *et al.* (2018) BDNF: A key factor with multipotent impact on brain signaling and synaptic plasticity. *Cell Mol Neurobiol* **38**:579–593.

54. Holt LM, Hernandez RD, Pacheco NL, *et al.* (2019) Astrocyte morphogenesis is dependent on BDNF signaling via astrocytic TrkB.T1. *Elife* **8**.

55. Hempstead BL. (2006) Dissecting the diverse actions of pro- and mature neurotrophins. *Curr Alzheimer Res* **3**:19–24.

56. Wisse BE, Schwartz MW. (2003) The skinny on neurotrophins. *Nat Neurosci* **6**:655–656.

57. Xu B, Xie X. (2016) Neurotrophic factor control of satiety and body weight. *Nat Rev Neurosci* **17**:282–292.

58. Barlohay B, Lebrun B, Moyse E, Jean A. (2005) Brain-derived neurotrophic factor plays a role as an anorexigenic factor in the dorsal vagal complex. *Endocrinology* **146**:5612–5620.

59. Pelleymounter MA, Cullen MJ, Wellman CL. (1995) Characteristics of BDNF-induced weight loss. *Exp Neurol* **131**:229–238.

60. Lyons WE, Mamounas LA, Ricaurte GA, *et al.* (1999) Brain-derived neurotrophic factor-deficient mice develop aggressiveness and

hyperphagia in conjunction with brain serotonergic abnormalities. *Proc Natl Acad Sci U S A* **96**:15239–15244.

61. Unger TJ, Calderon GA, Bradley LC, *et al.* (2007) Selective deletion of Bdnf in the ventromedial and dorsomedial hypothalamus of adult mice results in hyperphagic behavior and obesity. *J Neurosci* **27**:14265–14274.

62. Evans BA, Agar L, Summers RJ. (1999) The role of the sympathetic nervous system in the regulation of leptin synthesis in C57BL/6 mice. *FEBS Lett* **444**:149–154.

63. Bartness TJ, Song CK. (2007) Brain-adipose tissue neural crosstalk. *Physiol Behav* **91**:343–351.

64. Pedersen BK, Hoffman-Goetz L. (2000) Exercise and the immune system: Regulation, integration, and adaptation. *Physiol Rev* **80**:1055–1081.

65. Suzuki K, Tagami K. (2005) Voluntary wheel-running exercise enhances antigen-specific antibody-producing splenic B cell response and prolongs IgG half-life in the blood. *Eur J Appl Physiol* **94**:514–519.

66. Lavie CJ, Ozemek C, Carbone S, *et al.* (2019) Sedentary behavior, exercise, and cardiovascular health. *Circ Res* **124**:799–815.

67. Balducci S, Sacchetti M, Haxhi J, *et al.* (2014) Physical exercise as therapy for type 2 diabetes mellitus. *Diabetes Metab Res Rev* **30 Suppl 1**:13–23.

68. Hotting K, Roder B. (2013) Beneficial effects of physical exercise on neuroplasticity and cognition. *Neurosci Biobehav Rev* **37**: 2243–2257.

69. Karssemeijer EGA, Aaronson JA, Bossers WJ, *et al.* (2017) Positive effects of combined cognitive and physical exercise training on cognitive function in older adults with mild cognitive impairment or dementia: A meta-analysis. *Ageing Res Rev* **40**:75–83.

70. Deslandes A, Moraes H, Ferreira C, *et al.* (2009) Exercise and mental health: Many reasons to move. *Neuropsychobiology* **59**:191–198.

71. Ruegsegger GN, Booth FW. (2018) Health benefits of exercise. *Cold Spring Harb Perspect Med* **8**.

72. Brown JC, Winters-Stone K, Lee A, Schmitz KH. (2012) Cancer, physical activity, and exercise. *Compr Physiol* **2**:2775–2809.

73. Idorn M, Thor Straten P. (2017) Exercise and cancer: From "healthy" to "therapeutic"? *Cancer Immunol Immunother* **66**:667–671.

74. Hojman P, Gehl J, Christensen JF, Pedersen BK. (2018) Molecular mechanisms linking exercise to cancer prevention and treatment. *Cell Metab* **27**:10–21.

75. Suzuki K, Tagami K. (2005) Voluntary wheel-running exercise enhances antigen-specific antibody-producing splenic B cell response and prolongs IgG half-life in the blood. *Eur J Appl Physiol* **94**: 514–519.

76. Lu Y-P, Lou Y-R, Nolan B, *et al.* (2006) Stimulatory effect of voluntary exercise or fat removal (partial lipectomy) on apoptosis in the skin of UVB light-irradiated mice. *Proc Natl Acad Sci U S A* **103**:16301–16306.

77. McMurphy T, Huang W, Queen NJ, *et al.* (2018) Implementation of environmental enrichment after middle age promotes healthy aging. *Aging (Albany NY)* **10**:1698–1721.

78. Pedersen L, Idorn M, Olofsso GH, *et al.* (2016) Voluntary running suppresses tumor growth through epinephrine- and IL-6-dependent NK cell mobilization and redistribution. *Cell Metab* **23**:554–562.

79. Kempermann G, Fabel K, Ehninger D, *et al.* (2010) Why and how physical activity promotes experience-induced brain plasticity. *Front Neurosci* **4**:189.

80. Fabel K, Wolf SA, Ehninger D, *et al.* (2009) Additive effects of physical exercise and environmental enrichment on adult hippocampal neurogenesis in mice. *Front Neurosci* **3**:50.

81. Song Y, Gan Y, Wang Q, *et al.* (2017) Enriching the housing environment for mice enhances their NK cell antitumor immunity via sympathetic nerve-dependent regulation of NKG2D and CCR5. *Cancer Res* **77**:1611–1622.

82. Li G, Gan Y, Fan Y, *et al.* (2015) Enriched environment inhibits mouse pancreatic cancer growth and down-regulates the expression of mitochondria-related genes in cancer cells. *Sci Rep* **5**:7856–7856.

83. Garofalo S, D'Alessandro G, Chece G, *et al.* (2015) Enriched environment reduces glioma growth through immune and non-immune mechanisms in mice. *Nat Commun* **6**:6623–6623.

84. Nachat-Kappes R, Pinel A, Combe K, *et al.* (2012) Effects of enriched environment on COX-2, leptin and eicosanoids in a mouse model of breast cancer. *PLoS One* **7**:e51525.
85. Bice BD, Stephens MR, Georges SJ, *et al.* (2017) Environmental enrichment induces pericyte and IgA-dependent wound repair and lifespan extension in a colon tumor model. *Cell Rep* **19**:760–773.
86. Arnold KM, Opdenaker LM, Flynn D, Sims-Mourtada J. (2015) Wound healing and cancer stem cells: Inflammation as a driver of treatment resistance in breast cancer. *Cancer Growth Metastasis* **8**:1–13.
87. D'Errico I, Moschetta A. (2008) Nuclear receptors, intestinal architecture and colon cancer: An intriguing link. *Cell Mol Life Sci* **65**: 1523–1543.

3

Environment, Stress and Obesity: A Brain-Fat Axis for Prevention and Treatment of Obesity and Metabolic Syndromes

Worldwide Obesity Epidemic

The world is experiencing an epidemic of obesity and overweight clearly evidenced by the fact sheets from the World Health organization (WHO) (https://www.who.int/news-room/fact-sheets/detail/obesity-and-overweight). Obesity and overweight are defined as abnormal or excessive accumulation of fat that can impair health. Body mass index (BMI) is a simple index most commonly used to classify overweight and obesity in adults (**Table 3.1**). BMI is defined as a person's weight in kilograms divided by the square of one's height in meters (kg/m^2). For adults, WHO classifies a BMI $\geq$25 kg/m^2 as overweight, and a BMI $\geq$30 kg/m^2 as obesity. For children, age should be considered and WHO has charts and tables for defining overweight and obesity for children under 5 years of age and children aged between 5 and 19 years. BMI provides a simple and useful measure to estimate overweight and obesity at population level. Because it applies to both sexes, across all ages of adults, and demographic, BMI may not serve as a good indicator of fatness in different individuals but rather a rough guide.

The global rise of overweight and obesity is alarming. According to WHO's recent estimates, worldwide obesity has almost tripled between 1975 and 2016. In 2016, greater than 1.9 billion adults, 18 years and older, were overweight, among which more than 650 million were obese. The prevalence of overweight is astonishing, 39% of adults aged 18 years and older were overweight (39% of men

Table 3.1   Obesity Classification for Adults

BMI	Class
< 18.5	Underweight
18.5 to < 25.0	Normal weight
25.0 to < 30.0	Overweight
30.0 to < 35.0	Class 1 obesity
35.0 to < 40.0	Class 2 obesity
≥ 40.0	Class 3 obesity (also known as extreme, severe, or morbid obesity)

and 40% of women) in 2016. Obesity rate was approximately 13% of the world's adult population (11% of men and 15% of women).

Children are greatly affected as well, 38.2 million children under the age of 5 years estimated to be overweight or obese in 2019. The prevalence of overweight and obesity among children and adolescence (age 5–19 years) has risen 4.5 folds from merely 4% in 1975 to 18% in 2016. Meanwhile, over 124 million children and adolescents were obese in 2016.

Overweight and obesity were first considered a problem for wealthy western countries. However, their prevalence is rising fast in low- and middle-income countries, particularly in cities. Globally, more people are obese than underweight. And more deaths worldwide are linked to overweight and obesity than to underweight.

Overweight and obesity are the major risk factors for many serious diseases and health conditions (**Fig. 3.1**), including coronary heart disease, hypertension, type 2 diabetes, stroke, gallbladder disease, osteoarthritis, and many types of cancer (endometrial, breast, ovarian, prostate, liver, gallbladder, kidney, and colon).[1–3] Obesity is also associated with increased risk of mental illnesses such as clinical depression, anxiety, and other mental disorders.[4,5] In fact, obesity is a risk factor for all causes of death,[6] one in five death in the United States is thought to be related to obesity.

Medical complications of obesity

Heart disease	**Type II diabetes**
• Abnormal lipid profile	**Pancreatitis**
• High blood pressure	**Kidney disease**
Liver disease	**Gallstones**
• Fatty liver	**Gout**
• Cirrhosis	**Arthritis**
Lung disease	
• Asthma	**Female disorders**
• Pulmonary blood clots	• Abnormal periods
Cancer	• Infertility
• Breast	**Inflamed veins**
• Colon	**Stroke**
• Esophagus	
• Kidney	**Sleep apnea & snoring**
• Pancreas	**Depression**
• Prostate	
• Uterus	

Fig. 3.1. Obesity is associated with increased risk of serious diseases and health conditions.

The United States has the highest obesity prevalence among rich countries. According to Centers for Disease Control and Prevention (CDC), the prevalence of obesity was 42.4% in 2017–2018 for adults and 18.5% for children and adolescents (https://www.cdc.gov/nchs/products/databriefs/db360.htm). Olshansky and colleagues forecast a potential decline in life expectancy in the United States in the 21st century, largely based on the high prevalence of obesity.[7] There is evidence supporting the prediction. Studies have documented a slowdown in rates of mortality improvement in the United States and an increasing US mortality disadvantage relative to other high-income countries.[8,9] Middle-aged white populations have actually experienced rising mortality over much of the past several decades.[10,11] Preston and colleagues analyzed the data obtained from cohorts of the National Health and Nutrition Examination Survey (NHANES) and from the NHANES linked mortality files through December 2011. They estimate that rising BMI has reduced the annual rate of improvement in US death rates between 1988 and 2011 by more than half a percentage point, which is equivalent to a 23% relative reduction in the rate of mortality decline. This effect is large relative to international mortality trends. The increase in BMI has reduced life expectancy at age of 40 by 0.9 years, and accounted for 186,000 excess deaths in 2011.[12] The rise of obesity has stripped the United States the full benefits of factors working to lower mortality, including advances in medical technology and reduction in smoking. The link between obesity and cancer is discussed in Chapter 5.

The fundamental cause of overweight and obesity is a sustained imbalance of energy between calorie intake and energy expenditure. However, what is beneath this energy imbalance is complicated, and the etiology of obesity continues to evolve (**Table 3.2**). Obesity

Table 3.2   Potential Contributors or Influencers to Obesity

	Inside the Person	Outside the Person
Biological	Genetic and epigenetic factors	Environmental/chemical toxins
	Chronic inflammation (*Altered insulin signaling and glucose homeostasis*)	Infection (*human adenovirus 36*)
		Weight gain-inducing drugs
		Smoking
		Sleep deficits
	Central and peripheral regulators of appetite and adipose tissue	
	Pathological sources of endocrine dysregulation (*thyroid dysfunction, Cushing's syndrome*)	
	Age-related changes (*menopause, mobility decline, hormones*)	
	Thermogenesis	
	Gut microbiota	
	Hyper-reactivity to food cues	
	Heightened hunger response	
	Delayed satiety	
	Physical disabilities	
	Pain sensitivity	

Table 3.2 (*Continued*)

	Inside the Person	Outside the Person
Psychological	Disordered eating (*night eating syndrome, binge eating*) Emotional coping Mood disturbance (*depression, anxiety, bipolar etc.*) Mental disabilities Trauma history Self-regulatory and coping deficits Social anxiety (*exercise avoidance*)	Stress Child maltreatment Weight cycling (*yo-yo dieting*)
Developmental/ Maternal	Gestational diabetes	Maternal obesity, smoking, stress, employment Breastfeeding and related factors Delayed prenatal care Maternal overnutrition during pregnancy Birth by C-section Birth order (*first-born in family*) Having children (*for women*) Nonparental childcare Prenatal air pollution
Economic		Market economy Food surplus Pervasive food advertising Westernization and economic development Low nutrition support
Social		Family conflict Social networks Lack of healthcare provider support or inadequate access to care Weight bias and stigma (*avoidance of medical care, self-esteem, teasing history*) Lack of employer preparedness to assist with obesity Entering into a romantic relationship

(*Continued*)

Table 3.2   (*Continued*)

	Inside the Person	Outside the Person
Environmental Pressure on Physical Activity		Increased sedentary time (*inactive leisure "screen" time, inactive job requirements*) Labor saving devices Decreased opportunity for nonexercised based physical activity (*driving vs. walking to school and work, sedentary jobs*) Consistent temperature (*air conditioning/heating*) Built environment (*stairwell design/access, building design, absence of sidewalks*)
Food and Beverage Behavior/ Environment		Increased availability of energy dense, nutrient poor foods and beverages Larger portion sizes Eating as recreation, snacking, special occasions Skipping meals Food insecurity Lack of family meals Eating away from home Diet patterns Lack of nutritional education

Source: Obesity Society (www.obesity.org) educational material 2015. Potential contributors indicate anything that has been put forth in the research literature as a question of investigation and is not intended to be a verification of whether or not, or the extent to which, each may or may not contribute.

and related noncommunicable disease are largely preventable and reversible if the energy imbalance can be effectively addressed. It supposes to be straightforward, reducing energy intake and increasing physical activity, thereby normalizing the calorie-in/calorie-out balance. Unfortunately, the millions constantly struggling with weight can attest how difficult to lose weight and even harder to maintain a healthy weight.

The popular TV show, The Biggest Losers, illuminates the hardship. Morbid obese contestants competed on TV to lose the most weight guided by personal trainers. They went through strict dieting and vigorous physical exercise to achieve enormous weight loss, on average, 128 pounds over the course of the 30-week reality show. However, the happy ending did not last long. Many of the winners regained the weight. A study followed 14 contestants of The Biggest Losers for 6 years and found only one weighed less than when the show ended. More devastating, 4 out of 14 were heavier than they were on the show. The failure of maintaining weight loss is not because of lacking willpower or efforts. Instead, the winners of The Biggest Losers meticulously kept a healthy lifestyle, eating less, and moving more. The culprit turns out to be a dramatically reduced metabolic rate. The body has many means to regress back to a "set point," an individual's preferred weight. This set point is disturbed in obese individuals compared to those of healthy weight. When contestants of The Biggest Losers lost enormous weight (40%), their basal metabolic rate dialed down dramatically to counter the weight loss. And the slowed metabolism did not bounce back 6 years after The Biggest Loser competition.[13] As a result, for those who have achieved weight loss to maintain the lower weight, they have to eat hundreds of calories less each day than people of a comparable weight all along. This story does not imply weight loss is doomed because the persistent metabolic adaption was not universal. Some studies show gastric bypass patients had no negative effects on metabolism or recovered slowed metabolic rate after a year.[14,15] Nevertheless, the experience of The Biggest Losers underscores how difficult to reverse obesity. It is always the best not to disturb the set point at first place and thereby preventing obesity. But the reality of the obesity epidemic highlights the urgent need for effective therapeutic interventions. Understanding the biology of energy balance is essential for obesity prevention and treatment.

Environment, Mental State, and Obesity

Obesity has been recognized as a complex acquired disease with both environmental and genetic factors. Changes in dietary and physical activity patterns are often the result of environmental and societal changes (**Table 3.2**). There is strong evidence that social and environmental factors have profound effects on body weight and the development of obesity and associated metabolic disorders.[16–18]

From an evolutionary perspective, obesity and associated metabolic disorders can be seen as a maladaptive consequence of an initially successful adaptation to high environmental demands. In current human society, calorie-rich and usually palatable food is abundant meanwhile the energy-demanding actions (e.g., hunt, fight, flight) are no longer required. As such, the biological mechanisms adaptive successfully to prehistoric times can easily become maladaptive, triggering obesity and associated metabolic disorders.[17]

Psychological factors play a role in the development and propagation of obesity and metabolic syndromes particularly among individuals under psychosocial pressure or chronic stress.[19,20] Moreover, social networks appear to influence weight gain and weight loss while the underlying mechanisms remain unclear.[21,22] However, many studies of the etiology of obesity and related metabolic syndromes utilize animals (including the genetically modified rodents) in laboratory conditions without adequate social interactions. Because the external environment can impact the internal environment in profound ways ultimately altering body weight and body composition, it is imperative for investigators to take physical and social environments of laboratory animals into consideration not only for studies aiming to identify regulation pathways of energy balance, but also to evaluate potential therapeutics of obesity and associated metabolic syndromes.

Many Colors of Adipose Tissue: White, Brown, and In-between

Not all fat tissues are created equal. Instead, distinct adipose tissues are found in all mammals (**Table 3.3**).[23,24] The most well-known types

Table 3.3   Characteristics of Brown, Beige/Brite, and White Adipose Tissue

	Brown Adipose Tissue	Beige/Brite Adipose Tissue	White Adipose Tissue
Depots	• Interscapular • Cervical • Paravertebral • Perirenal • Supraclavicular	Emerges in white adipose depots upon appropriate stimuli ("browning")	• Subcutaneous • Intra-abdominal • Gonadal • Epicardial
Adipocyte Morphology	Elliptical	Spherical	Spherical
Cell Composition	• Multilocular lipid droplets • Oval central nucleus • High mitochondria density	• Multilocular lipid droplets • Medium mitochondria density	• Unilocular lipid droplet • Flattened peripheral nucleus • Low mitochondria density • Little endoplasmic reticulum
Function	• Energy expenditure (nonshivering thermogenesis) • Endocrine (e.g., FGF21) • Cardioprotective	• Thermogenic competent (adaptive thermogenesis) • Endocrine (e.g., FGF21) • Cardioprotective	• Energy storage • Endocrine (a variety of adipokines, cytokines, lipid molecules, etc.)

(Continued)

Table 3.3   (Continued)

	Brown Adipose Tissue	Beige/Brite Adipose Tissue	White Adipose Tissue
UCP1	Positive	Positive upon induction	Negative
Thermogenic Mechanism	UCP1-dependent	• UCP1-dependent • Creatine cycling • Ca^{++} cycling	
Progenitor	Myogenic origin Myf5+, En-1+, Pax7+	Vascular smooth muscle origin with specific transcription factors expression (Zic1, Tbx15, etc.)	CD24+, CD34+, PDGFRα+
Immune	Low infiltration of pro-inflammatory immune cells	Low infiltration of pro-inflammatory immune cells	High infiltration of pro-inflammatory immune cells during obesity
Correlation to Obesity/ Insulin Resistance	Negative	Negative	Positive for visceral depots

are white adipose tissue (WAT) and brown adipose tissue (BAT), comprising white adipocytes and brown adipocytes, respectively. White adipocytes are large spherical cells with a unilocular droplet containing energy-dense lipids that occupies approximately 90% of the cell volume. WAT depots are distributed in two anatomical body compartments — visceral and subcutaneous.[25] WAT was previously viewed as a passive organ with relatively simple functions such as storage of excessive energy (as triacylglycerols), heat insulation, and mechanical cushioning. Developments in the past several decades have demonstrated that WAT exerts many functions far beyond energy balance, and the versatile and complex WAT is highly adaptive to internal and external stimuli.

Brown adipocytes are polygonal cells, smaller in size, and multilocular in which lipids are partitioned into multiple droplets occupying ~50% of the volume of cell. In humans at normal conditions, BAT is found primarily around the large blood vessels, particularly in the supraclavicular region. Rather than storing energy, BAT dissipates energy as heat. Brown adipocyte activity is controlled by the sympathetic nervous system (SNS).[26] BAT is densely innervated by noradrenergic nerve fibers that are in direct contact with brown adipocytes.[27] Upon SNS activation, noradrenaline acts on adipocytes through specific receptors, mainly β3-adrenergic receptor (AR), to stimulate brown adipocyte activities including lipolysis, mitochondrial biogenesis, and the synthesis and activity of uncoupling protein 1 (UCP1). UCP1 is a mitochondrial protein uniquely found in brown adipocytes, and uncouples fatty acid oxidation from adenosine triphosphate (ATP) production thereby dissipating energy as heat.[25] In small mammals, BAT is vital for the regulation of body temperature[28] and is also involved in the control of body weight.[29]

WAT and BAT are widely different at morphological and molecular levels, and develop from different origins (**Table 3.3**). Classical brown adipocytes are thought to derive from myogenic factor 5 (Myf5)-positive precursors.[30] Despite their different anatomy and functions, brown and white adipocytes exist together in fat depots supplied by specific blood vessels and nerves. In most adult mammals, WAT is prevalent, but the WAT/BAT ratio varies with genetic background, sex, age, nutritional status, and environmental conditions. Propensity to obesity in certain rodent models correlates with decreased BAT activity while resistance to obesity correlates with increased BAT function or the emergence of brown adipocyte-like cells (beige or brite cells) in WAT depots.[31,32] The concept of an adipose organ has been proposed mostly by Cinti and colleagues referring to a multi-depot organ characterized by two adipose tissues with different anatomy and functional roles.[27,33] BAT and WAT act cooperatively to satisfy the different physiological roles required for optimal adaptation to environmental changes.[25]

Adipose organ exhibits considerable plasticity — capacity for reciprocal conversion between brown and white adipocytes. Numerous studies have documented the opposing phenomena of browning versus whitening. Some adipocytes in each population can reversibly turn into one another. In basal conditions, the adipose organ employs the two tissues to meet the two physiological requirements of heat production via BAT and energy storage via WAT. In case of chronic energy surplus, BAT is able to transform to WAT to store more energy molecules (whitening), whereas, in the event of sustained heat requirement (i.e. chronic cold exposure), WAT can convert to BAT (browning).[33] The brown-like cells (UCP1-positive, multilocular, thermogenic) in predominantly white fat depots are considered to a new type of brown adipocyte and referred to various terms such as beige cell, brite cell (brown in white), and inducible brown-like adipocytes.[34–37] These adipocytes will be referred to beige adipocytes here after.

Beige adipocytes are not derived from the same Myf5-positive precursors that give rise to the typical intrascapular and perirenal brown adipocytes.[30] A subset of beige adipocytes originates from smooth muscle–like cells.[38] In addition, beige adipocytes can be induced by selected stimuli in addition to chronic cold exposure, such as fibroblast growth factor 21 (FGF-21),[39] bone morphogenetic protein 4 (BMP4)[40] and 7 (BMP7),[41] and irisin (a myokine released from skeletal muscles after exercise).[42,43] Some evidence suggests that adult human BAT is primarily composed of beige adipocytes,[43–45] drawing more attention to the beige cells as a therapeutic target for combating obesity.

The nature of this white-to-brown conversion is not entirely clear. Two theories are proposed: adipocyte transdifferentiation and precursor differentiation. Several data support the notion that browning occurs through direct transformation of adult adipocytes, i.e. via physiological reversible transdifferentiation[46–48] accompanied by tissue reorganization with changes in the density of capillaries and parenchymal nerve fibers.[49] On the other hand, more recent data suggest that the beige adipocytes emerging in WAT depots derive from *de novo* differentiation of stem cells or committed precursor cells.[36,38,50,51] These beige cells are thermogenic competent but are developmental and molecular distinct from classical brown adipocyte.[34]

The identity of the adipocyte precursor is controversial with several conflicting hypotheses. There is evidence that both brown and white adipocyte progenitor cells reside in the blood vessel wall and may be pericytes or endothelial cells of adipose capillaries.[52–54] Other studies suggest fully differentiated adipocytes may arise from mesothelial cells or neural crest cells in certain adipose depots.[55,56] It is plausible that adipocyte precursors may derive from diverse developmental pathways depending on the age (pre- and postnatal developing versus adults), the species (humans versus rodents), location of the fat deposit (subcutaneous versus visceral), and diet (normal versus a high-fat diet).

The astonishing progress in adipose biology clearly illuminates adipose organ a highly complex, dynamic, and convertible organ. Indeed, fat is so fascinating, not boring at all. Many of the anatomo-physiological features of murine fat depots can apply to humans.[27,33]

Boosting Adaptive Thermogenesis to Combat Obesity

Raising metabolic rate has always been the "holy grail" for treating obesity and related metabolic syndromes. In early 20th century, dinitrophenol, an agent that increases metabolism, was aggressively marketed as a drug for weight loss. Dinitrophenol was later banned because of serious toxicities, including death from hyperpyrexia. Unfortunately, hundreds of thousands patients had been treated with this toxic chemical before it was pulled from market.[57] Dinitrophenol is an uncoupler that dissociates the processes of respiration and oxidative phosphorylation. During respiration, chemical energy is coupled to the production of ATP, otherwise, energy is released as heat. Therefore, stimulating this uncoupling of oxidation from ATP synthesis can increase energy expenditure. Strategies capable of promoting mitochondrial uncoupling safely may represent an effective treatment for obesity by increasing the metabolic rate. Uncoupling proteins are a natural target for boosting thermogenesis as these mitochondrial membrane proteins leak protons across the inner mitochondrial membrane. Among the three different, yet closely related, uncoupling proteins described up to date, UCP1 is the classic uncoupler driving adaptive thermogenesis upon β-AR activation. UCP1 is expressed exclusively in BAT, the main site of thermogenesis in mammals, and thermogenic beige cells in certain WAT depots upon stimulation. UCP2 (expressed broadly) and UCP3 (expressed primarily in skeletal muscle) may be involved in protection against oxidative damage.[58]

BAT has become a potential target for pharmacological and genetic manipulation to curb human obesity because position emission tomography has provided evidence that adult humans retain considerable amounts of metabolically active BAT depots that can be stimulated by cold exposure and SNS activation.[59–61] BAT dissipates the energy provided by triglycerides directly as heat through UCP1.[28,29] Comparing to restricting food intake, boosting energy expenditure is understandably preferred to counteract obesity. But is such a small amount of BAT, roughly 0.05%–1% of body weight in adult humans in contrast to 5%–10% in mouse, enough to make a metabolic difference? It is estimated that 40–50 g of maximally stimulated BAT in humans can account for up to 20% of energy expenditure, equivalent to 20 kg of body weight, over a year.[62] Such significant energy expenditure of BAT could be highly relevant in terms of human energy balance. Furthermore, even a small but consistent imbalance in the energy input versus energy output equation can ultimately dictate obesity versus leanness. Cannon and Nedergaard conclude that modifying thermogenesis through chronic cold exposure or manipulating UCP1 can alter energy balance and body weight that are not fully compensated by changes in food intake.[63] Indeed, studies have demonstrated an inverse correlation between BAT activity in adult humans and body fat.[60,61,64–67] For morbid obese subjects with an extremely wide range of body composition, BAT activity is found to be highly correlated reversely with BMI and body fat percentage.[68] Moreover, histological studies have reported brown adipocytes dispersed among white fat depots in 24% of adult humans' biopsies and reaching 50% of cases with exclusion of people older than 50 years.[65] In addition, studies of human fat cell dynamics reveal a high turnover rate of adipocytes — approximately 10% of fat cells being renewed annually across all adult ages and levels of BMI.[69] Human white adipocytes obtained from subcutaneous fat tissues can be genetically manipulated *in vitro* to develop "brown" characteristics by overexpressing transcription coactivator PGC-1α.[70,71] These findings collectively point to therapeutic potential of BAT-oriented strategies to raise metabolic rate by facilitating brown adipocyte maintenance, stimulating preexisting brown precursors, and inducing white-to-brown conversion.[33,72,73]

However, Nedergaard and Cannon point out the potential flaw of the strategies solely based on increasing the total amount of BAT or UCP1. The UCP1 in intact brown adipocytes is constantly inhibited by purine nucleotides in the cytosol. In other words, the UCP1 is not automatically active and its inhibition must be overcome through a process initiated physiologically by SNS stimulation.[74] Indeed, there are no indications that the amount of UCP1, representing the capacity for thermogenesis, influences basal brown adipocyte metabolic rate or whole-body metabolic rate. Chronic cold exposure leads to substantial browning in rodents. But BAT activity is turned off immediately after mice are transferred to warm conditions, within seconds.[74] Thus, an individual constantly decides how much combustion is needed to meet environmental demand and that is independent of the thermogenic capacity. In this sense, BAT and UCP1 are like furnace and fuel, while the SNS stimulation is the igniter to spark a fire. Indeed, BAT is densely innervated by sympathetic nerve fibers that are in direct contact with brown adipocytes through synaptoid junctions. These junctions are responsible for activating brown adipocyte. Although the sympathetic stimulus is selectively delivered to a few adipocytes, gap junctions among adjacent brown adipocytes can amplify this stimulus, thereby enabling a simultaneous, synchronized activation of a large number of brown adipocytes including those not reached directly by sympathetic nerve.[27,75] It is plausible that the brain plays a commanding role in the adaptive thermogenesis. Our work has revealed a new avenue to induce beige cells and continuous but preferential SNS activation in WAT through a specific brain-adipocyte axis.

Environmental Enrichment Induces Leanness and White Fat Browning via the HSA Axis

EE Reduces Adiposity More Effectively than Physical Exercise Alone

During our investigations on how EE influences cancer growth, we noticed that mice living in EE housing appeared leaner. We then set out to examine the metabolic phenotypes in a separate study.[76] We randomized the male C57BL/6 mice to three housing groups: standard environment (SE) — standard grouped housing, environmental enrichment (EE) — larger space with running wheels, and regularly reconfigured toys and mazes (Chapter 1, Figure 1.1), voluntary running — specialty cage with free access to a running wheel. All animals had free access to food and water under an ambient temperature of 22°C. After 4-week living in respective housing, the EE mice had slightly lower body weights than the SE mice but a remarkable decrease of intra-abdominal fat mass by ~50%. All of the WAT pads from EE mice shrank markedly: decrease in inguinal WAT (iWAT) and epididymal WAT (eWAT) mass by ~47%, and retroperitoneal WAT (rWAT) by ~74%.

Was this loss of body fat simply caused by physical exercise? The answer is no according to the wheel running results. Four-week of voluntary running decreased body weight similarly to EE, but was substantially less effective in reducing adiposity compared to EE. The decrease of various WAT pads weight in runners ranged from 25% to 40%, approximately half of the reductions observed in EE. Both EE and running increased gastrocnemius mass by 23% and 13%, respectively. Of note, we previously traced the traveling distance of EE mice plus the wheel running distance excluding activity within the feeding cage (the regular mouse cage)[77] (more details in Chapter 2). The total distance traveled by the EE mice was 0.86 km/day more than the SE mice but approximately 66% lower than runner's average traveling distance 2 km/day/mouse indicating the further reduction of adiposity found in EE was not due to greater overall motor activity.

To further investigate the extent to which physical activity accounts for the lean phenotype induced by EE, we repeated the experiment and added another group of mice housed in the regular EE cage but without the running wheels. In addition, instead of being housed in the specialty running wheel cages equipped to measure running distance in the previous experiment, the voluntary running group in this experiment was housed in the regular SE cages provided with the same wheels as used in the EE setting. We monitored body weight over 9 weeks. In contrast to the 4-week EE with minimal handling, the runners were the only group that showed a significant decrease in body weight while the body weight of EE mice with no access to running wheels was identical to the SE mice (**Fig. 3.2(a)**). However, the standard EE (with access to wheels) led to the largest reduction in adiposity, with iWAT, eWAT, and rWAT decreased by 46%, 58%, and 70%, respectively. The EE no wheel mice showed a trend toward greater iWAT and eWAT mass reduction than the wheel running mice when fat mass was calibrated to body weight. These data indicate wheel running not essential for the EE-induced leanness (**Fig. 3.2(b)**).[76]

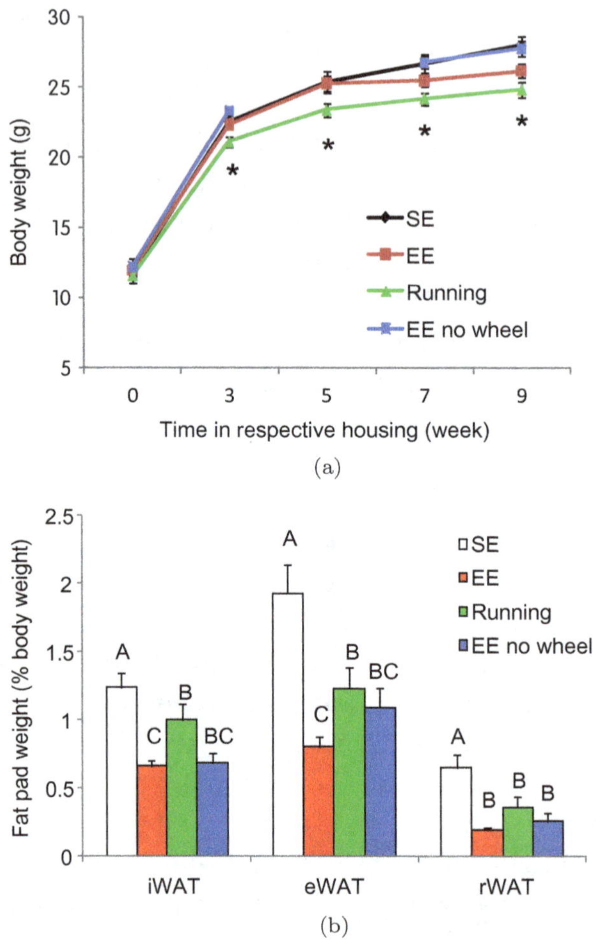

Fig. 3.2. EE reduces adiposity of mice fed on normal chow diet. (a) EE and EE no wheel did not decrease body weight, whereas voluntary wheel running decreased body weight ($n = 10$–20 per group).*$P < 0.05$ for running. (b) WAT mass calibrated to body weight after 10-week respective housing ($n = 10$–19 per group). Data are mean ± SEM. Bars not connected by same letter are significantly different. Reprinted from Cell Metab Vol 14, Cao *et al.* White to brown fat phenotypic switch induced by genetic and environmental activation of a hypothalamic-adipocyte axis, 324–338, Copyright (2011), with permission from Elsevier.

EE Elevates Energy Expenditure

Interestingly, the alteration of body composition upon EE exposure was not associated with lower food intake. In fact, EE mice consumed more food than SE mice. Thus, we reasoned that the increase in energy expenditure may cause the lean phenotype. We first attempted to measure the whole-body metabolism of mice after 5-week EE using the indirect calorimetry for 3 days at room temperature of 22°C. No difference in oxygen consumption was found in the EE mice compared to the SE mice. Notably, the EE mice, upon removal from their complex environment, showed significantly lower physical activity in the metabolic chambers. The acute change of environment from EE to single housing in the metabolic chamber may elicit coping behaviors which in turn affects metabolism and complicates the evaluation of energy expenditure. Therefore, the routine protocol of indirect calorimetry assay may not properly represent the energy expenditure in the EE.[76]

We then adopted an alternative approach to measure whole-body metabolism for 3 hours starting immediately upon removal from the EE cage. The EE mice showed increased basal resting oxygen consumption at thermoneutrality of 29°C (**Fig. 3.3(a)**).[29] Next, we measured the oxygen consumption of dissected fat tissues *ex vivo*. The rWAT collected from EE mice showed higher oxygen consumption compared to their counterparts from SE mice by approximately 50% (**Fig. 3.3(b)**). These data together with increased food intake indicate that elevated energy expenditure rather than appetite suppression underlies the lean phenotype.[76]

EE Induces Browning of Selective WAT Depot

BAT and WAT perform opposing functions with WAT accumulating surplus energy while BAT dissipating chemical energy as heat. We examined the impact of EE on BAT and WAT gene expression profiles by quantitative reverse transcription polymerase chain reaction

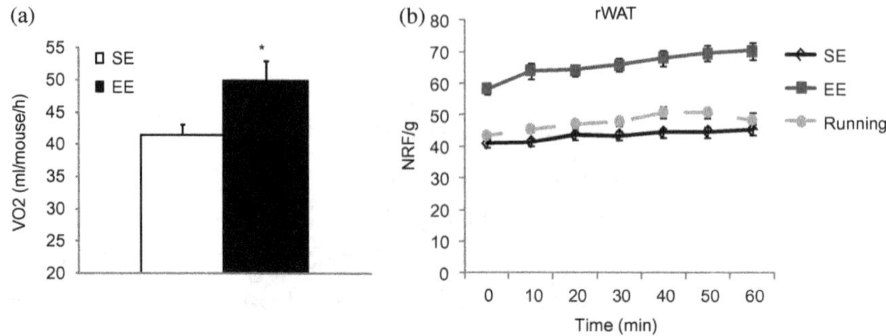

Fig. 3.3. EE elevates energy expenditure. (a) Basal oxygen consumption at thermoneutrality. n = 18 per group, *P < 0.05. (b) Oxygen consumption in rWAT ex vivo. n = 3 per group, P < 0.05 EE compared to SE and Running, NRF, normalized relative fluorescence. Data are mean ± SEM. Reprinted from Cell Metab Vol 14, Cao *et al.* White to brown fat phenotypic switch induced by genetic and environmental activation of a hypothalamic-adipocyte axis, 324–338, Copyright (2011), with permission from Elsevier.

(RT-PCR) after 4-week EE. Limited gene expression changes were observed in BAT with 6 out of the 19 genes profiled showing significant change (**Fig. 3.4**).

In contrast, rWAT, the depot shrinking the most, was far more responsive to the EE with 15 out of the 19 genes profiled showing altered expression (**Fig. 3.5**).[76] *Prdm16* (encoding PR-domain-containing 16), the genetic switch determining the formation and function of brown adipocytes,[30] was significantly upregulated by 2.8-fold in rWAT of EE mice. The stimulation of *Prdm16* was accompanied by a robust induction of a brown adipocyte molecular signature including *Cidea* (13.6-fold), *Elovl3* (27.4-fold), *Ucp1*, and *Ppargc1a* (encoding PGC-1α), all of which are brown adipocyte or beige adipocyte selective markers and positively regulated by *Prdm16*.[30] PGC-1α has been shown to induce mitochondrial biogenesis and thermogenic genes and whereby switching cells from energy storage to energy expenditure phenotype.[78] Several transcriptional regulators, such as RIP140,[79] SRC2,[80] Rb,[81] and Twist1,[82] are thought to control brown adipocyte development and function, at least in part,

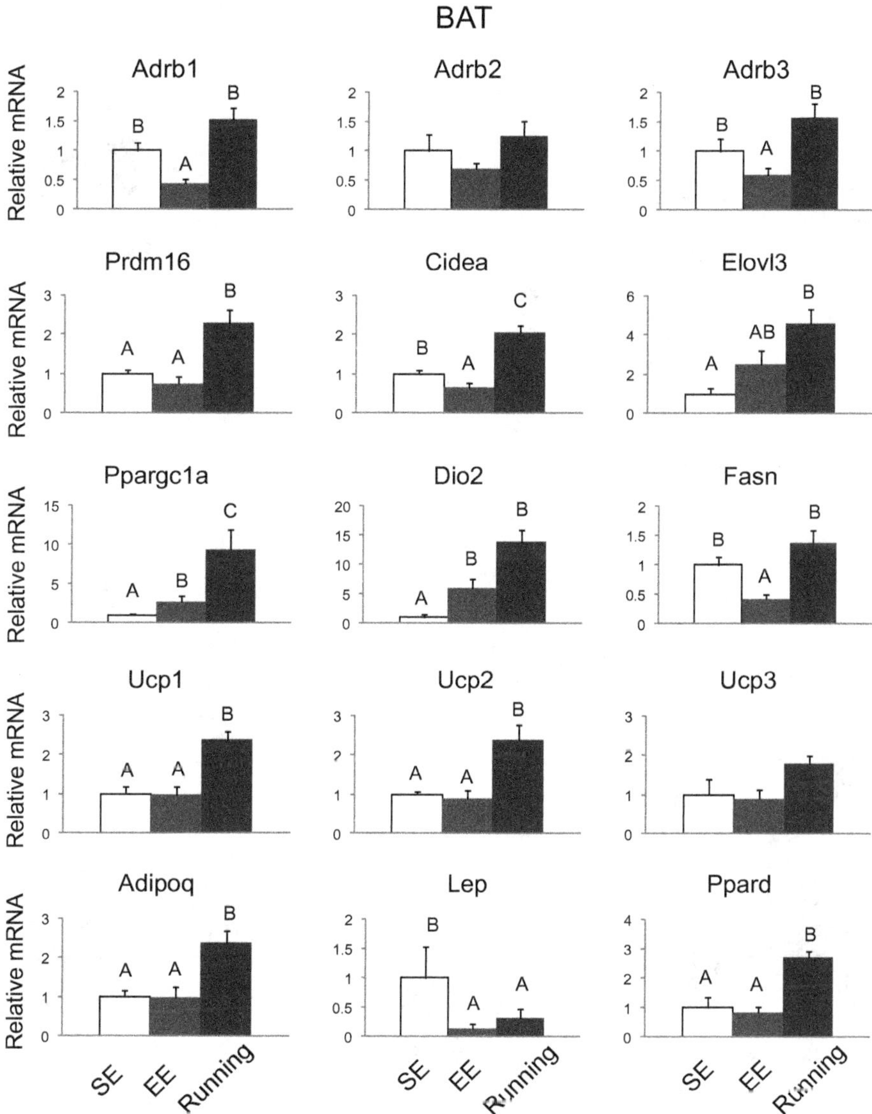

Fig. 3.4. Gene expression profile of brown adipose tissue (BAT) after 4-week respective housing, $n = 5$ per group. Bars not connected by the same letter are significantly different. Data are mean ± SEM. Reprinted from Cell Metab Vol 14, Cao *et al.* White to brown fat phenotypic switch induced by genetic and environmental activation of a hypothalamic-adipocyte axis, 324–338, Copyright (2011), with permission from Elsevier.

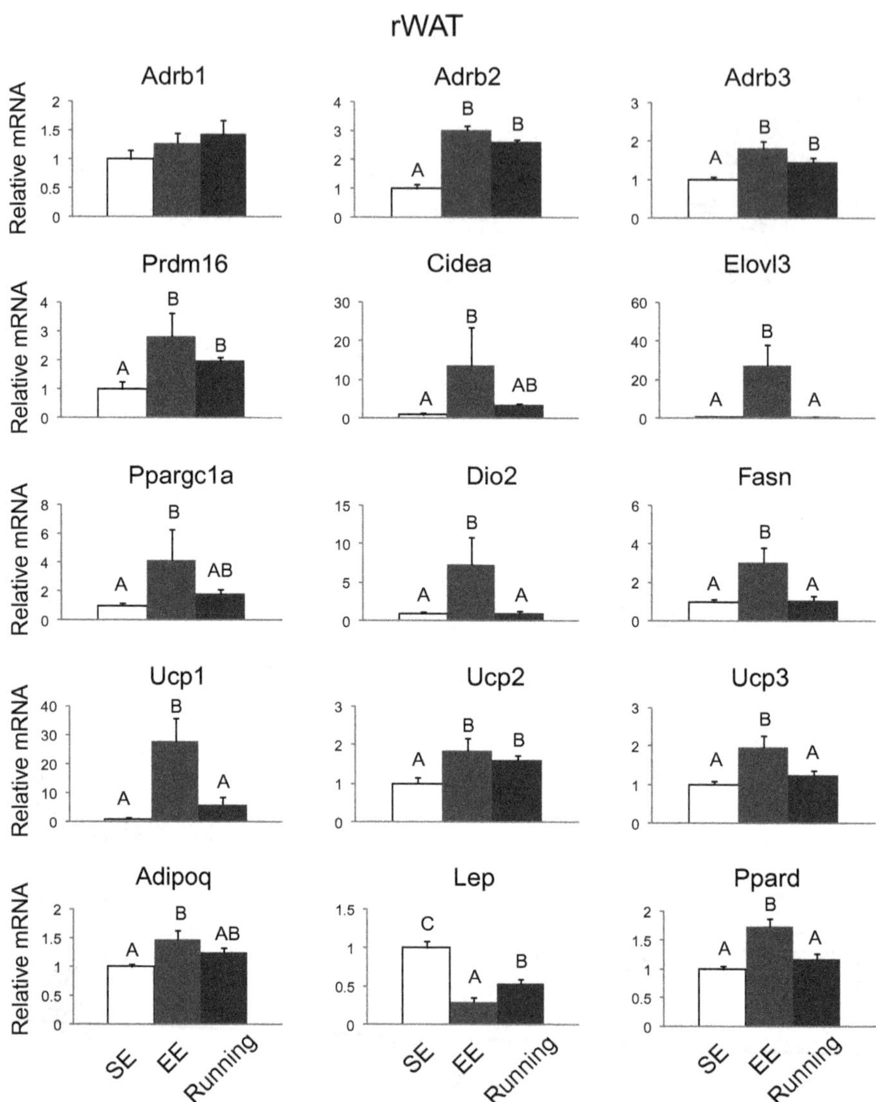

Fig. 3.5. Gene expression profile of retroperitoneal white adipose tissue (rWAT) after 4-week respective housing, $n = 5$ per group. Bars not connected by the same letter are significantly different. Data are mean ± SEM. Reprinted from Cell Metab Vol 14, Cao *et al*. White to brown fat phenotypic switch induced by genetic and environmental activation of a hypothalamic-adipocyte axis, 324–338, Copyright (2011), with permission from Elsevier.

through regulating the transcriptional activity or gene expression of PGC-1α. EE upregulated *Ppargc1a* expression in rWAT by 4.1-fold. Thermogenesis is primarily mediated by UCP 1 (*Ucp1*), which is a specific BAT marker.[83] *Ucp1* expression was increased 28-fold in rWAT of EE mice. Other uncoupling proteins involving in protection against oxidative damage, *Ucp2* and *Ucp3*, were also upregulated. Moreover, the two genes involved in oxidative metabolism, *Dio2* (encoding type 2 5′ deiodinase) and *Ppard* (encoding peroxisome proliferator-activated receptor δ), were upregulated by 7.3-fold and 1.7-fold, respectively. β-adrenergic signaling is essential to the activation of BAT and induction of beige cells in response to cold and the regulation of adiposity.[84–86] Both *Adrb2* and *Adrb3* encoding β-AR 2 and 3 were upregulated in rWAT of EE mice while *Adrb1* and *Adrb3* were downregulated in BAT. Contrary to the strong induction of the brown adipocyte gene program in rWAT, EE suppressed the expression of the white adipocyte-enriched gene resistin and had no effect on adipocyte markers shared by both brown and white adipocytes such as adipogenic transcription factor *Pparg* (encoding peroxisome proliferator-activated receptor γ) and adipocyte differentiation marker *Ap2* (encoding adipocyte protein 2).[87]

Histology analyses showed that the rWAT adipocytes of EE mice were smaller than those in the SE mice (**Fig. 3.6(a)**).[76] The shrink of fat mass was unlikely due to damage to adipocytes because no increase in apoptosis measured by TUNEL was found in EE mice. Consistent with the robust induction of brown adipocyte gene signature, pockets of cells with the multilocular morphology characteristic of brown adipocytes[88] were observed in rWAT of EE mice (**Fig. 3.6(a)**). Immunohistochemical staining revealed markedly higher level of UCP1 protein not only in the cells with typical brown adipocyte morphology but also in some cells with unilocular white adipocyte morphology surrounding the cluster of brown-like/beige adipocytes (**Fig. 3.6(a)**).[88]

Western blotting showed significant increase of UCP1, mitochondrial protein HSP60, β3-AR, and PGC-1α levels in EE rWAT

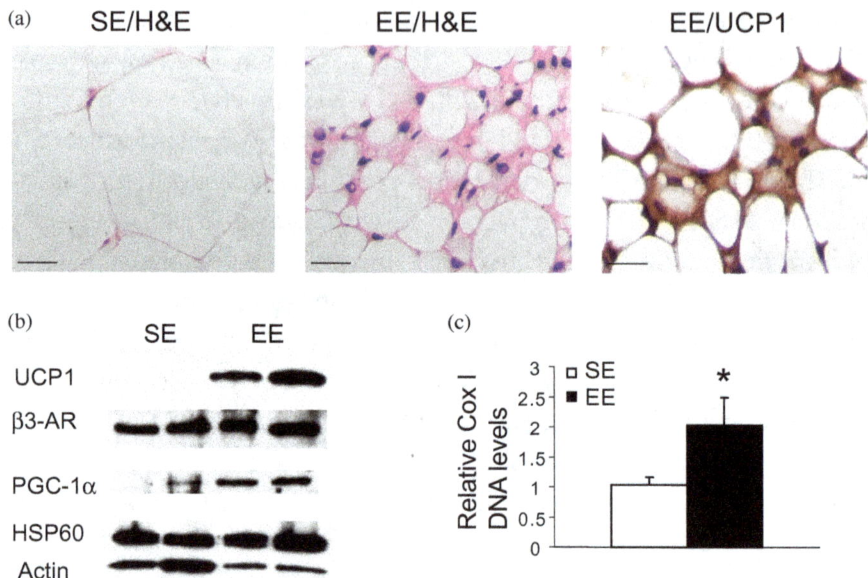

Fig. 3.6.   EE induces beige cells in selective white adipose tissue depot. (a) H&E staining and UCP1 immunohistochemistry of rWAT after 4-week respective housing. Scale bar, 20 μm. (b) Western blotting of rWAT. (c) Mitochondrial DNA content of rWAT. $n = 4$ per group. $*P < 0.05$. Data are mean ± SEM. Reprinted from Cell Metab Vol 14, Cao *et al.* White to brown fat phenotypic switch induced by genetic and environmental activation of a hypothalamic-adipocyte axis, 324–338, Copyright (2011), with permission from Elsevier.

(**Fig. 3.6(b)**) consistent with the upregulation of messenger RNAs (mRNAs).[76] Furthermore, the mitochondrial DNA content (using a mitochondrial gene Cox I as a surrogate) of EE rWAT was increased by 2-fold, indicating enhanced mitochondrial biogenesis (**Fig. 3.6(c)**).[86]

The other two WAT pads eWAT and iWAT displayed fewer genetic changes than rWAT, and did not show substantial induction of beige cells. However, expression of the major adipokine, leptin (*Lep*), was highly suppressed in all fat depots (BAT, iWAT, eWAT, and rWAT) consistent with the observed 64% drop in circulating leptin levels.[76]

Four-week of voluntary wheel running induced gene expression profiles in BAT and rWAT distinctive to those of EE. Running resulted in more robust changes in BAT than EE while less beige gene signature in rWAT (**Figs. 3.4, 3.5**). In addition, we analyzed the

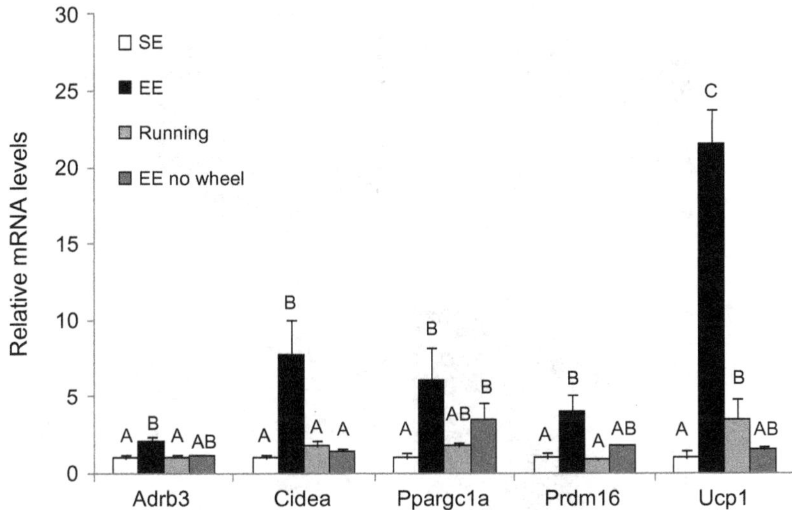

Fig. 3.7.   Gene expression profile of retroperitoneal white adipose tissue (rWAT) after 9-week respective housing, $n = 4$ per group. Bars not connected by the same letter are significantly different. Data are mean ± SEM. Reprinted from Cell Metab Vol 14, Cao *et al*. White to brown fat phenotypic switch induced by genetic and environmental activation of a hypothalamic-adipocyte axis, 324–338, Copyright (2011), with permission from Elsevier.

rWAT gene expression profiles after 10 weeks of EE, wheel-running, and EE no wheel. No surprise, the standard EE induced the most robust beige gene program. The effects of wheel-running and EE no wheel were not additive (**Fig. 3.7**). These data suggest that EE and running reduces adiposity through distinct molecular mechanisms.

Extended EE Leads to More Prominent Browning

We then examined the effect of long-term EE for 3 months.[76] The color changes of fat pads could not be missed by the naked eyes so that no microscope was needed: WAT turning brown and BAT going even darker (**Fig. 3.8(a)**). Brown adipocyte-like/beige cells were found in eWAT of 3-month EE mice (**Fig. 3.8(b)**), which was rare in 4-week EE mice.

The expressions of brown adipocyte gene markers were highly upregulated in eWAT (**Fig. 3.9(a)**). In contrast to clusters of

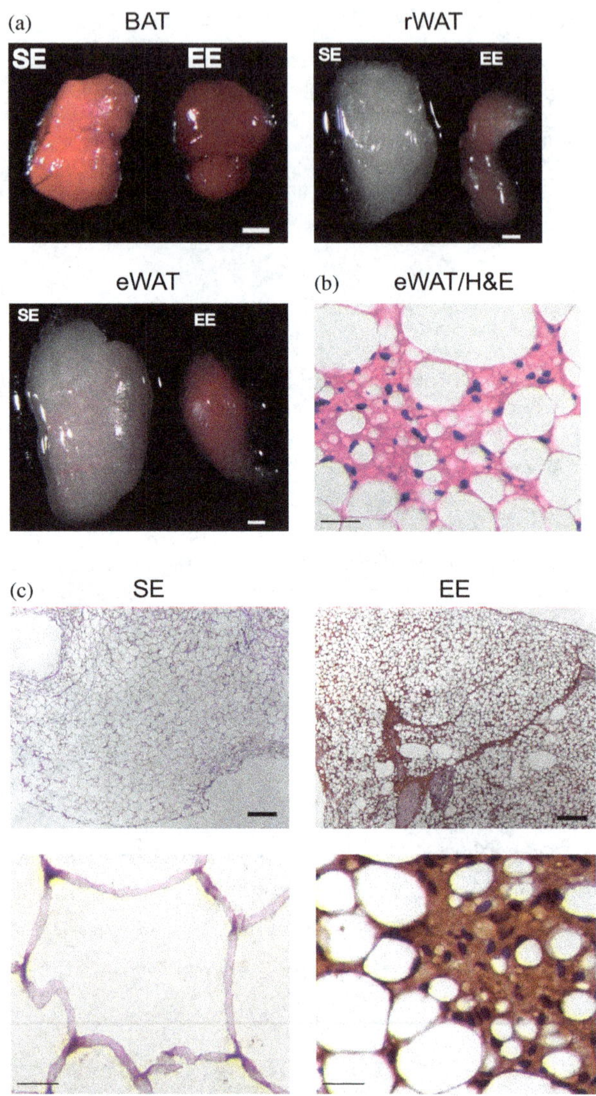

Fig. 3.8. Long-term EE leads to stronger white fat browning. (a) Representatives of BAT, eWAT, and rWAT of SE or EE mice after 3-month respective housing. Scale bar, 1 mm. (b) H&E staining of eWAT. Scale bar, 20 μm. (c) UCP1 immunohistochemistry of rWAT. Scale bar, 200 μm in the upper panels, 20 μm in the lower panels. Reprinted from Cell Metab Vol 14, Cao *et al.* White to brown fat phenotypic switch induced by genetic and environmental activation of a hypothalamic-adipocyte axis, 324–338, Copyright (2011), with permission from Elsevier.

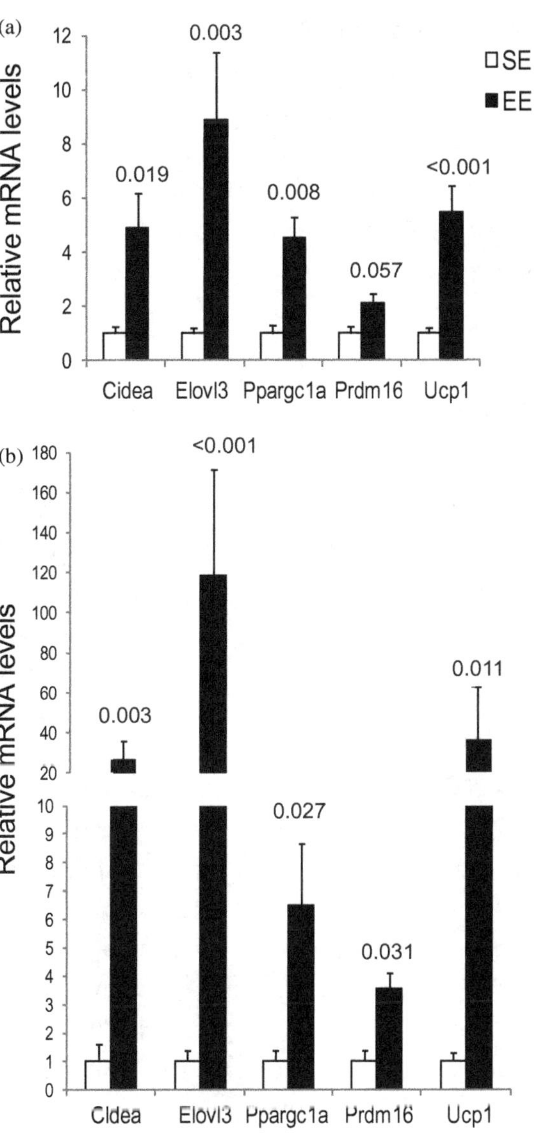

Fig. 3.9. Gene expression profile of eWAT in (a) and rWAT in (b) after 3-month respective housing, $n = 4$ per group. *P* values are shown above the bars. Data are mean ± SEM. Reprinted from Cell Metab Vol 14, Cao *et al.* White to brown fat phenotypic switch induced by genetic and environmental activation of a hypothalamic-adipocyte axis, 324–338, Copyright (2011), with permission from Elsevier.

UCP1[+] beige cells found in rWAT of 4-week EE mice, widespread and stronger staining of UCP1 was observed in 3-month EE mice (**Fig. 3.8(c)**) associated with more robust induction of the beige gene signature (**Fig. 3.9(b)**). For example, *Elovl3* was upregulated by 118-fold after 3-month EE while by 27-fold after 4-week EE. Moreover, the BAT depot became darker after 3-month EE suggesting enhanced thermogenic activity that requires further investigation.

EE Inhibits Diet-Induced Obesity

EE-induced WAT browning and elevated energy expenditure in mice fed a normal chow diet. Next, we investigated whether this white-to-brown transformation could protect animals against diet-induced obesity (DIO). We randomized the mice to live in EE or SE, and changed the normal chow to a high-fat diet (HFD, 45% kcal from fat, caloric density 4.73 kcal/g). EE mice showed slower weight gain as early as 2-week EE. After 4-week HFD feeding, the weight gain of EE mice was 29% less than that of SE mice. EE mice remained lean with over 60% smaller WAT depots compared to SE mice (**Fig. 3.10(a)**). No change in food intake was observed. The core body temperature of EE mice was increased (EE: $34.86 \pm 0.20°C$ versus SE: $34.17 \pm 0.14°C$, $P = 0.01$) supporting the notion that elevated energy expenditure, rather than appetite suppression, giving rise to the resistance to obesity. Moreover, EE prevented DIO-associated metabolic disturbance including hyperinsulinemia, hyperleptinemia, hyperglycemia, and dyslipidemia (**Fig. 3.10(b)**). Resembling the observations in normal chow-fed mice, EE also induced the beige gene signature in HFD mice (**Fig. 3.10(c)**). And the levels of *Ppargc1a* and *Prdm16* were inversely correlated with rWAT mass (**Fig. 3.10(d), (e)**), implicating a robust functional effect of these molecular changes.[76]

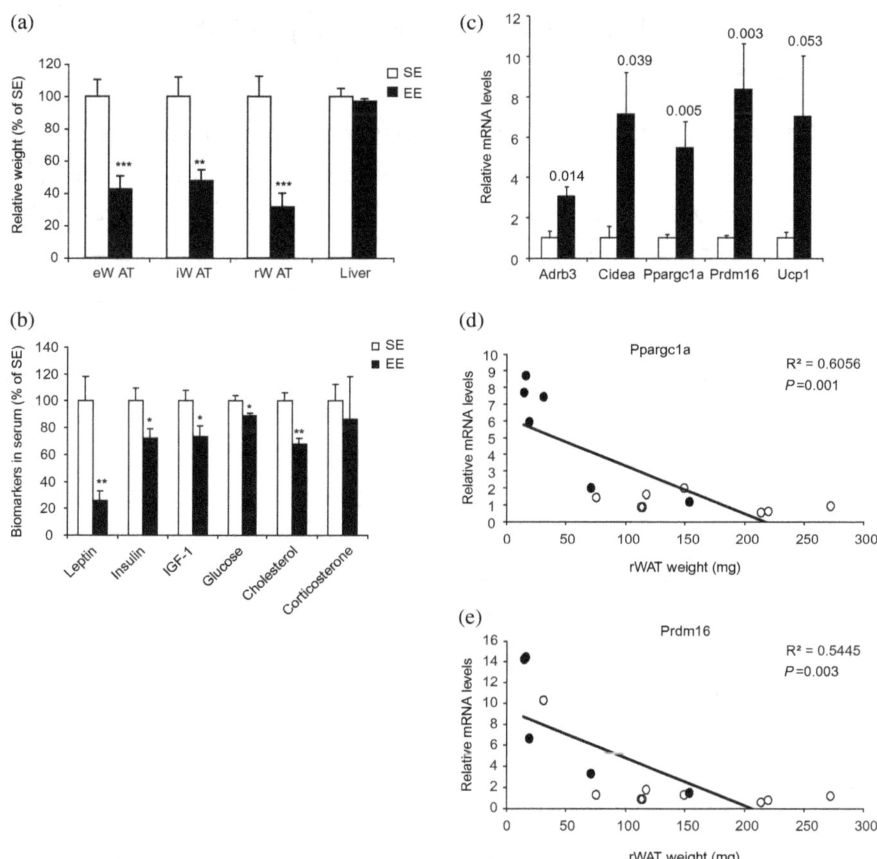

Fig. 3.10. EE inhibits high fat diet (HFD)-induced obesity. (a) Relative tissue mass after 4-week HFD feeding and respective housing. (b) Serum biomarkers. $n = 10$ per group for (a) and (b). $*P < 0.05$, $**P < 0.01$, $***P < 0.001$. (c) Gene expression profile of rWAT. $n = 5$ per group. P values are shown above the bars. Data are mean ± SEM. (d) and (e) Ppargc1a and Prdm16 mRNA levels were inversely correlated to rWAT weight. Filled circles, individual EE mouse; unfilled circles, individual SE mouse. Reprinted from Cell Metab Vol 14, Cao *et al.* White to brown fat phenotypic switch induced by genetic and environmental activation of a hypothalamic-adipocyte axis, 324–338, Copyright (2011), with permission from Elsevier.

EE Enhances WAT Response to Sympathetic Stimulus

Intact sympathetic stimulation is essential to the thermogenic activity of BAT[89] and the induction of brown adipocyte-like cells in WAT depots.[31] BAT is profusely innervated by sympathetic nerve terminals with norepinephrine (NE) while WAT is to a lesser degree.[90,91] In mice fed on normal chow, EE resulted in approximate 2-fold increase of NE selectively in WAT whereas no significant increase in serum, muscle, or BAT. Although NE content *per se* is not an index of NE release or sympathetic tone, the coordinated increase of β-ARs expression and NE levels in WAT strongly point to a change in β-AR signaling and might partially explain EE's preferential regulation of WAT.

Given the fact that EE led to substantial reduction of fat mass, we sought to test whether this fat loss could influence animal's response to cold exposure. Mice, after 3-month EE or SE housing, were randomized to stay at 4°C or 22°C. After 3-hour acute cold exposure, the EE mice maintained a similar body temperature as SE mice. We examined the expression of genes involved in thermogenesis and known to be activated by cold in both BAT and WAT. Both *Dio2* and *Ppargc1a* expression levels were higher in BAT of EE mice than SE mice at 22°C, and their expression was upregulated after cold exposure. In rWAT of SE mice, neither *Dio2* nor *Ppargc1a* was altered after cold exposure consistent with the understanding that WAT does not take part in acute cold response (**Fig. 3.11**). In contrast, *Dio2* expression in rWAT of EE mice was over 5-fold higher than SE mice at 22°C, and its expression was further upregulated by additional 2.6-fold in response to cold (**Fig. 3.11**), indicating an enhanced molecular response of the EE rWAT to acute cold exposure.[76]

We further examined whether EE affects the sensitivity of rWAT to NE stimulation at thermoneutrality of 30°C. We injected

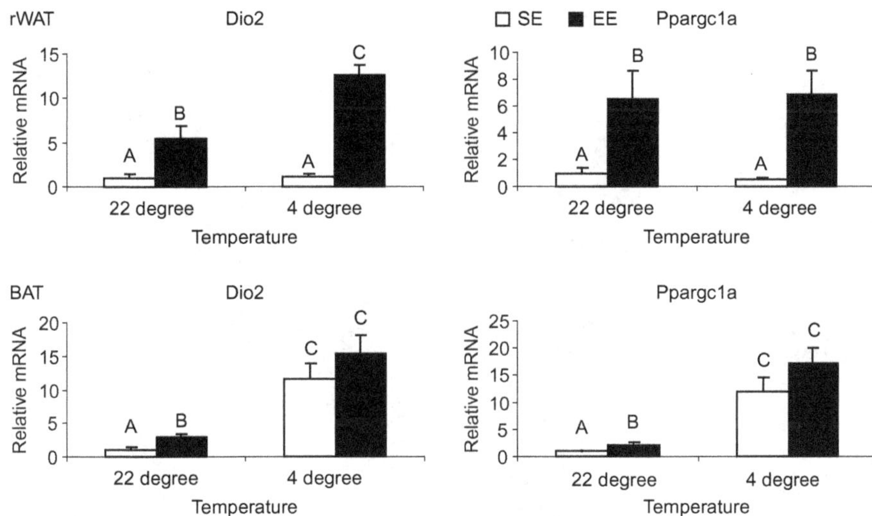

Fig. 3.11. EE leads to efficient cold response. Mice of 3-month EE or SE housing were randomized to acute cold exposure for 3 hr. Gene expression of Dio2 and Ppargc1a in rWAT and BAT, n = 4 per group. Bars not connected by the same letter are significantly different. Data are mean ± SEM. Reprinted from Cell Metab Vol 14, Cao *et al*. White to brown fat phenotypic switch induced by genetic and environmental activation of a hypothalamic-adipocyte axis, 324–338, Copyright (2011), with permission from Elsevier.

subcutaneously a low dose of NE (0.3 mg/kg) to mice after 10-week EE and examined the expression of genes known to be regulated by NE.[34] Four hours after NE injection, no significant gene expression changes were found in SE rWAT. In contrast, the EE rWAT was highly responsive to the low-dose NE stimulation. *Lep* that was sharply downregulated in EE rWAT compared to SE mice was further reduced significantly after NE injection. *Ucp1* was robustly induced by NE in the EE rWAT (**Fig. 3.12**). These data suggest EE is likely linked with an elevated sympathetic tone to WAT, and sensitizes rWAT to acute cold exposure or NE stimulation.[76]

Conversely, β-blocker propranolol supplied in drinking water efficiently blocked the molecular features associated with EE underscoring the essential involvement of the SNS.[76]

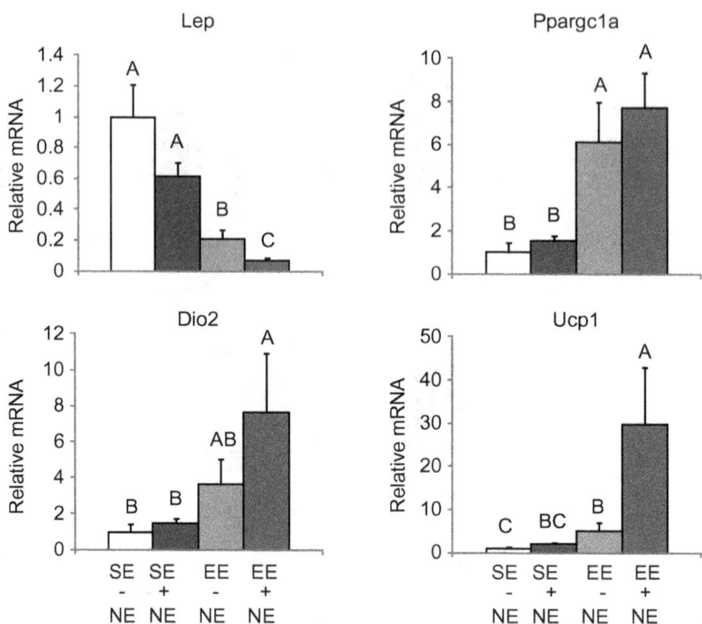

Fig. 3.12. EE enhances the sensitivity of rWAT to norepinephrine (NE) stimulation at thermoneutrality. Mice of 10-week EE or SE housing were randomized to receive NE or vehicle. Gene expression of rWAT, $n = 4$ per group. Bars not connected by the same letter are significantly different. Data are mean ± SEM. Reprinted from Cell Metab Vol 14, Cao *et al*. White to brown fat phenotypic switch induced by genetic and environmental activation of a hypothalamic-adipocyte axis, 324–338, Copyright (2011), with permission from Elsevier.

Hypothalamic BDNF is the Key Brain Mediator of EE-induced WAT Browning

We previously observed a remarkable anticancer effect induced by EE, which was mediated by hypothalamic brain-derived neurotrophic factor (BDNF) via activation of the hypothalamic-sympathoneural-adipocyte (HSA) axis.[77] Thus, we hypothesized that this brain-adipocyte axis could also regulate the browning of WAT and adiposity. BDNF has been identified as a key element in energy homeostasis.[92–94] Our previous studies had demonstrated that hypothalamic gene transfer of BDNF leads to marked weight loss and alleviation of obesity and diabetes.[95] In this study,[76] we further investigated the role of BDNF in EE-induced WAT browning.

A rAAV vector expressing the human BDNF gene was injected to the hypothalamus of DIO mice with a yellow fluorescent protein (YFP) as a control.[95] The transgene expression level, location (mainly in arcuate nucleus of hypothalamus (ARC) and ventromedial hypothalamus (VMH)) and duration were similar to the previous studies.[77,95] Hypothalamic BDNF gene transfer led to marked weight loss and fat loss (**Fig. 3.13**), reproducing the impact of EE on DIO mice but to a greater degree (**Fig. 3.10**). Moreover, BDNF overexpression induced a beige gene signature in rWAT resembling that of EE (**Fig. 3.14(a)**), together with robust increase in proteins involved in thermogenesis and mitochondrial function (UCP1 and HSP60) (**Fig. 3.14(b)**). All WAT depots dissected from BDNF mice showed substantially higher oxygen consumption *ex vivo* compared to their counterparts from YFP mice (**Fig. 3.14(c)**).

Next, we investigated whether β-blockade could attenuate hypothalamic BDNF's regulation of WAT. rAAV-BDNF or empty (carrying no transgene) viral vectors were injected to the hypothalamus bilaterally. At 8 weeks after viral vector injection, BDNF-overexpressing mice lost weight on average 3.8 g while control mice gained 2.9 g. Meanwhile, BDNF mice consumed more food than control mice (AAV-BDNF: 4.77 ± 0.13 g/day versus AAV-Empty: 4.04 ± 0.18 g/day, $P = 0.004$). Then, mice were randomly assigned to receive the combination of the β1/β2 blocker propranolol and β3 blocker SR59230A or vehicle delivered by osmotic minipumps. The β-blockade efficiently attenuated the induction of beige gene signature induced by hypothalamic BDNF overexpression.[76]

Similar to our mechanistic studies on cancer, we conducted several experiments to define the role of BDNF in regulating WAT browning. First, BDNF heterozygous mice (BDNF+/−) develop adult-onset obesity associated with hypothalamic BDNF protein levels approximately 40% lower than wild type.[92] We found a substantial increase in the fat pad mass of BDNF+/− mice before a significant body weight difference occurred compared to wild type mice. The

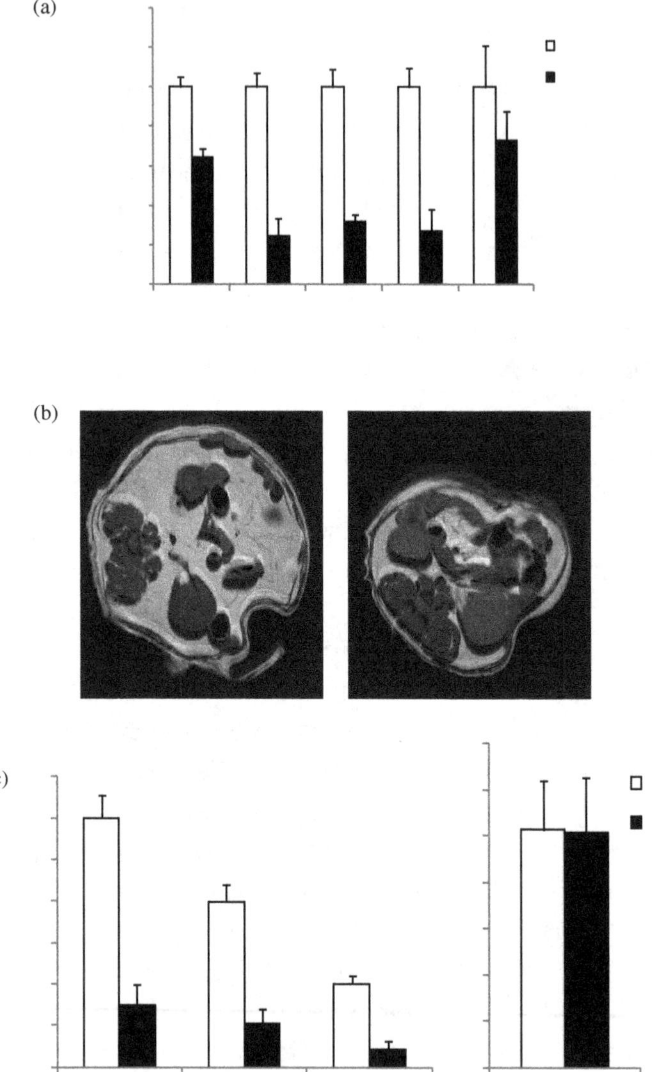

Fig. 3.13. Hypothalamic BDNF gene transfer reproduces EE-associated inhibition of diet-induced obesity. (a) rAAV-mediated gene delivery of BDNF to hypothalamus reduced adiposity. (b) Representative MRI images. White area, adipose tissues. (c) MRI analysis of fat mass and lean mass. $n = 4$–5 per group. *$P < 0.05$, **$P < 0.01$. Data are mean $\pm$ SEM. intra-ab, intra-abdominal; subcu, subcutaneous. Reprinted from Cell Metab Vol 14, Cao *et al*. White to brown fat phenotypic switch induced by genetic and environmental activation of a hypothalamic-adipocyte axis, 324–338, Copyright (2011), with permission from Elsevier.

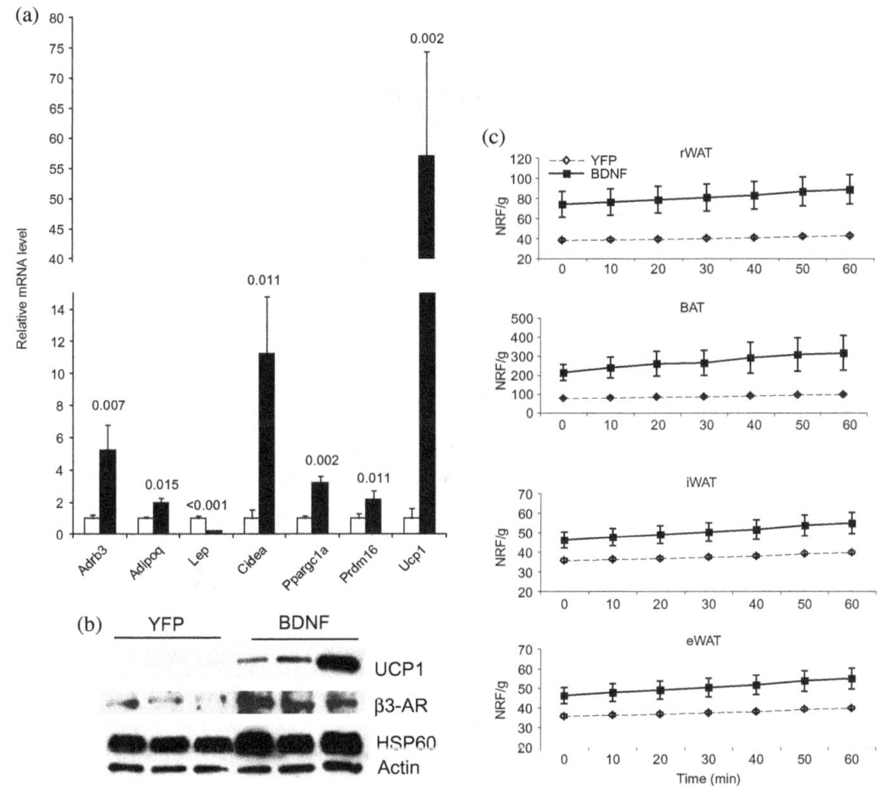

Fig. 3.14. Hypothalamic BDNF gene transfer mimics EE-induced browning of white adipose tissue. (a) Hypothalamic gene transfer of BDNF induced a gene signature in rWAT similar to EE. n = 4–5 per group. *P* values are shown above bars. (b) Western blotting of rWAT of BDNF-overexpressing mice and YFP-expressing mice. (c) *ex vivo* oxygen consumption of dissected fat depots (triplicate each fat depot, n = 3 per group, P < 0.05). Data are mean ± SEM. Reprinted from Cell Metab Vol 14, Cao *et al.* White to brown fat phenotypic switch induced by genetic and environmental activation of a hypothalamic-adipocyte axis, 324–338, Copyright (2011), with permission from Elsevier.

molecular features of rWAT in BDNF+/− mice were a complete reversal of that found with EE or BDNF-overexpressing mice, namely a suppression of β-ARs and beige gene program.[76]

Second, instead of global BDNF deficiency, we used a dominant negative truncated form of the high affinity BDNF receptor (TrkB.T1) to specifically inhibit BDNF signaling in the hypothalamus of adult mice. Mice receiving rAAV-TrkB.T1 injection to the hypothalamus consumed more food and gained more weight than AAV-YFP controls (**Fig. 3.15(a)**). Similar to DIO mice, rWAT was enlarged in TrkB. T1 mice on normal chow diet, and had a molecular signature similar

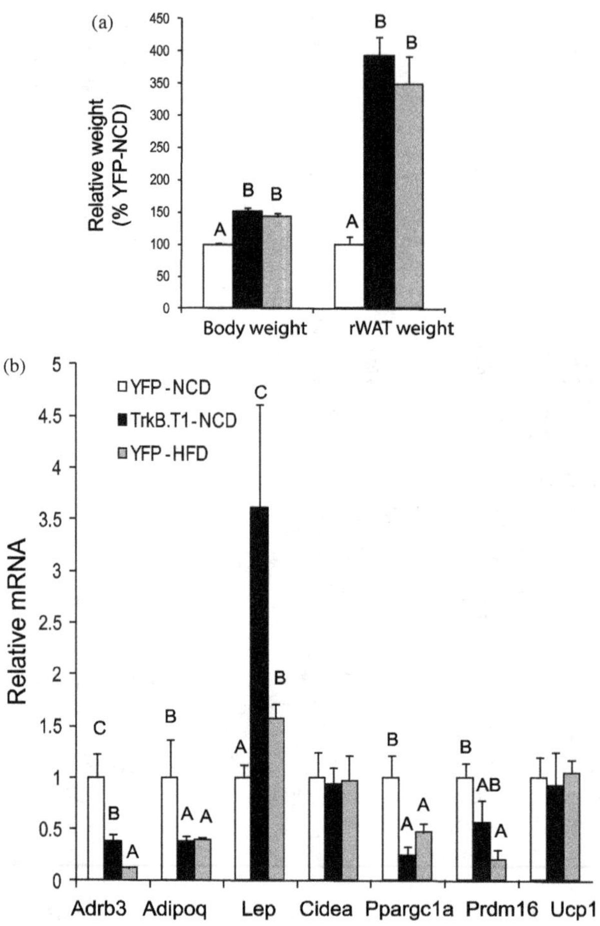

Fig. 3.15. Hypothalamic gene transfer of a dominant negative BDNF receptor (TrkB.T1 leads to obesity and a reversal of the EE-associated gene signature in rWAT. (a) TrkB.T1-expressing mice were equally obese as DIO mice expressing YFP. (b) rWAT gene expression profile of TrkB.T1-expressing mice fed with normal chow diet (NCD) compared to lean YFP-expressing mice fed with NCD and YFP-expressing mice fed with high fat diet (HFD). $n = 5$ per group. Data are mean ± SEM. Bars not connected by the same letter are significantly different. Reprinted from Cell Metab Vol 14, Cao *et al.* White to brown fat phenotypic switch induced by genetic and environmental activation of a hypothalamic-adipocyte axis, 324–338, Copyright (2011), with permission from Elsevier.

to BDNF+/− mice (**Fig. 3.15(b)**). Taken together, both global and hypothalamic-specific inhibition of BDNF led to a complete reversal of the EE-associated molecular features in rWAT, indicating BDNF's critical involvement in regulating WAT gene program.[76]

Third, we investigated whether BDNF mediated the EE-induced rWAT browning by using microRNA to block EE-induced BDNF upregulation in hypothalamus.[95] MicroRNA knockdown of BDNF led to accelerated weight gain by approximately 2-fold, and completely abolished the molecular changes in rWAT associated with EE (**Fig. 3.16**).[76]

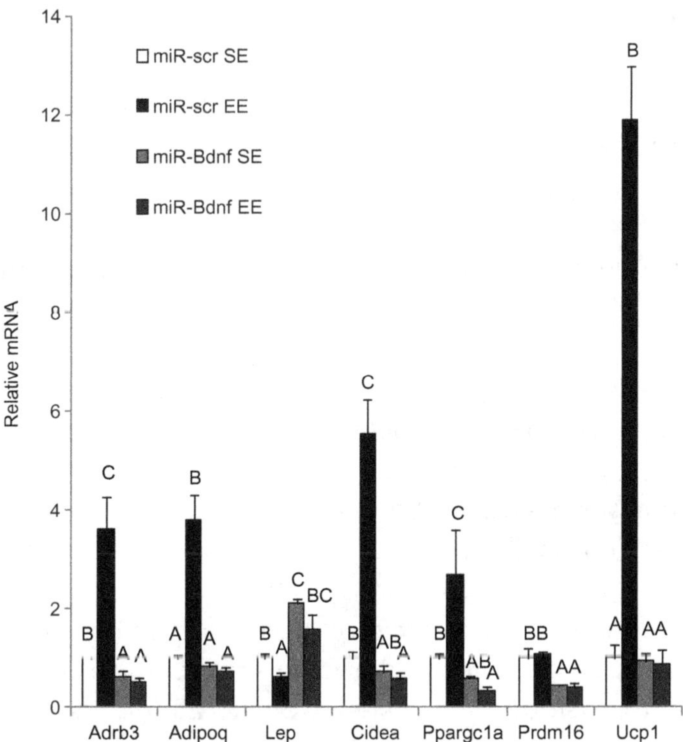

Fig. 3.16. Hypothalamic gene transfer of a microRNA targeting Bdnf blocks EE-associated molecular features of rWAT. *n* = 4 per group. Data are mean ± SEM. Bars not connected by the same letter are significantly different. scr, scramble sequence. Reprinted from Cell Metab Vol 14, Cao *et al*. White to brown fat phenotypic switch induced by genetic and environmental activation of a hypothalamic-adipocyte axis, 324–338, Copyright (2011), with permission from Elsevier.

EE Represents a Novel and Unique Model to Study WAT Browning

Our studies have revealed a new type of thermogenesis that contributes to the profound impact on body composition and metabolism in mice living in EE housing, in the absence of chronic cold exposure or prolonged pharmacological β-adrenergic stimulation.[76] The characteristics of EE-induced WAT browning include:

1. Intra-abdominal WAT is most responsive[76] whereas wheel running induces browning mostly in the subcutaneous depot.[42]
2. Physical activity alone does not account for the EE effects on adipose tissue.[76]
3. A brain-fat pathway — the HSA axis has been revealed with BDNF as a key mediator in the hypothalamus.[76]
4. EE provides a model to study social factors in metabolism.

The induction of beige genetic program by EE is remarkable when compared to some of the most effective physiological and pharmacological approaches to induce browning. The emergence of beige cells is under genetic control with large variabilities among inbred strains of mice.[96] C57BL/6 mice, the strain we used in the EE experiments, respond poorly to SNS stimulation probably due to low β-AR expression levels.[86,96] Studies have shown that cold exposure at 5°C for 7 days fails to induce beige cells in rWAT with only low induction of *Ucp1* expression.[96] In contrast, 4-week EE leads to a 27-fold induction of *Ucp1*, which is more effective compared to the 9-fold induction observed in the same strain of mice acclimated to 5°C cold temperature for 4 weeks, or the 23-fold induction after injection of β agonist CL316243 for 11–12 days.[97] Of interest, EE significantly upregulates both β2 and β3 AR gene expression and protein levels in rWAT. This phenomenon is opposite to the desensitization of β-ARs after extended exposure to β agonist,[98] which is worthy of further investigation.

The first report on EE-induced WAT browning and the underlying mechanism was published in Cell Metabolism. A cover art depicts how EE regulates adiposity. A complex and engaging environment induces BDNF expression in the hypothalamus and subsequently elevating the sympathetic tone preferentially to the WAT. NE releasing from sympathetic nerve terminals acts on the adipocyte β-ARs to induce beige cells contributing to burning out energy. Consequently, increase in energy expenditure instead of appetite suppression leads to reduction of adiposity and protection against obesity.[76]

Adipose VEGF is Downstream of the HSA Axis Controlling WAT Browning

Since the original publication on EE's metabolic benefits, we have continued to search for players among the regulatory network linking social and physical environment to energy balance regulation. We have identified adipose vascular endothelial growth factor (VEGF) as a key component of the HSA axis underlying the browning effect of EE.[99] VEGF is the only *bona fide* endothelial cell growth factor and its presence is essential for initiation of the angiogenic program.[100,101]

The adipose tissue is comprised of many types of cells, in which ~60% are adipocytes and the rest are endothelial cells, fibroblasts, precursors, and multiple types of immune cells.[102] In order to examine additional consequences of EE-induced adipose remodeling, we profiled molecular features in the rWAT[103] brought by short-term EE of 6 days including markers of angiogenesis (*Vegf*, *Hif1a*), macrophages (*Emr1* encoding F4/80, *Mgll*), peripheral nerve (*Uchl1* encoding PGP95),[104] all previously implicated in adipose remodeling,[105] brown adipocyte markers (*Prdm16*, *Ucp1*, *Ppargc1a*), β3-AR, and leptin. Six-day EE upregulated β3-AR expression and downregulated leptin expression. Interestingly, Vegf expression was upregulated significantly by 70% whereas no changes in macrophage markers or peripheral nerve markers. No induction of the beige gene program was observed at the 6-day timepoint. And the source of the *Vegf* upregulation was the mature adipocytes but not the stromal vascular fractions (SVF). VEGF caught our eyes because it appears among the earliest molecular events triggered in rWAT by EE prior to the emergence of beige cells. We next further characterized EE regulation of adipose VEGF and found the following features:[99]

1. With progression of EE by the 4-week timepoint, VEGF expression was increased to a larger extent (by ~3.5-fold), and sustained at least for 3 months in contrast to the transient upregulation of VEGF by cold exposure.[106]

2. Immunohistochemistry showed increased VEGF and its receptor kinase insert domain receptor (KDR) as well as the vascular marker CD31 in rWAT of EE mice.

3. Other members of the VEGF family (VEGF-B and placental growth factor) showed no change.

4. No *Vegf* or *Cd31* upregulation was observed in iWAT by 4-week EE concomitant of no beige gene induction in iWAT.[76]

5. Leptin expression was decreased by ~77% in iWAT, suggesting the dissociation of leptin suppression from the browning effect of EE.

6. VEGF plays a direct role in the maintenance, activation, and expansion of BAT.[107,108] However, EE did not change the expression of *Vegf* and its receptors in BAT, liver, or skeletal muscle.

7. EE-induced *Vegf* upregulation was hypoxia-independent.

8. In DIO mice, EE increased *Vegf* expression to a greater degree than that observed in mice fed a normal chow diet. And the mRNA level of *Vegf* was inversely correlated with the rWAT mass,

while positively correlated with beige cell markers *Ppargc1a* and *Prdm16*.

These data suggest an organ-specific, and even an adipose depot-specific regulation of VEGF and angiogenesis by EE coincident with induction of beige cells.

To investigate whether SNS tone drives VEGF upregulation by EE, we conducted unilateral sympathetic denervation of the rWAT by local injection of the neural toxin 6-hydroxydopamine (6OHDA).[109] 6OHDA denervation led to approximately 40% decrease of NE in rWAT and prevented the increase of NE associated with EE. Partial sympathetic denervation blocked the upregulation of *Vegf*, increase of angiogenesis, and induction of beige gene program induced by EE. Additional studies by genetically manipulating hypothalamic BDNF signaling also demonstrated VEGF downstream of the HSA axis.[99]

For a gain-of-function study of the role of VEGF in WAT browning, we employed an engineered serotype of AAV, Rec2 that can sufficiently deliver transgene to adipose tissues.[110] We injected Rec2 vector harboring human VEGF directly to the rWAT and housed the mice in SE. AAV-mediated VEGF overexpression (4.5-fold increase of VEGF level in rWAT) reproduced the WAT browning effect of EE. Beige cells were observed in rWAT receiving VEGF vector adjacent to the areas of increased vasculature (**Fig. 3.17**). Of note, adipose VEGF overexpression did not significantly suppress leptin expression, a molecular feature induced by EE, suggesting VEGF signaling was specifically involved in the browning effect of EE but may not be involved in the regulation of leptin expression.

Conversely, adipose-specific VEGF knockout or pharmacological VEGF blockade by antibody abolished the beige cell recruitment induced by EE (**Fig. 3.18**). Furthermore, VEGF may have actions independent of angiogenesis[99] (**Fig. 3.19**).

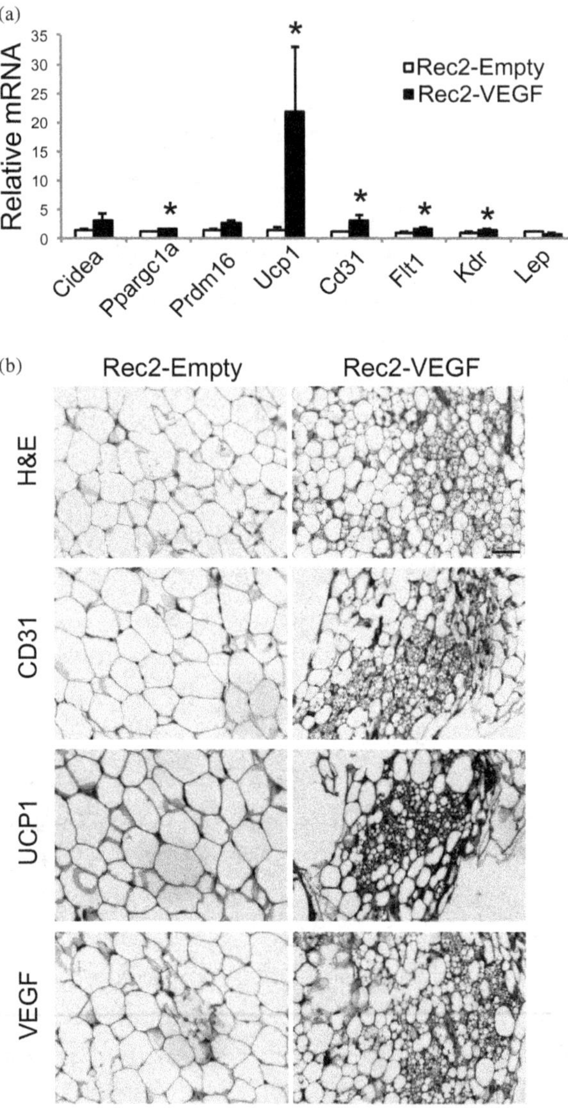

Fig. 3.17. rAAV-mediated gene transfer of VEGF to the rWAT reproduces the WAT browning effect of EE. (a) rWAT gene expression profile 4-week post Rec2-VEGF injection. Rec2-Empty carries the same expression cassette but without a transgene. $n = 8$ per group. Data are mean ± SEM. $*P < 0.05$. (b) Immunohistochemistry of rWAT. Scale bar, 50 μm. Reprinted from During *et al*. Adipose VEGF links the white-to-brown fat switch with environmental, genetic, and pharmacological stimuli in male mice. Endocrinology 2015, 156 (6), 2059–2073, by permission of Oxford University Press/Endocrine Society.

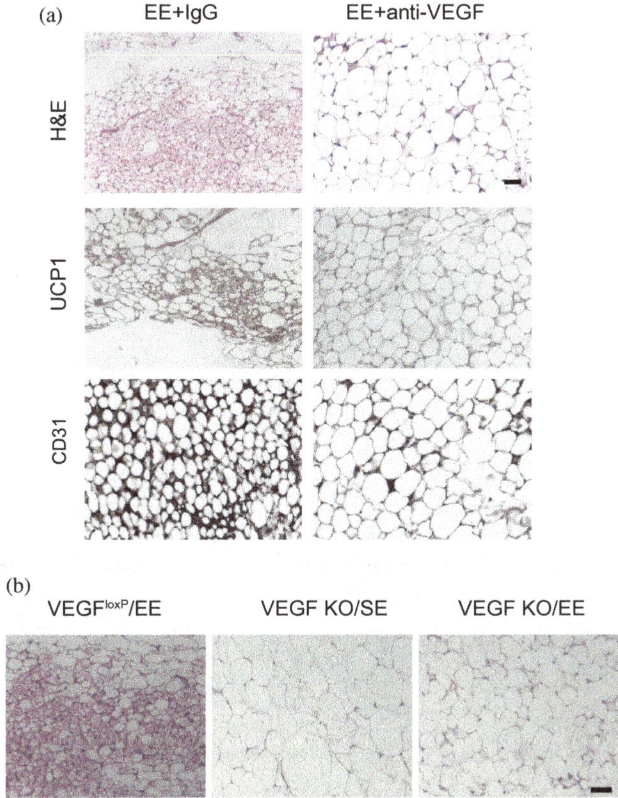

Fig. 3.18. VEGF blockade abolishes EE-induced WAT browning. (a) Anti-VEGF antibody blocked the induction of beige cells associated with EE. Representative immunohistochemistry images after 4-week EE and anti-VEGF antibody treatment. (b) Adipose-specific VEGF knockout mice showed no EE-induced rWAT browning. Representative immunohistochemistry of rWAT after 4-week EE. Scale bar, 50 µm. Reprinted from During *et al.* Adipose VEGF links the white-to-brown fat switch with environmental, genetic, and pharmacological stimuli in male mice. Endocrinology 2015, 156 (6), 2059–2073, by permission of Oxford University Press/Endocrine Society.

An interesting finding of this study is that VEGF integrates multiple upstream stimulations to a common pathway that is essential to the emergence of beige cells. In addition to EE, blockade of VEGF could substantially abrogate the browning

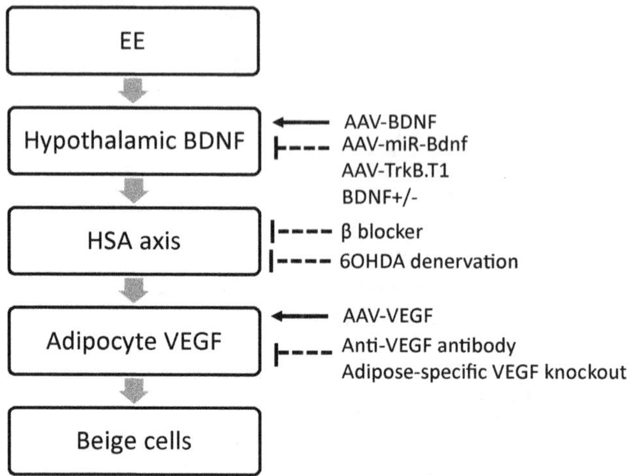

Fig. 3.19. Mechanism of EE-induced WAT browning. EE upregulates BDNF expression in the hypothalamus, leading to the activation of the HSA axis. The preferential increase of sympathetic tone to the WAT upregulates VEGF expression in adipocytes, resulting in the induction of beige cells. Gain- and loss-of-function studies identify each major component of the brain BDNF-HSA-adipocyte VEGF pathway.

effects induced by the β3-adrenergic agonist CL-316,243,[84] the PPARγ ligand rosiglitazone,[34,111] and voluntary running.[42] UCP1 was particularly sensitive to the anti-VEGF antibody whose upregulation by EE, running, or rosiglitazone was completely abolished (**Fig. 3.20**).[99] Thus, adipose VEGF signaling is likely a downstream pathway shared by diverse physiological and pharmacological interventions that all lead to the induction of beige cells. Targeting this common pathway important for coordination between angiogenesis and the browning may have therapeutic potential.

Adipose PTEN Acts as a Downstream Mediator of the HSA Axis Regulating Adipocyte Size

Adipose tissue, particularly WAT, is a reliable responder to the EE paradigm. EE-induced metabolic remodeling is characterized by

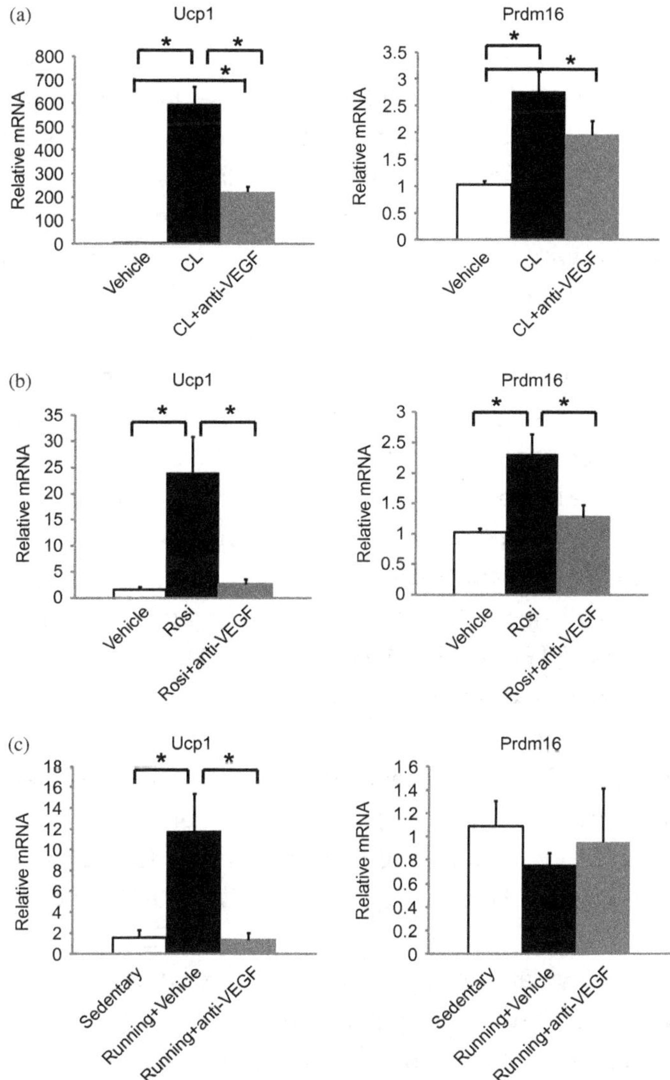

Fig. 3.20. VEGF blockade inhibits WAT browning induced by diverse physiological and pharmacological approaches. (a) rWAT gene expression after chronic injection of ß3-agonist CL-316243 and anti-VEGF antibody. (b) rWAT gene expression after chronic injection of rosiglitazone and anti-VEGF antibody. (c) rWAT gene expression after 3-week wheel running and anti-VEGF antibody treatment. $n = 5$ per group. Data are mean ± SEM. *$P < 0.05$ between groups as indicated. Reprinted from During *et al.* Adipose VEGF links the white-to-brown fat switch with environmental, genetic, and pharmacological stimuli in male mice. Endocrinology 2015, 156 (6), 2059–2073, by permission of Oxford University Press/ Endocrine Society.

reduced adiposity, drop of circulating leptin level, improved glycemic control, higher metabolic rate, and induction of beige cells in selective fat depots. Almost all fat pads, subcutaneous and visceral, are smaller in EE mice including those where beige cells are rare. Therefore, EE might reduce the size of adipocyte through a mechanism shared among all WAT depots independent of browning. In a recent study, we have identified PTEN as such a key mediator.[112]

Phosphatase and tensin homolog deleted on chromosome ten (PTEN) is a well-known tumor suppressor.[113] PTEN can serve as a potent regulator of cellular growth, survival, and insulin-mediated glucose uptake via its lipid phosphatase actions,[114–116] and is implicated in adipose remodeling processes.[117] In fact, loss- and gain-of-function studies in genetically modified mouse models have shown that PTEN plays a pivotal role in the development of mature adipose tissue, serving to control the size and/or mass of adipocytes and thereby fat distribution.[118–122] Moreover, the transgenic mice globally overexpressing PTEN (PTEN[tg]) display smaller body size, leanness, elevated energy expenditure, hyper-activation of BAT function, obesity resistance, anti-cancer state, and extended lifespan.[121,122] Additionally, similar results have been observed in fat-specific insulin receptor knock-out (FIRKO) mice.[123–125] Our research on how EE influences aging in older mice has shown that EE confers many of these physiological benefits across various murine models[126] (see Chapter 7), promoting us to explore whether EE regulates adipose PTEN expression and how PTEN modulation contributes to the EE-induced WAT remodeling process.

In a series of experiments, we found that EE upregulated adipose PTEN expression in both subcutaneous and visceral WAT depots independent of sex and age. The PTEN upregulation was associated with smaller adipocyte size and higher lipolysis and suppression of Protein kinase B also known as AKT, and extracellular signal-regulated kinase (ERK) phosphorylation. No surprise, PTEN regulation was found to be controlled by the HSA axis. Overexpressing PTEN in adipose tissue, independent of housing, recapitulated some aspects of EE adipose phenotype including suppression of AKT and ERK phosphorylation, increased hormone-sensitive lipase (HSL) phosphorylation, and decreased adipose mass. Conversely, genetically knocking down adipose PTEN blocked the EE-induced reduction of adipocyte size. These data suggest adipose PTEN may serve as one downstream factor of the EE-induced WAT remodeling, likely contributing to increased lipolysis and reduced adipocyte size.[112]

One Brain-Fat Axis Regulates Multiple Downstream Processes

A decade of research by our lab has characterized downstream processes within the HSA axis, finding that several aspects of EE-induced adipose remodeling are all driven by a single brain-fat axis through activating the β-adrenergic signaling. Some changes in downstream actors are not necessarily linked. For example, activating the HSA axis both suppresses leptin expression — contributing to anticancer effects,[127] and induces VEGF expression — resulting in beige cell induction and rising energy expenditure.[100] However, the leptin suppression and VEGF stimulation are dissociated. Interference with one downstream actor does not abrogate the other as long as the HSA axis is functional.[76,77] PTEN seems to be another downstream actor of the HSA axis that contributes to regulating adipocyte size and lipolysis. There is certainly much more to learn about the adipose remodeling processes in response to environmental stimuli. It is likely that the HSA axis is just one component of a complex regulatory network. Nevertheless, available evidence suggests a central role of the hypothalamic BDNF driving multiple downstream processes within the adipose tissue in a coordinated way leading to various health benefits. **Figure 3.21** summarizes the adipose mediators identified up to date.

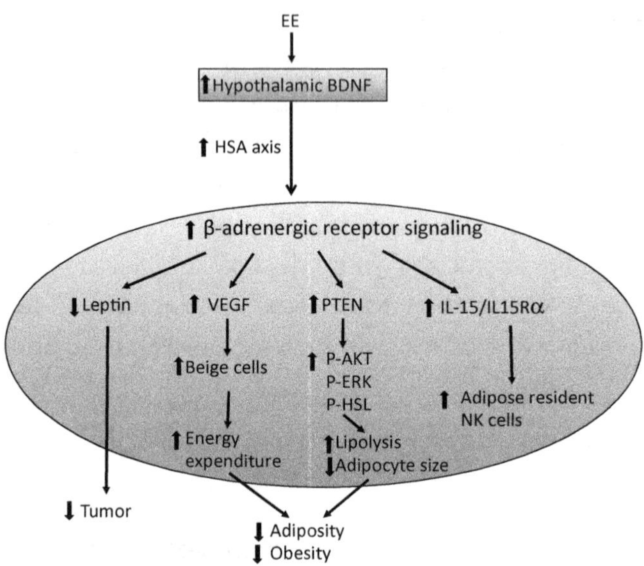

Fig. 3.21.   EE-induced remodeling of WAT driven by the HSA axis. See Chapter 6 for the adipose resident natural killer (NK) cell modulation. P-AKT/ERK/HSL, phosphorylation; HSL, hormone-sensitive lipase.

Adipose PTEN Regulates Fat Homeostasis and Redistribution

This section tells a story of accidental discovery from our investigation on EE remodeling of fat. When we found EE upregulated PTEN expression in the WAT, we sought to conduct a loss-of-function study by Cre-loxP depletion of PTEN in selected fat depot. To test the conditional knockdown efficacy, we injected the rAAV vector harboring Cre recombinase (AAV-Cre) to one iWAT pad of PTEN^{flox} mice and the rAAV carrying no transgene (AAV-empty) to the contralateral side of iWAT depot. The results were interesting and surprising. The iWAT depot receiving AAV-Cre where PTEN was depleted, was enlarged massively compared to naïve PTEN^{flox} mice while the contralateral side of iWAT depot receiving AAV-empty shrank dramatically with visibly apparent browning **(Fig. 3.22)**. Total intra-abdominal WAT and BAT were substantially reduced in AAV-Cre-treated mice. No significant changes were seen in body weight, total fat mass, or

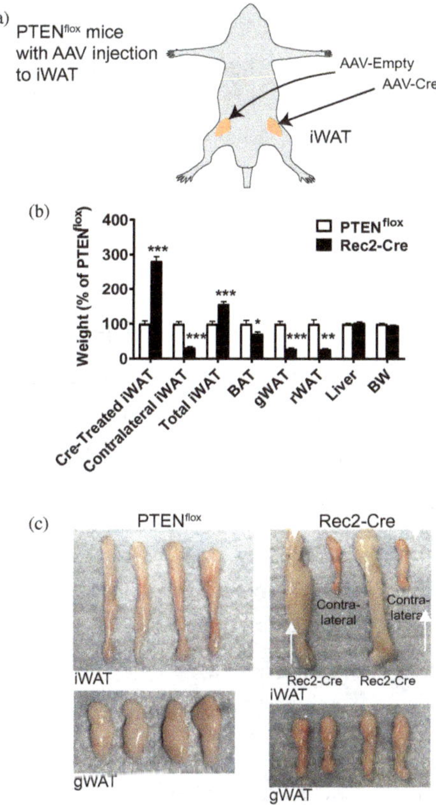

Fig. 3.22. Knockdown PTEN in individual fat depot leads to massive expansion of the affected depot associated with a compensatory reduction of other fat depots. (a) Study design. (b) Relative tissue mass 7-week post AAV injection. PTEN^{flox}, naive mice ($n = 5$); Rec2-Cre, PTEN^{flox} mice receiving AAV to iWAT ($n = 6$). Data are mean $\pm$ SEM. $*P < 0.05$, $**P < 0.01$, $***P < 0.001$. (c) Representatives of inguinal WAT (iWAT) and gonadal WAT (gWAT). Reprinted from Mol Metab Vol 30, Huang *et al.* Adipose PTEN regulates adult adipose tissue homeostasis and redistribution via a PTEN-leptin-sympathetic loop, pages 48–60, copyright (2019), with permission from Elsevier.

liver. The data suggest PTEN knockdown in one fat depot alters whole body fat distribution but not adiposity. This PTEN-triggered fat redistribution was observed in both sexes, and independent of the location of fat in which PTEN was deleted. (e.g., visceral fat PTEN knockdown enlarging the visceral depot while browning and shrinking the subcutaneous fat).[128]

We then utilized genetic and pharmacological approaches to elucidate the mechanism of this PTEN-driven adipose remodeling and redistribution. The following findings reveal a novel regulatory feedback loop.

1. Injection of AAV-Cre to individual fat pad of PTEN^{flox} mice resulted in PTEN deficiency in the transduced depot leading to massive expansion of the affected fat depot through activation of AKT pathway together with suppression of lipolysis. This hypertrophic expansion of one individual fat pad led to upregulation of PTEN in other fat depots and the compensatory shrink of these depots to achieve a set point of whole-body adiposity.
2. Administration of an AKT inhibitor prevented the effects associated with adipose PTEN knockdown, indicating AKT signaling downstream of PTEN knockdown and a mechanistic drive for the observed adipose redistribution feedback loop.
3. A deficiency of PTEN in individual fat depot caused a surge of leptin level in the circulation (3–4 folds). Chemical denervation study demonstrated that sympathetic innervation was essential for PTEN knockdown-induced adipose redistribution. Moreover, knockdown of leptin receptor in the hypothalamus attenuated the adipose redistribution induced by PTEN deficiency in individual fat pad.

Collectively, our studies uncover a feedback loop "adipose PTEN-leptin-SNS" that regulates adipose homeostasis. Specifically, loss of PTEN in one fat pad leads to hypertrophic expansion of affected depot and a surge of leptin level that at least partially acts on the hypothalamus to elevate sympathetic tone. The rise of sympathetic tone subsequently upregulates the PTEN expression, enhances lipolysis, induces beige cells in other fat depots whereby reducing mass of these fat depots to counteract the expansion of PTEN-deficient fat depot and maintain a stable whole-body adiposity (**Fig. 3.23**).[128]

This study not only demonstrates new function of adipose PTEN but also illuminates the bidirectional crosstalk between fat and brain.

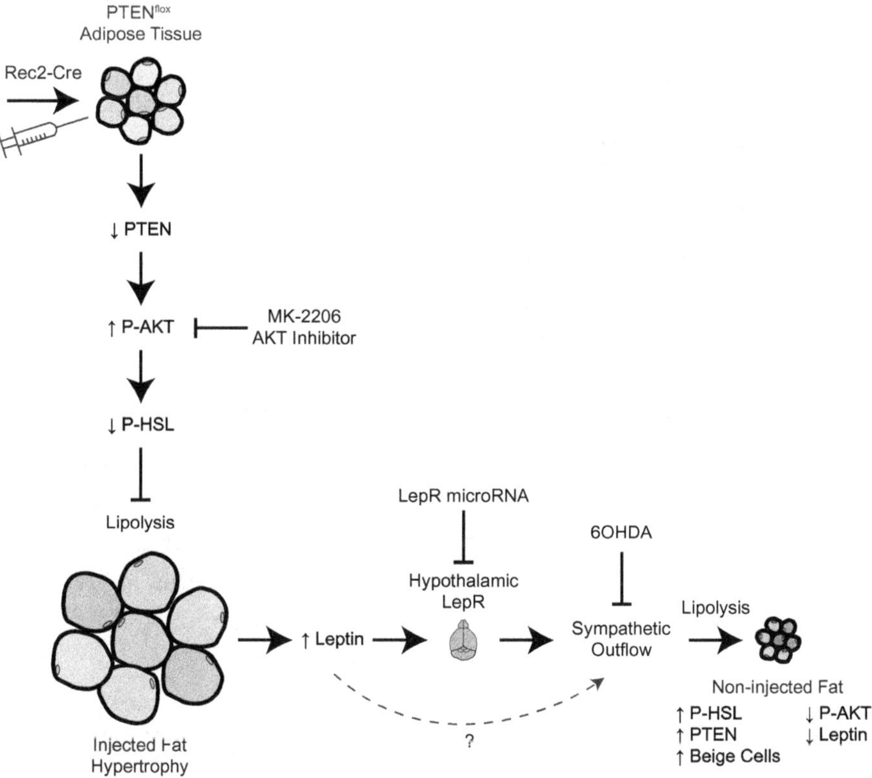

Fig. 3.23. Mechanim of PTEN knockdown-induced adipose redistribution. Knockdown PTEN in individual fat depot results in hypertrophy of the affected fat depot through activation of AKT signaling associated with suppression of lipolysis and induction of leptin. The rise of circulating leptin acts on hypothalamic leptin receptor, leading to elevated sympathetic outflow to other fat depots. The rise of sympathetic tone subsequently upregulates the PTEN expression, increases lipolysis, induces beige cells in other depots.This adipose PTEN-leptin-SNS feedback loop reduces the mass of PTEN-intact fat depots to counteract the expansion of PTEN-deficient fat depot, and maitains a set point of adipose PTEN level and whole body adiposity. Reprinted from Mol Metab Vol 30, Huang *et al.* Adipose PTEN regulates adult adipose tissue homeostasis and redistribution via a PTEN-leptin-sympathetic loop, pages 48–60, copyright (2019), with permission from Elsevier.

The body has such a marvelous way to maintain homeostasis. But in certain circumstances, these delicate but resilient feedback pathways might become hurdles. For example, removing selective fat depot might not be sufficient to alleviate overall obesity because of these compensatory responses regressing toward the preexisting setpoint of whole-body adiposity.

Exploring Additional Upstream Players of the HSA Axis

Our exploration of the HSA axis does not stop at the adipose tissue. In fact, we attempted to identify other functional molecules in the hypothalamus on top of the HSA, and found VGF closely associated with the HSA axis activation.[129] VGF (nonacronymic) was originally identified as a nerve growth factor (NGF)-inducible transcript in PC12 pheochromocytoma cells and is expressed widely throughout the nervous system, and its highest expression occurs in the hypothalamus.[130–134] In addition to NGF, VGF can be induced by BDNF.[135] *Vgf* gene produces a peptide precursor that is further processed to generate several mature peptides with distinct functions.[136,137] Evidence suggests that VGF acts in the melanocortin pathway that regulates energy balance and glucose homeostasis through its sympathetic and parasympathetic innervation to the BAT, WAT, and pancreas.[104,138–142]

We observed that both EE and hypothalamic overexpression of BDNF stimulated *Vgf* expression in the hypothalamus. Then we used the Cre-loxP system to knockdown *Vgf* specifically in the hypothalamus of adult mice.[129] This approach allows investigation on the role of VGF in energy balance and metabolic adaption to EE in adult mice and meanwhile avoids the compensatory responses during development that may confound the germline knockout.

Our pharmacological and genetic studies suggest that VGF in the hypothalamus is responsive to environmental cue, likely downstream of BDNF, and involved in the melanocortin pathway regulating homeostasis. However, hypothalamic VGF is not a major player of the HSA axis in contrast to the critical role of BDNF. The conclusion is supported by the following results from this study.[129]

1. EE upregulated *Vgf* expression in the hypothalamus following the upregulation of *Bdnf*.

2. In addition to EE, *Vgf* expression was regulated by food deprivation, leptin, and melanocortin receptor agonist in the hypothalamus but not the cortex, often parallel to the changes of *Bdnf*.

3. Acute infusion of BDNF protein or long-term overexpression of BDNF in the hypothalamus upregulated *Vgf* expression.

4. Conversely, inhibition of BDNF signaling via heterozygous knockout, microRNA-mediated *Bdnf* knockdown, or dominant negative TrkB.T1 all downregulated *Vgf* expression. These data collectively suggest BDNF regulates hypothalamic Vgf expression.

5. Hypothalamic *Vgf* knockdown had no significant impact on *Bdnf* expression indicating VGF acts downstream of BDNF.

6. We previously showed that inhibiting the hypothalamic *Bdnf* upregulation completely abolished EE-induced metabolic phenotypes. In contrast, preventing EE-induced *Vgf* upregulation failed to attenuate the decrease of adiposity or *Bdnf* upregulation suggesting a minor role of VGF in the HSA axis, with respect to EE.[129]

Although hypothalamic VGF not essential to EE metabolic outcomes, this study provides interesting evidence with regards to the biological functions of VGF. Specific knockdown of hypothalamic VGF in male adult mice resulted in increased adiposity, decreased core body temperature, reduced energy expenditure, impaired glycemic control, and disturbance of molecular features of BAT and WAT with no effect on food intake.[129] This metabolic phenotype is the contrary to the lean and hypermetabolic phenotype of germline VGF knockout mice.[143–145] The inconsistency might originate from the compensatory changes during development when VGF is knockout in germline or the heterogeneous expression of VGF peptides in extrahypothalamic neuro-endocrine tissues such as the stomach and pancreas.[137,146] Of note, the phenotype of hypothalamic VGF knockdown was largely consistent to the functions of a VGF-derived peptide observed in the adult animals.[147] Moreover, the metabolic disturbances (reduced metabolic rate, impairment of glucose tolerance) were not observed in female mice although the degree of VGF knockdown in the hypothalamus was equivalent to that in the male mice. These results clearly highlight the complexity of VGF functions and the necessity for tissue specific manipulation studies.

EE Alleviates Obesity and Associated Metabolic Disorders in a Variety of Animal Models

Since the discovery of the metabolic phenotype of EE and the underlying HSA axis, we have generalized EE intervention to a variety of mouse models predisposed to obesity and associated metabolic syndromes.

The BTBR Mouse Model of Autism

Autism spectrum disorder (ASD) is a complex neurodevelopmental disorder causing significant social, communication, learning, and behavioral challenges. Hallmark symptoms of ASD include persistent impaired social/communication skills and restrictive/repetitive behaviors.[148] The impaired social interaction of ASD is characterized by deficits in social-emotional reciprocity, nonverbal communicative behaviors, as well as developing, maintaining, and understanding relationships. The ASD-associated restrictive/repetitive behaviors include stereotyped or repetitive motor movements, speech, or use of objects; insistence on sameness; highly restricted or fixated interests; and hyper- or hyporeactivity to sensory inputs.[149] Epidemiological studies performed by the CDC conclude ASD presents with a frequency of 1 in every 59 children, with boys 4 times more likely than girls to be diagnosed with ASD.[150] The etiology of the disorder remains a topic of debate — genetic, biologic, and environmental factors are all thought to play a part.[148,151]

Currently there is no cure for ASD. However, research has shown that some intervention treatments can improve a child's development and ameliorate symptoms in ASD patients.[152] For example, a personalized online therapy has been shown to achieve improvements in learning, memory, anxiety, attention span, motor skills, eating, sleeping, sensory processing, self-awareness, communication, social skills, and mood.[153] Early intensive behavioral intervention administered to autistic children at a young age has been shown to improve social behavior.[154] A recent meta-analysis suggests that cognitive behavioral therapy may be effective to alleviate anxiety in some ASD presentations.[155] These human intervention successes, although limited, underscore the potential benefit of developing analogous treatments in animal models to elucidate mechanisms underlying ASD treatments.

BTBR mice exhibit some behavioral and physiological deficits similar to those observed in ASD patients. The BTBR strain has disturbed endocrine function and was originally bred for studies on abdominal obesity, insulin resistance, diabetes-induced nephropathy, and phenylketonuria.[148,156] Studies have shown that the BTBR strain consistently manifests ASD-like behaviors.[148] BTBR mice display reduced social approach, low reciprocal social interactions, impaired juvenile play, repetitive behaviors, and communication deficits.[157] This strain is also used as a model of generalized anxiety, and has been used to study psychiatric comorbidities present in ASD.[158–160] On the other hand, there is evidence that HFD feeding exacerbates cognitive rigidity and social deficiency in BTBR mice, suggesting a link between the aforementioned metabolic deficiencies and behavior deficits.[161]

How EE may influence behaviors has been explored in a variety of ASD murine models. Encouraging results from animal studies have promoted translation to human treatment.[162–166] This topic is discussed in Chapter 9. However, few studies assess the metabolic outcome of EE in an animal model of ASD. Therefore, we attempted to fill this gap by investigating the metabolic and behavioral effects of EE in the BTBR mice with a perspective of the HSA axis.[167]

Juvenile BTBR mice were randomized to SE or EE housing and maintained on normal chow diet. EE was initiated at a juvenile age (4–5 weeks old) to mimic early-age interventions. For the duration of 17-week EE study, mice were subjected to a battery of metabolic and behavioral assessments (**Fig. 3.24**). EE exerted significant metabolic benefits in male BTBR mice characterized as reduced adiposity by ~70%, increased lean mass, improved glycemic control, and decreased circulating leptin, all typical metabolic improvement seen in C57BL/6 mice. EE upregulated BDNF expression in the hypothalamus by ~25% but not in the amygdala and hippocampus. Interestingly, BDNF receptor TrkB (*Ntrk2*) was upregulated in all three brain regions profiled to greater extent (3~6 folds) than *Bdnf*

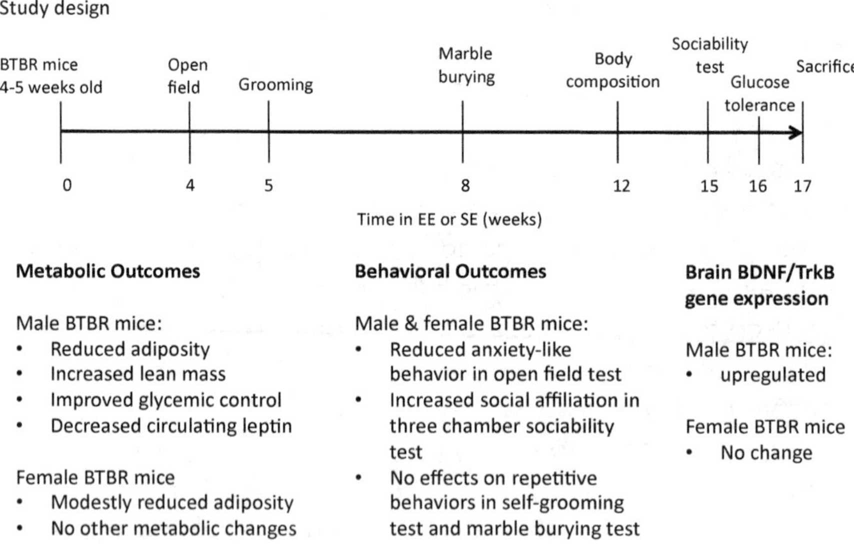

Fig. 3.24. EE improves metabolic and behavioral health in the BTBR mouse model of autism.

in male BTBR mice living in EE. BTBR females were less responsive to EE intervention displaying reduction of adiposity by ~60% but no changes in glycemic control, circulating leptin, or *Bdnf/Ntrk2* gene expression. Notably, both male and female BTBR mice living in EE had higher food intake when calibrated to body weight, once again indicating the lean phenotype induced by EE not due to appetite suppression.[167]

After 4-week EE, BTBR mice were subjected to the open field test.[168] Based on mouse prey tendencies and their desire to avoid open areas, the open field test is often used to assess anxiety and other measures such as general locomotion and exploratory behavior. An increase of proportional time and/or distance traveled in the center portion of the open arena is thought to reflect lower level of anxiety. EE mice showed increased proportional time spent in the center indicating amelioration of BTBR anxiety-like symptoms.[167] However, EE did not alter BTBR repetitive behaviors as assessed by self-grooming test.[169,170] and marble burying test.[170,171]

BTBR mice display reduced social approach and low reciprocal social interactions.[157] The Three-Chamber Sociability (TCS) test has been used to study social affiliation and novel social engagement in mouse models. Mice are given the opportunity to wander three chambers while investigating social stimuli. The test subject is placed in an apparatus consisting of three connected plexiglass chambers with removable dividers between each chamber. In the first phase to examine social affiliation, the test subject is exposed to a novel confined peer and an opposing empty chamber. The wire cage restricts social or aggressive interactions between the two mice beyond nose contact. After habituation period, chamber dividers are lifted to allow the test subject to move freely around all three chambers for a 10-min observation period. A second 10-min test is conducted immediately afterward to assess social novelty engagement. In the second phase, the familiar mouse (the "novel confined peer" from the first phase test) and a new unfamiliar mouse are placed in the opposite chamber.[172] The time spent in each chamber and number of chamber entries of the test subject are analyzed blindly. The social preference index is defined as the ratio of time spent in the mouse chamber over the time spent in the empty chamber. BTBR mice living in EE showed significantly increased social preference index compared to their counterparts living in SE, indicating improvement in social affiliation by EE housing. However, during the second phase of TCS test, EE mice showed no preference for a novel social peer. The social novelty index is defined as the ratio of time spent in the novel mouse chamber over the familiar mouse chamber. The social novelty index was not different between EE and SE mice, suggesting no EE-mediated improvements in social novelty engagement.

Taken together, these results demonstrate that like-peer EE improves metabolic and behavioral health in BTBR mice in a sex-dependent fashion. The positive correlation between upregulation of BDNF signaling genes (*Bdnf* and *Ntrk2*) and more robust metabolic improvement has promoted us to investigate whether manipulating this signaling pathway can recapitulate the benefits of EE.

The *db/db* Mouse of Genetic Obesity and Type II Diabetes

Leptin is a hormone regulating appetite and energy expenditure, and mutations in either the leptin gene (*Lep*) or its receptor (*Lepr*) lead to hyperphagia and subsequent obesity and diabetes. Mice homozygous for obese (Lep^{ob}, commonly known as *ob/ob*) and the diabetes (Lepr^{db}, commonly known as *db/db*) mutations were the earliest characterized mouse models of diabetes.[173] Both *ob/ob* and *db/db* mice remain popular and have been widely used in obesity and diabetes research. We have reported that EE lessens obesity in leptin-deficient *ob/ob* mice (also mentioned in Chapters 2 and 5).[77] Here we show unpublished data of EE effects on leptin receptor-deficient *db/db* mice generated mostly by Grant Foglesong, then a graduate student of the lab.

db/db mice become apparently obese around 3–4 weeks of age. Plasma insulin begins to rise at 10–14 days after birth and blood glucose is elevated at 4–8 weeks of age. We randomized female *db/db* mice (B6 *db*, The Jackson Laboratory stock No:000697), 6 weeks of age, to live in EE (10 mice in a large EE bin, see Chapter 1, Fig. 1.1) or SE (five mice in a standard mouse cage). *db/db* mice living in SE gained weight fast and became extremely obese (**Fig. 3.25(a)**). EE housing slowed the pace of weight gain

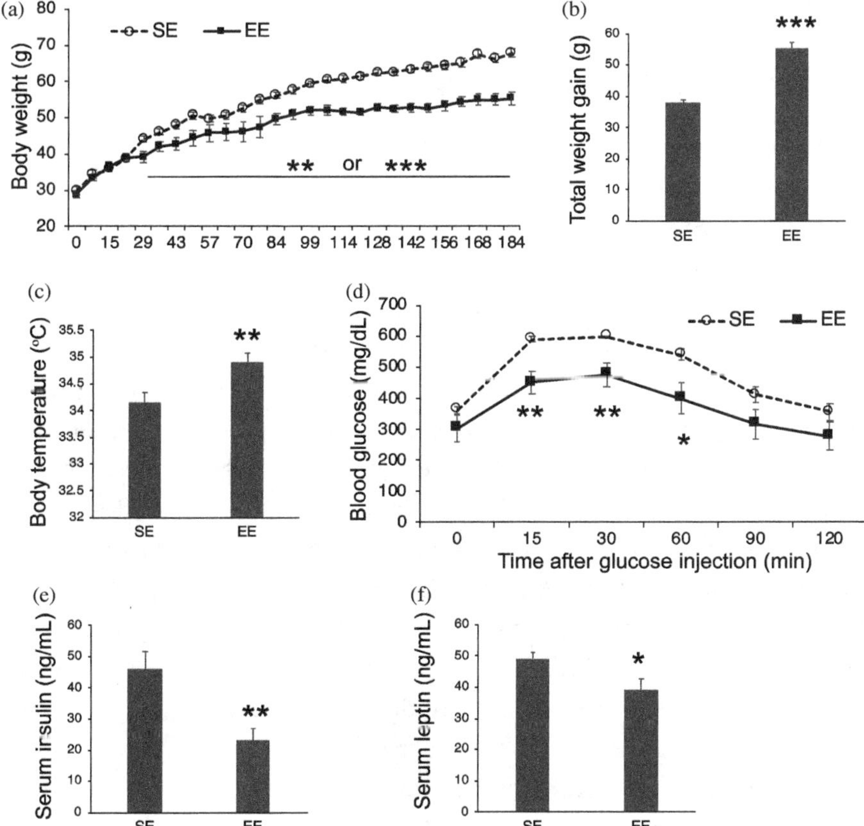

Fig. 3.25. EE exerts metabolic benefits in obese and diabetic *db/db* mice. (a) Body weight. (b) Total weight gain of 184 days. (c) Rectal temperature at 90-day EE. (d) Glucose tolerance test at 100-day EE. (e) Serum insulin. (f) Serum leptin at the end of the experiment. Data are mean ± SEM, *n* = 10 per group. *$P < 0.05$, **$P < 0.01$, ***$P < 0.001$.

and attenuated obesity throughout the course of the experiment of 184 days (**Fig. 3.25(b)**). EE *db/db* mice had higher core body temperature compared to SE mice measured at 90-day EE time-point (**Fig. 3.25(c)**). EE markedly improved glucose tolerance at 100-day EE (**Fig. 3.25(d)**). *db/db* mice have skyrocketing insulin level in the circulation. EE dropped the serum insulin level by half (**Fig. 3.25(e)**). Circulating leptin level was also reduced significantly in EE mice (**Fig. 3.25(f)**). Together, these data demonstrate that EE is highly effective to remedy obesity and diabetes in the genetic model of *db/db* mice.

Postmenopausal Obesity

Menopause brings about many concerns to women. One of the most important is weight gain and central obesity. In fact, the risk of developing obesity and metabolic syndrome in menopausal women is three times higher than before menopause.[174] These metabolic dysfunctions emerging post menopause — weight gain, central obesity, insulin resistance, glucose and lipid metabolic disturbances, are caused clearly if not all by the natural decrease in estrogen levels. Indeed, animal studies suggest the propensity to developing obesity differs between the two sexes, which is directly due to sex hormones.[175] Female animals gain less weight compared to males when being fed a high-fat diet. Experimentally induced menopause by ovariectomy abolishes this protection against DIO in females.[176]

Estrogens act to suppress food intake by enhancing the potency of other anorectic signals (e.g., leptin, BDNF, cholecystokinin) while inhibiting the potency of orexigenic signals (ghrelin, melanin-concentrating hormone).[177–180] On the other hand, estrogens increase energy expenditure. Rodent studies suggest that activating estrogen receptors in the ventral medial nucleus of the hypothalamus results in elevated energy expenditure.[181,182] Human studies show menopause is associated with decreased whole body fat oxidation and lower metabolic rate during sleep and physical exercise.[183,184]

Moreover, estrogen replacement therapy has been shown to prevent postmenopausal weight gain and reduction in energy expenditure.[185]

We have observed sexual dimorphism in response to EE intervention. Generally speaking, EE results in more pronounced metabolic effects in male mice (C57BL/6 strain and BTBR strain) than females at least up to middle age. There are some metabolic effects shared between estrogens and EE such as increasing energy expenditure, resistance to DIO, browning of adipose tissues.[60,186] Of interest, estrogens act on estrogen receptor α (ERα) to regulate the gene and protein expression of BDNF in the brain.[187] Hypothalamic BDNF has been identified as the upstream brain mediator driving EE-induced adipose remodeling including induction of beige cells. Therefore, the female brain is more sensitive to the signaling molecules critical to energy homeostasis such as leptin and BDNF. This ERα signaling may protect female mice against DIO, but on the other hand, might partially explain the relatively modest metabolic response to EE compared to male mice because females have a fitter baseline.

To investigate whether EE influences the development of postmenopausal obesity, Grant Foglesong and others of our lab used ovariectomy to induce menopause in young female mice. Ovariectomized mice, 6 weeks of age, were randomized to live in SE or EE (15 mice in large EE bin, see Chapter 1, Fig. 1.1) for 7 weeks. The diet was switched to HFD (60% calories from fat). Ovariectomized mice living in SE quickly developed obesity upon HFD feeding, gaining weight by ~50% over 7 weeks. In contrast, ovariectomized mice living in EE maintained normal weight (**Fig. 3.26(a)**). By the end of the 7-week experiment, SE mice gained on average 15.3 g while EE mice gained only 4.4 g, over 70% less weight gain. EE mice had higher core body temperature (**Fig. 3.26(b)**) consistent with higher energy expenditure. EE mice showed markedly improved glucose tolerance (**Fig. 3.26(c)**) and substantially reduced serum insulin levels during the glucose tolerance test indicating significant enhancement of insulin sensitivity (**Fig. 3.26(d)**). Circulating leptin and IGF-1

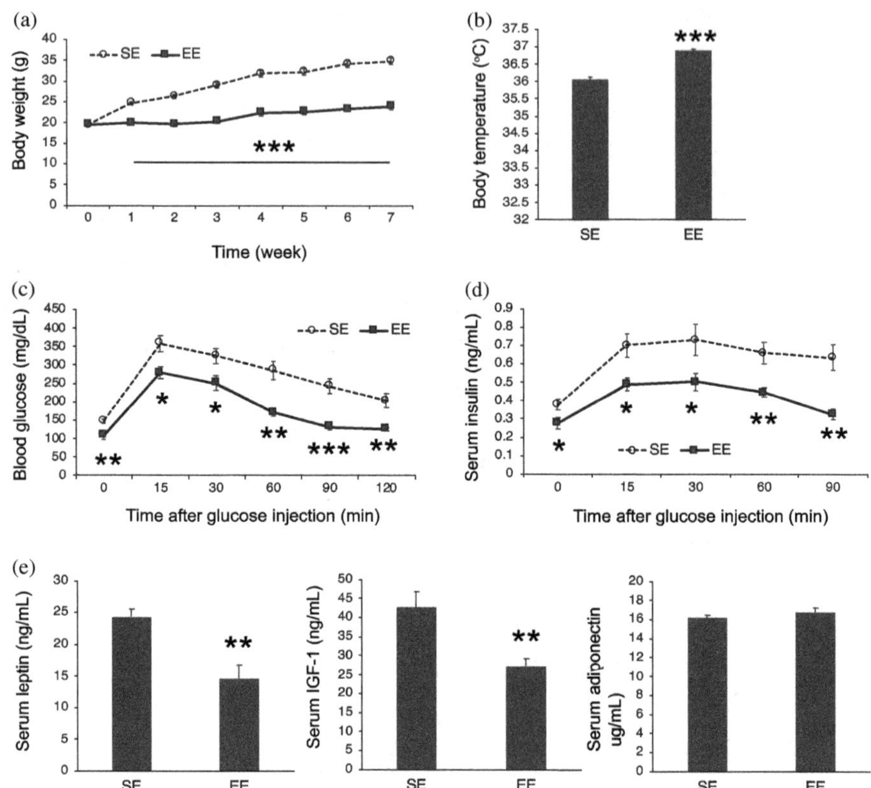

Fig. 3.26. EE prevents obesity and insulin resistance in ovariectomized mice on HFD. (a) Body weight. (b) Rectal temperature at 4-week EE. (c) Glucose tolerance test at 4-week EE. (d) Serum insulin levels during glucose tolerance test. (e) Serum biomarkers at 5-week EE Data are mean ± SEM, $n = 15$ per group for a, b, e; $n = 10$ per group for c and d. $*P < 0.05$, $**P < 0.01$, $***P < 0.001$.

levels were reduced in EE mice but adiponectin was not changed (**Fig. 3.26(e)**).

These preliminary data demonstrate the striking efficacy of EE to prevent obesity and associated metabolic disturbances after menopause. We find these results intriguing and encouraging because they suggest a bio-behavioral intervention (or lifestyle intervention) may be highly effective for postmenopausal obesity and associated metabolic syndromes and therefore provide an alternative to hormone replacement therapy that has considerable adverse effects for long-term treatment. Moreover, the data shown in **Fig. 3.26** is in line with previous findings suggesting estrogens help mice resist DIO. In our published study,[128] normal female mice at the same age were subjected to the same EE protocol and same HFD feeding. SE mice gained ~10 g weight by 7-week HFD feeding in contrast to ~15 g weight gain of ovariectomized mice at the same timepoint **(Fig. 3.26(a))**. The weight gains were not different between EE and SE housing groups during this period in normal female mice. Significant lower weight gain was observed in EE mice after longer HFD feeding. As such, EE appears more effective in the absence of estrogens, a condition susceptible to obesity. We are interested in understanding the interplay between estrogen and EE within the brain and adipose tissue in future research.

Summary

A decade of work has demonstrated a consistent metabolic phenotype induced by EE including reduced adiposity without suppression of food intake, elevated energy expenditure associated with induction of beige cells in selective WAT depots, improved glycemic control, and resistance to obesity and associated metabolic syndromes in a variety of mouse models of genetic forms or DIO. Adipose remodeling is among the earliest and most prominent adaptive responses to EE. A specific brain-fat axis, the HSA axis, plays a critical role in linking environmental stimuli to phenotypic changes in the adipose tissue through which modulating systemic metabolism. Downstream of the HSA axis, several signaling molecules have been identified to mediate different aspects of adipose remodeling — connected or dissociable, but all controlled by sympathetic tone. Upstream of the HSA axis is the hypothalamic BDNF whose upregulation drives adipose remodeling and other diverse systemic effects associated with EE. It is increasingly recognized that EE can recapitulate the metabolic benefits of a healthy lifestyle in animal research and facilitate discovery and validate therapeutic targets for obesity and associated metabolic disorders. However, we have just scratched the surface regarding phenotypic characterizations, and mechanistic studies are lagging behind. Some areas are particularly of interest such as epigenetic changes, crosstalk among adipose tissue and other metabolic active tissues (liver, muscle, and pancreas), bottom-up signaling pathways from fat to brain, influence on preference to palatable foods, and interplay between stress hormones and EE. What's utterly important is to raise the awareness among researchers of the marked impact of physical and social environments on the physiology and pathology of laboratory animals not only for the well-being of animals but also for the sake of science.

References

1. Bhaskaran K, Douglas I, Forbes H, *et al.* (2014) Body-mass index and risk of 22 specific cancers: A population-based cohort study of 5.24 million UK adults. *Lancet* **384**:755–765.
2. Lloyd-Jones D, Adams R, Carnethon M, *et al.* (2009) Heart disease and stroke statistics — 2009 update: A report from the American heart association statistics committee and stroke statistics subcommittee. *Circulation* **119**:480–486.
3. Bornfeldt KE, Tabas I. (2011) Insulin resistance, hyperglycemia, and atherosclerosis. *Cell Metab* **14**:575–585.
4. Kasen S, Cohen P, Chen H, Must A. (2008) Obesity and psychopathology in women: A three decade prospective study. *Int J Obes (Lond)* **32**:558–566.
5. de Wit L, Luppino F, van Straten A, *et al.* (2010) Depression and obesity: A meta-analysis of community-based studies. *Psychiatry Res* **178**:230–235.

6. Xu H, Cupples LA, Stokes A, Liu CT. (2018) Association of obesity with mortality over 24 years of weight history: Findings from the Framingham heart study. *JAMA Netw Open* **1**:e184587.

7. Olshansky SJ, Passaro DJ, Hershow RC, *et al.* (2005) A potential decline in life expectancy in the United States in the 21st century. *N Engl J Med* **352**:1138–1145.

8. Institute of Medicine, National Research Council (2013) *U.S. Health in International Perspective: Shorter Lives, Poorer Health.* The National Academies Press, Washington, DC.

9. National Research Council. (2011) *Explaining Divergent Levels of Longevity in High-Income Countries.* The National Academies Press, Washington, DC.

10. Squires D, Blumenthal D. (2016) Mortality trends among working-age whites: The untold story. *Issue Brief (Commonw Fund)* **3**:1–11.

11. Case A, Deaton A. (2015) Rising morbidity and mortality in midlife among white non-Hispanic Americans in the 21st century. *Proc Natl Acad Sci U S A* **112**:15078–15083.

12. Preston SH, Vierboom YC, Stokes A. (2018) The role of obesity in exceptionally slow US mortality improvement. *Proc Natl Acad Sci U S A* **115**:957–961.

13. Fothergill E, Guo J, Howard L, *et al.* (2016) Persistent metabolic adaptation 6 years after "The Biggest Loser" competition. *Obesity (Silver Spring)* **24**:1612–1619.

14. Knuth ND, Johannsen DL, Tamboli RA, *et al.* (2014) Metabolic adaptation following massive weight loss is related to the degree of energy imbalance and changes in circulating leptin. *Obesity (Silver Spring)* **22**:2563–2569.

15. Das SK, Roberts SB, McCrory MA, *et al.* (2003) Long-term changes in energy expenditure and body composition after massive weight loss induced by gastric bypass surgery. *Am J Clin Nutr* **78**:22–30.

16. Bessesen DH. (2011) Regulation of body weight: What is the regulated parameter? *Physiol Behav* **104**:599–607.

17. van Dijk G, Buwalda B. (2008) Neurobiology of the metabolic syndrome: An allostatic perspective. *Eur J Pharmacol* **585**:137–146.

18. Caballero B. (2019) Humans against obesity: Who will win? *Adv Nutr* **10**:S4–S9.

19. Bjorntorp P. (1992) Abdominal obesity and the metabolic syndrome. *Ann Med* **24**:465–468.

20. Brunner EJ, Hemingway H, Walker BR, *et al.* (2002) Adrenocortical, autonomic, and inflammatory causes of the metabolic syndrome: Nested case-control study. *Circulation* **106**:2659–2665.

21. Smith NR, Zivich PN, Frerichs L. (2020) Social influences on obesity: Current knowledge, emerging methods, and directions for future research and practice. *Curr Nutr Rep* **9**:31–41.

22. Powell K, Wilcox J, Clonan A, *et al.* (2015) The role of social networks in the development of overweight and obesity among adults: A scoping review. *BMC Public Health* **15**:996.

23. El Hadi H, Di Vincenzo A, Vettor R, Rossato M. (2018) Food ingredients involved in white-to-brown adipose tissue conversion and in calorie burning. *Front Physiol* **9**:1954.

24. Koenen M, Hill MA, Cohen P, Sowers JR. (2021) Obesity, adipose tissue and vascular dysfunction. *Circ Res* **128**:951–968.

25. Giordano A, Frontini A, Cinti S. (2016) Convertible visceral fat as a therapeutic target to curb obesity. *Nat Rev Drug Discov* **15**:405–424.

26. Morrison SF, Madden CJ, Tupone D. (2014) Central neural regulation of brown adipose tissue thermogenesis and energy expenditure. *Cell Metab* **19**:741–756.

27. Cinti S. (1999) *The Adipose Organ.* Editrice Kurtis, Milan.

28. Enerback S, Jacobsson A, Simpson EM, *et al.* (1997) Mice lacking mitochondrial uncoupling protein are cold-sensitive but not obese. *Nature* **387**:90–94.

29. Feldmann HM, Golozoubova V, Cannon B, Nedergaard J. (2009) UCP1 ablation induces obesity and abolishes diet-induced thermogenesis in mice exempt from thermal stress by living at thermoneutrality. *Cell Metab* **9**:203–209.

30. Seale P, Bjork B, Yang W, *et al.* (2008) PRDM16 controls a brown fat/ skeletal muscle switch. *Nature* **454**:961–967.

31. Cannon B, Nedergaard J. (2004) Brown adipose tissue: Function and physiological significance. *Physiol Rev* **84**:277–359.

32. Seale P, Conroe HM, Estall J, *et al.* (2011) Prdm16 determines the thermogenic program of subcutaneous white adipose tissue in mice. *J Clin Invest* **121**:96–105.
33. Frontini A, Cinti S. (2010) Distribution and development of brown adipocytes in the murine and human adipose organ. *Cell Metab* **11**:253–256.
34. Petrovic N, Walden TB, Shabalina IG, *et al.* (2010) Chronic peroxisome proliferator-activated receptor gamma (PPARgamma) activation of epididymally derived white adipocyte cultures reveals a population of thermogenically competent, UCP1-containing adipocytes molecularly distinct from classic brown adipocytes. *J Biol Chem* **285**:7153–7164.
35. Schulz TJ, Huang P, Huang TL, *et al.* (2013) Brown-fat paucity due to impaired BMP signalling induces compensatory browning of white fat. *Nature* **495**:379–383.
36. Harms M, Seale P. (2013) Brown and beige fat: Development, function and therapeutic potential. *Nat Med* **19**:1252–1263.
37. Wu J, Cohen P, Spiegelman BM. (2013) Adaptive thermogenesis in adipocytes: Is beige the new brown? *Genes Dev* **27**:234–250.
38. Long JZ, Svensson KJ, Tsai L, *et al.* (2014) A smooth muscle-like origin for beige adipocytes. *Cell Metab* **19**:810–820.
39. Fisher FM, Kleiner S, Douris N, *et al.* (2012) FGF21 regulates PGC-1alpha and browning of white adipose tissues in adaptive thermogenesis. *Genes Dev* **26**:271–281.
40. Qian SW, Tang Y, Li X, *et al.* (2013) BMP4-mediated brown fat-like changes in white adipose tissue alter glucose and energy homeostasis. *Proc Natl Acad Sci U S A* **110**:E798–E807.
41. Schulz TJ, Huang TL, Tran TT, *et al.* (2011) Identification of inducible brown adipocyte progenitors residing in skeletal muscle and white fat. *Proc Natl Acad Sci U S A* **108**:143–148.
42. Bostrom P, Wu J, Jedrychowski MP, *et al.* (2012) A PGC1-alpha-dependent myokine that drives brown-fat-like development of white fat and thermogenesis. *Nature* **481**:463–468.
43. Wu J, Boström P, Sparks LM, *et al.* (2012) Beige adipocytes are a distinct type of thermogenic fat cell in mouse and human. *Cell* **150**:366–376.

44. Sharp LZ, Shinoda K, Ohno H, *et al.* (2012) Human BAT possesses molecular signatures that resemble beige/brite cells. *PLoS One* **7**:e49452.

45. Shinoda K, Luijten IHN, Hasegawa Y, *et al.* (2015) Genetic and functional characterization of clonally derived adult human brown adipocytes. *Nat Med* **21**:389–394.

46. Himms-Hagen J, Melnyk A, Zingaretti MC, *et al.* (2000) Multilocular fat cells in WAT of CL-316243-treated rats derive directly from white adipocytes. *Am J Physiol Cell Physiol* **279**:C670–681.

47. Granneman JG, Li P, Zhu Z, Lu Y. (2005) Metabolic and cellular plasticity in white adipose tissue I: Effects of beta3-adrenergic receptor activation. *Am J Physiol* **289**:E608–616.

48. Lee YH, Petkova AP, Konkar AA, Granneman JG. (2015) Cellular origins of cold-induced brown adipocytes in adult mice. *FASEB J* **29**:286–299.

49. Murano I, Barbatelli G, Giordano A, Cinti S. (2009) Noradrenergic parenchymal nerve fiber branching after cold acclimatisation correlates with brown adipocyte density in mouse adipose organ. *J Anat* **214**:171–178.

50. Ravussin E, Kozak LP. (2009) Have we entered the brown adipose tissue renaissance? *Obes Rev* **10**:265–268.

51. Gesta S, Tseng YH, Kahn CR. (2007) Developmental origin of fat: Tracking obesity to its source. *Cell* **131**:242–256.

52. Tang W, Zeve D, Suh JM, *et al.* (2008) White fat progenitor cells reside in the adipose vasculature. *Science* **322**:583–586.

53. Gupta RK, Mepani RJ, Kleiner S, *et al.* (2012) Zfp423 expression identifies committed preadipocytes and localizes to adipose endothelial and perivascular cells. *Cell Metab* **15**:230–239.

54. Tran KV, Gealekman O, Frontini A, *et al.* (2012) The vascular endothelium of the adipose tissue gives rise to both white and brown fat cells. *Cell Metab* **15**:222–229.

55. Chau YY, Bandiera R, Serrels A, *et al.* (2014) Visceral and subcutaneous fat have different origins and evidence supports a mesothelial source. *Nat Cell Biol* **16**:367–375.

56. Billon N, Iannarelli P, Monteiro MC, *et al.* (2007) The generation of adipocytes by the neural crest. *Development* **134**:2283–2292.

57. Colman E. (2007) Dinitrophenol and obesity: An early twentieth-century regulatory dilemma. *Regul Toxicol Pharmacol* **48**: 115–117.
58. Lodhi IJ, Semenkovich CF. (2009) Why we should put clothes on mice. *Cell Metab* **9**:111–112.
59. Cypess AM, Lehman S, Williams G, *et al.* (2009) Identification and importance of brown adipose tissue in adult humans. *New Engl J Med* **360**:1509–1517.
60. van Marken Lichtenbelt WD, Vanhommerig JW, Smulders JM, *et al.* (2009) Cold-activated brown adipose tissue in healthy men. *New Engl J Med* **360**:1500–1508.
61. Virtanen KA, Lidell ME, Orava J, *et al.* (2009) Functional brown adipose tissue in healthy adults. *New Engl J Med* **360**:1518–1525.
62. Rothwell NJ, Stock MJ. (1983) Luxuskonsumption, diet-induced thermogenesis and brown fat: The case in favour. *Clin Sci (Lond)* **64**:19–23.
63. Cannon B, Nedergaard J. (2009) Thermogenesis challenges the adipostat hypothesis for body-weight control. *Proc Nutr Soc* **68**: 401–407.
64. Saito M, Okamatsu-Ogura Y, Matsushita M, *et al.* (2009) High incidence of metabolically active brown adipose tissue in healthy adult humans: Effects of cold exposure and adiposity. *Diabetes* **58**:1526–1531.
65. Nedergaard J, Bengtsson T, Cannon B. (2007) Unexpected evidence for active brown adipose tissue in adult humans. *Am J Physiol* **293**:E444–452.
66. Zingaretti MC, Crosta F, Vitali A, *et al.* (2009) The presence of UCP1 demonstrates that metabolically active adipose tissue in the neck of adult humans truly represents brown adipose tissue. *Faseb J* **23**:3113–3120.
67. Yoneshiro T, Aita S, Matsushita M, *et al.* (2011) Brown adipose tissue, whole-body energy expenditure, and thermogenesis in healthy adult men. *Obesity (Silver Spring)* **19**:13–16.
68. Vijgen GH, Bouvy ND, Jaap Teule GJ, *et al.* (2011) Brown adipose tissue in morbidly obese subjects. *PLoS One* **6**:e17247.
69. Spalding KL, Arner E, Westermark PA, *et al.* (2008) Dynamics of fat cell turnover in humans. *Nature* **453**:783–787.

70. Tiraby C, Tavernier G, Lefort C, *et al.* (2003) Acquirement of brown fat cell features by human white adipocytes. *J Biol Chem* **278**:33370–33376.

71. Mazzucotelli A, Viguerie N, Tiraby C, *et al.* (2007) The transcriptional coactivator peroxisome proliferator activated receptor (PPAR) gamma coactivator-1 alpha and the nuclear receptor PPAR alpha control the expression of glycerol kinase and metabolism genes independently of PPAR gamma activation in human white adipocytes. *Diabetes* **56**:2467–2475.

72. Enerback S. (2010) Brown adipose tissue in humans. *Int J Obes (Lond)* **34 Suppl 1**:S43–46.

73. Kajimura S, Seale P, Spiegelman BM. (2010) Transcriptional control of brown fat development. *Cell Metab* **11**:257–262.

74. Nedergaard J, Cannon B. (2010) The changed metabolic world with human brown adipose tissue: Therapeutic visions. *Cell Metab* **11**:268–272.

75. Barbatelli G, Heinzelmann M, Ferrara P, *et al.* (1994) Quantitative evaluations of gap junctions in old rat brown adipose tissue after cold acclimation: A freeze-fracture and ultra-structural study. *Tissue Cell* **26**:667–676.

76. Cao L, Choi EY, Liu X, *et al.* (2011) White to brown fat phenotypic switch induced by genetic and environmental activation of a hypothalamic-adipocyte axis. *Cell Metab* **14**:324–338.

77. Cao L, Liu X, Lin E-JD, *et al.* (2010) Environmental and genetic activation of a brain-adipocyte BDNF/leptin axis causes cancer remission and inhibition. *Cell* **142**:52–64.

78. Puigserver P, Wu Z, Park CW, *et al.* (1998) A cold-inducible coactivator of nuclear receptors linked to adaptive thermogenesis. *Cell* **92**:829–839.

79. Leonardsson G, Steel JH, Christian M, *et al.* (2004) Nuclear receptor corepressor RIP140 regulates fat accumulation. *Proc Natl Acad Sci U S A* **101**:8437–8442.

80. Picard F, Géhin M, Annicotte J-S, *et al.* (2002) SRC-1 and TIF2 control energy balance between white and brown adipose tissues. *Cell* **111**:931–941.

81. Hansen JB, Jørgensen C, Petersen RK, *et al.* (2004) Retinoblastoma protein functions as a molecular switch determining white versus brown adipocyte differentiation. *Proc Natl Acad Sci U S A* **101**:4112–4117.

82. Pan D, Fujimoto M, Lopes A, Wang YX. (2009) Twist-1 is a PPARdelta-inducible, negative-feedback regulator of PGC-1alpha in brown fat metabolism. *Cell* **137**:73–86.

83. Nicholls DG, Locke RM. (1984) Thermogenic mechanisms in brown fat. *Physiol Rev* **64**:1–64.

84. Himms-Hagen J, Cui J, Danforth E Jr, *et al.* (1994) Effect of CL-316,243, a thermogenic beta 3-agonist, on energy balance and brown and white adipose tissues in rats. *Am J Physiol* **266**:R1371–1382.

85. Bachman ES, Dhillon H, Zhang C-Y, *et al.* (2002) betaAR signaling required for diet-induced thermogenesis and obesity resistance. *Science (New York, N.Y)* **297**:843–845.

86. Xue B, Rim J-S, Hogan JC, *et al.* (2007) Genetic variability affects the development of brown adipocytes in white fat but not in interscapular brown fat. *J Lipid Res* **48**:41–51.

87. Kajimura S, Seale P, Tomaru T, *et al.* (2008) Regulation of the brown and white fat gene programs through a PRDM16/CtBP transcriptional complex. *Genes Dev* **22**:1397–1409.

88. Tsukiyama-Kohara K, Poulin F, Kohara M, *et al.* (2001) Adipose tissue reduction in mice lacking the translational inhibitor 4E-BP1. *Nat Med* **7**:1128–1132.

89. Landsberg L, Young JB. (1984) The role of the sympathoadrenal system in modulating energy expenditure. *Clin Endocrinol Metab* **13**:475–499.

90. Slavin BG, Ballard KW. (1978) Morphological studies on the adrenergic innervation of white adipose tissue. *Anat Rec* **191**:377–389.

91. Youngstrom TG, Bartness TJ. (1995) Catecholaminergic innervation of white adipose tissue in Siberian hamsters. *Am J Physiol* **268**:R744–751.

92. Lyons WE, Mamounas LA, Ricaurte GA, *et al.* (1999) Brain-derived neurotrophic factor-deficient mice develop aggressiveness and hyperphagia in conjunction with brain serotonergic abnormalities. *Proc Natl Acad Sci USA* **96**:15239–15244.

93. Rios M, Fan G, Fekete C, *et al.* (2001) Conditional deletion of brain-derived neurotrophic factor in the postnatal brain leads to obesity and hyperactivity. *Mol Endocrinol* **15**:1748–1757.

94. Xu B, Goulding EH, Zang K, *et al.* (2003) Brain-derived neurotrophic factor regulates energy balance downstream of melanocortin-4 receptor. *Nat Neurosci* **6**:736–742.

95. Cao L, Lin E-JD, Cahill MC, *et al.* (2009) Molecular therapy of obesity and diabetes by a physiological autoregulatory approach. *Nat Med* **15**:447–454.

96. Guerra C, Koza RA, Yamashita H, *et al.* (1998) Emergence of brown adipocytes in white fat in mice is under genetic control. Effects on body weight and adiposity. *J Clin Invest* **102**:412–420.

97. Vegiopoulos A, Müller-Decker K, Strzoda D, *et al.* (2010) Cyclooxygenase-2 controls energy homeostasis in mice by de novo recruitment of brown adipocytes. *Science* **328**:1158–1161.

98. Arner P. (1992) Adrenergic receptor function in fat cells. *Am J Clin Nutr* **55**:228S–236S.

99. During MJ, Liu X, Huang W, *et al.* (2015) Adipose VEGF links the white-to-brown fat switch with environmental, genetic, and pharmacological stimuli in male mice. *Endocrinology* **156**:2059–2073.

100. Papetti M, Herman IM. (2002) Mechanisms of normal and tumor-derived angiogenesis. *Am J Physiol Cell Physiol* **282**:C947–970.

101. Zhang QX, Magovern CJ, Mack CA, *et al.* (1997) Vascular endothelial growth factor is the major angiogenic factor in omentum: Mechanism of the omentum-mediated angiogenesis. *J Surg Res* **67**:147–154.

102. Riordan NH, Ichim TE, Min W-P, *et al.* (2009) Non-expanded adipose stromal vascular fraction cell therapy for multiple sclerosis. *J Transl Med* **7**:29.

103. Sackmann-Sala L, Berryman DE, Munn RD, *et al.* (2012) Heterogeneity among white adipose tissue depots in male C57BL/6J mice. *Obesity (Silver Spring)* **20**:101–111.

104. Giordano A, Frontini A, Murano I, *et al.* (2005) Regional-dependent increase of sympathetic innervation in rat white adipose tissue during prolonged fasting. *J Histochem Cytochem* **53**:679–687.

105. Sun K, Kusminski CM, Scherer PE. (2011) Adipose tissue remodeling and obesity. *J Clin Invest* **121**:2094–2101.

106. Xue Y, Petrovic N, Cao R, *et al.* (2009) Hypoxia-independent angiogenesis in adipose tissues during cold acclimation. *Cell Metab* **9**:99–109.

107. Sun K, Kusminski CM, Luby-Phelps K, *et al.* (2014) Brown adipose tissue derived VEGF-A modulates cold tolerance and energy expenditure. *Mol Metab* **3**:474–483.

108. Shimizu I, Aprahamian T, Kikuchi R, *et al.* (2014) Vascular rarefaction mediates whitening of brown fat in obesity. *J Clin Invest* **124**:2099–2112.

109. Rooks CR, Penn DM, Kelso E, *et al.* (2005) Sympathetic denervation does not prevent a reduction in fat pad size of rats or mice treated with peripherally administered leptin. *Am J Physiol Regul Integr Comp Physiol* **289**:R92–102.

110. Liu X, Magee D, Wang C, *et al.* (2014) Adipose tissue insulin receptor knockdown via a new primate-derived hybrid recombinant AAV serotype. *Mol Ther Methods Clin Dev* **1**:8.

111. Wilson-Fritch L, Nicoloro S, Chouinard M, *et al.* (2004) Mitochondrial remodeling in adipose tissue associated with obesity and treatment with rosiglitazone. *J Clin Invest* **114**:1281–1289.

112. Huang W, Queen NJ, McMurphy T, *et al.* (2020) Adipose PTEN acts as a downstream mediator of a brain-fat axis in environmental enrichment. *Compr Psychoneuroendocrinol* **4**:8.

113. Li J, Yen C, Liaw D, *et al.* (1997) PTEN, a putative protein tyrosine phosphatase gene mutated in human brain, breast, and prostate cancer. *Science* **275**:1943–1947.

114. Stambolic V, Suzuki A, de la Pompa JL, *et al.* (1998) Negative regulation of PKB/Akt-dependent cell survival by the tumor suppressor PTEN. *Cell* **95**:29–39.

115. Chalhoub N, Baker SJ. (2009) PTEN and the PI3-kinase pathway in cancer. *Annu Rev Pathol* **4**:127–150.

116. Ortega-Molina A, Serrano M. (2013) PTEN in cancer, metabolism, and aging. *Trends Endocrinol Metab* **24**:184–189.

117. Myers MP, Pass I, Batty IH, *et al.* (1998) The lipid phosphatase activity of PTEN is critical for its tumor supressor function. *Proc Natl Acad Sci U S A* **95**:13513–13518.

118. Kurlawalla-Martinez C, Stiles B, Wang Y, *et al.* (2005) Insulin hypersensitivity and resistance to streptozotocin-induced diabetes in mice lacking PTEN in adipose tissue. *Mol Cell Biol* **25**:2498–2510.

119. Morley TS, Xia JY, Scherer PE. (2015) Selective enhancement of insulin sensitivity in the mature adipocyte is sufficient for systemic metabolic improvements. *Nat Commun* **6**:7906.

120. Sanchez-Gurmaches J, Hung C-M, Sparks CA, *et al.* (2012) PTEN loss in the Myf5 lineage redistributes body fat and reveals subsets of white adipocytes that arise from Myf5 precursors. *Cell Metab* **16**:348–362.

121. Ortega-Molina A, Efeyan A, Lopez-Guadamillas E, *et al.* (2012) Pten positively regulates brown adipose function, energy expenditure, and longevity. *Cell Metab* **15**:382–394.

122. Garcia-Cao I, Song MS, Hobbs RM, *et al.* (2012) Systemic elevation of PTEN induces a tumor-suppressive metabolic state. *Cell* **149**: 49–62.

123. Katic M, Kennedy AR, Leykin I, *et al.* (2007) Mitochondrial gene expression and increased oxidative metabolism: Role in increased lifespan of fat-specific insulin receptor knock-out mice. *Aging Cell* **6**:827–839.

124. Bluher M, Michael MD, Peroni OD, *et al.* (2002) Adipose tissue selective insulin receptor knockout protects against obesity and obesity-related glucose intolerance. *Dev Cell* **3**:25–38.

125. Bluher M, Kahn BB, Kahn CR. (2003) Extended longevity in mice lacking the insulin receptor in adipose tissue. *Science* **299**:572–574.

126. Cao L, During MJ. (2012) What is the brain-cancer connection? *Annu Rev Neurosci* **35**:331–345.

127. Foglesong GD, Queen NJ, Huang W, *et al.* (2019) Enriched environment inhibits breast cancer progression in obese models with intact leptin signaling. *Endocr Relat Cancer* **26**:483–495.

128. Huang W, Queen NJ, McMurphy TB, *et al.* (2019) Adipose PTEN regulates adult adipose tissue homeostasis and redistribution via a PTEN-leptin-sympathetic loop. *Mol Metab* **30**:48–60.

129. Foglesong GD, Huang W, Liu X, *et al.* (2016) Role of hypothalamic VGF in energy balance and metabolic adaption to environmental enrichment in mice. *Endocrinology* **157**:983–996.

130. Levi A, Eldridge JD, Paterson BM. (1985) Molecular cloning of a gene sequence regulated by nerve growth factor. *Science* **229**:393–395.

131. van den Pol AN, Bina K, Decavel C, Ghosh P. (1994) VGF expression in the brain. *J Comp Neurol* **347**:455–469.

132. van den Pol AN, Decavel C, Levi A, Paterson B. (1989) Hypothalamic expression of a novel gene product, VGF: Immunocytochemical analysis. *J Neurosci* **9**:4122–4137.

133. Snyder SE, Pintar JE, Salton SR. (1998) Developmental expression of VGF mRNA in the prenatal and postnatal rat. *J Comp Neurol* **394**:64–90.

134. Snyder SE, Salton SR. (1998) Expression of VGF mRNA in the adult rat central nervous system. *J Comp Neurol* **394**:91–105.

135. Alder J, Thakker-Varia S, Bangasser DA, *et al.* (2003) Brain-derived neurotrophic factor-induced gene expression reveals novel actions of VGF in hippocampal synaptic plasticity. *J Neurosci* **23**:10800–10808.

136. Bartolomucci A, Possenti R, Levi A, *et al.* (2007) The role of the vgf gene and VGF-derived peptides in nutrition and metabolism. *Genes Nutr* **2**:169–180.

137. Brancia C, Cocco C, D'Amato F, *et al.* (2010) Selective expression of TLQP-21 and other VGF peptides in gastric neuroendocrine cells and modulation by feeding. *J Endocrinol* **207**:329–341.

138. Fan W, Dinulescu DM, Butler AA, *et al.* (2000) The central melanocortin system can directly regulate serum insulin levels. *Endocrinology* **141**:3072–3079.

139. Cone RD. (2005) Anatomy and regulation of the central melanocortin system. *Nat Neurosci* **8**:571–578.

140. Penn DM, Jordan LC, Kelso EW, *et al.* (2006) Effects of central or peripheral leptin administration on norepinephrine turnover in defined fat depots. *Am J Physiol Regul Integr Comp Physiol* **291**:R1613–1621.

141. Song CK, Jackson RM, Harris RB, *et al.* (2005) Melanocortin-4 receptor mRNA is expressed in sympathetic nervous system outflow neurons to white adipose tissue. *Am J Physiol Regul Integr Comp Physiol* **289**:R1467–1476.

142. Voss-Andreae A, Murphy JG, Ellacott KLJ, *et al.* (2007) Role of the central melanocortin circuitry in adaptive thermogenesis of brown adipose tissue. *Endocrinology* **148**:1550–1560.

143. Hahm S, Mizuno TM, Wu TJ, *et al.* (1999) Targeted deletion of the Vgf gene indicates that the encoded secretory peptide precursor plays a novel role in the regulation of energy balance. *Neuron* **23**:537–548.

144. Watson E, Fargali S, Okamoto H, *et al.* (2009) Analysis of knockout mice suggests a role for VGF in the control of fat storage and energy expenditure. *BMC Physiol* **9**:19.

145. Fargali S, Scherer T, Shin AC, *et al.* (2012) Germline ablation of VGF increases lipolysis in white adipose tissue. *J Endocrinol* **215**:313–322.

146. Stephens SB, Schisler JC, Hohmeier HE, *et al.* (2012) A VGF-derived peptide attenuates development of type 2 diabetes via enhancement of islet beta-cell survival and function. *Cell Metab* **16**:33–43.

147. Bartolomucci A, La Corte G, Possenti R, *et al.* (2006) TLQP-21, a VGF-derived peptide, increases energy expenditure and prevents the early phase of diet-induced obesity. *Proc Natl Acad Sci U S A* **103**:14584–14589.

148. Meyza KZ, Blanchard DC. (2017) The BTBR mouse model of idiopathic autism — Current view on mechanisms. *Neurosci Biobehav Rev* **76**:99–110.

149. American Psychiatric Association. (2013) *"Neurodevelopmental Disorders" in Diagnostic and Statistical Manual of Mental Disorders*. American Psychiatric Association, Washington, DC.

150. Baio J, Wiggins L, Christensen DL, *et al.* (2018) Prevalence of autism spectrum disorder among children aged 8 years — autism and developmental disabilities monitoring network, 11 sites, United States, 2014. *MMWR Surveill Summ* **67**:1–23.

151. Bai D, Yip BHK, Windham GC, *et al.* (2019) Association of genetic and environmental factors with autism in a 5-country cohort. *JAMA Psychiatry* **76**:1035–1043.

152. NR Council. (2001) *Educating Children with Autism*. National Academy Press, Washington, DC.

153. Aronoff E, Hillyer R, Leon M. (2016) Environmental enrichment therapy for autism: Outcomes with increased access. *Neural Plast* **2016**:2734915.

154. Waters CF, Amerine Dickens M, Thurston SW, *et al.* (2018) Sustainability of early intensive behavioral intervention for children with autism spectrum disorder in a community setting. *Behav Modif* **44**:3–26.

155. Perihan C, Burke M, Bowman-Perrott L, *et al.* (2019) Effects of cognitive behavioral therapy for reducing anxiety in children with high functioning ASD: A systematic review and meta-analysis. *J Autism Dev Disord* **50**:1958–1972.

156. Clee SM, Nadler ST, Attie AD. (2005) Genetic and genomic studies of the BTBR ob/ob mouse model of type 2 diabetes. *Am J Ther* **12**:491–498.

157. McFarlane HG, Kusek GK, Yang M, *et al.* (2008) Autism-like behavioral phenotypes in BTBR T+tf/J mice. *Genes Brain Behav* **7**:152–163.

158. Miller BH, Schultz LE,Gulati A, *et al.* (2010) Phenotypic characterization of a genetically diverse panel of mice for behavioral despair and anxiety. *PLoS One* **5**:e14458.

159. Chao OY, Yunger R, Yang YM. (2018) Behavioral assessments of BTBR T+ltpr3tf/J mice by tests of object attention and elevated open platform: Implications for an animal model of psychiatric comorbidity in autism. *Behav Brain Res* **347**:140–147.

160. Wang Y, Zhao S, Liu X, *et al.* (2018) Oxytocin improves animal behaviors and ameliorates oxidative stress and inflammation in autistic mice. *Biomed Pharmacother* **107**:262–269.

161. Zilkha N, Kuperman Y, Kimchi T. (2017) High-fat diet exacerbates cognitive rigidity and social deficiency in the BTBR mouse model of autism. *Neuroscience* **345**:142–154.

162. Yamaguchi H, Hara Y, Ago Y, *et al.* (2017) Environmental enrichment attenuates behavioral abnormalities in valproic acid-exposed autism model mice. *Behav Brain Res* **333**:67–73.

163. Hulbert SW, Bey AL, Jiang YH. (2018) Environmental enrichment has minimal effects on behavior in the Shank3 complete knockout model of autism spectrum disorder. *Brain Behav* **8**:e01107.

164. Lewis MH, Lindenmaier Z, Boswell K, *et al.* (2018) Subthalamic nucleus pathology contributes to repetitive behavior expression and is reversed by environmental enrichment. *Genes Brain Behav* **17**:e12468.

165. Lonetti G, Angelucci A, Morando L, *et al.* (2010) Early environmental enrichment moderates the behavioral and synaptic phenotype of MeCP2 null mice. *Biol Psychiatry* **67**:657–665.
166. Kerr B, Silva PA, Walz K, Young JI. (2010) Unconventional transcriptional response to environmental enrichment in a mouse model of Rett syndrome. *PLoS One* **5**:e11534.
167. Queen NJ, Boardman AA, Patel RS, *et al.* (2020) Environmental enrichment improves metabolic and behavioral health in the BTBR mouse model of autism. *Psychoneuroendocrinology* **111**:104476.
168. Gould TD. (2009) *Mood and Anxiety Related Phenotypes in Mice: Characterization Using Behavioral Tests.* Neuromethods. Humana Press, New York, NY.
169. Kalueff AV, Aldridge JW, LaPorte JL, *et al.* (2007) Analyzing grooming microstructure in neurobehavioral experiments. *Nat Protoc* **2**:2538–2544.
170. Ellegood J, Crawley JN. (2015) Behavioral and neuroanatomical phenotypes in mouse models of autism. *Neurotherapeutics* **12**:521–533.
171. Angoa-Perez M, Kane MJ, Briggs DI, *et al.* (2013) Marble burying and nestlet shredding as tests of repetitive, compulsive-like behaviors in mice. *J Vis Exp* (82):50978.
172. Kaidanovich-Beilin O, Lipina T, Vukobradovic I, *et al.* (2011) Assessment of social interaction behaviors. *J Vis Exp* (4):2473.
173. Coleman DL. (1978) Obese and diabetes: Two mutant genes causing diabetes-obesity syndromes in mice. *Diabetologia* **14**:141–148.
174. Kwasniewska M, Pikala M, Kaczmarczyk-Chałas K, *et al.* (2012) Smoking status, the menopausal transition, and metabolic syndrome in women. *Menopause* **19**:194–201.
175. Palmer BF, Clegg DJ. (2015) The sexual dimorphism of obesity. *Mol Cell Endocrinol* **402**:113–119.
176. Stubbins RE, Holcomb VB, Hong J, Nunez NP. (2012) Estrogen modulates abdominal adiposity and protects female mice from obesity and impaired glucose tolerance. *Eur J Nutr* **51**:861–870.
177. Clegg DJ, Brown LM, Woods SC, Benoit SC. (2006) Gonadal hormones determine sensitivity to central leptin and insulin. *Diabetes* **55**:978–987.

178. Clegg DJ, Brown LM, Zigman JM, *et al.* (2007) Estradiol-dependent decrease in the orexigenic potency of ghrelin in female rats. *Diabetes* **56**:1051–1058.

179. Messina MM, Boersma G, Overton JM, Eckel LA. (2006) Estradiol decreases the orexigenic effect of melanin-concentrating hormone in ovariectomized rats. *Physiol Behav* **88**:523–528.

180. Zhu Z, Liu X, Senthil Kumar SP, *et al.* (2013) Central expression and anorectic effect of brain-derived neurotrophic factor are regulated by circulating estradiol levels. *Horm Behav* **63**:533–542.

181. Musatov S, Chen W, Pfaff DW, *et al.* (2007) Silencing of estrogen receptor alpha in the ventromedial nucleus of hypothalamus leads to metabolic syndrome. *Proc Natl Acad Sci U S A* **104**:2501–2506.

182. Xu Y, Nedungadi TP, Zhu L, *et al.* (2011) Distinct hypothalamic neurons mediate estrogenic effects on energy homeostasis and reproduction. *Cell Metab* **14**:453–465.

183. Abildgaard J, Pedersen AT, Green CJ, *et al.* (2013) Menopause is associated with decreased whole body fat oxidation during exercise. *Am J Physiol Endocrinol Metab* **304**:E1227–1236.

184. Lovejoy JC, Champagne CM, de Jonge L, *et al.* (2008) Increased visceral fat and decreased energy expenditure during the menopausal transition. *Int J Obes (Lond)* **32**:949–958.

185. Gambacciani M, Ciaponi M, Cappagli B, *et al.* (1997) Body weight, body fat distribution, and hormonal replacement therapy in early postmenopausal women. *J Clin Endocrinol Metab* **82**:414–417.

186. Nookaew I, Svensson P-A, Jacobson P, *et al.* (2013) Adipose tissue resting energy expenditure and expression of genes involved in mitochondrial function are higher in women than in men. *J Clin Endocrinol Metab* **98**:E370–378.

187. Solum DT, Handa RJ. (2002) Estrogen regulates the development of brain-derived neurotrophic factor mRNA and protein in the rat hippocampus. *J Neurosci* **22**:2650–2659.

Gene Therapy for Obesity and Associated Metabolic Syndrome

Introduction

Environmental enrichment (EE) has been demonstrated to induce beneficial effects in animal models of a wide variety of brain disorders and recently metabolic syndromes and cancer. We are always mindful of our ultimate goal: harnessing the knowledge gained from animal research to improve human health, disease prevention, and treatment. Our research on EE and the hypothalamic-sympatho-neural-adipocyte (HSA) axis has promoted us to develop molecular therapy for obesity and associated metabolic syndromes as well as technologies to improve gene therapy.

Adeno-Associated Viral Vectors

Adeno-associated viral (AAVs) vectors are attractive vehicles for gene therapy and versatile tools for biomedical research because they can transduce both dividing and postmitotic tissues with low immunogenicity and long-lasting transgene expression.[1] In 2012, the first gene therapy product using AAV vector — Glybera — was approved in Europe to treat hereditary lipoprotein lipase (LPL) deficiency. In 2017, the US FDA approved the first AAV-based gene therapy — Luxturna (Spark Therapeutics, Inc.) — for a genetic retinal disorder.[2] In 2019, another AAV-based gene therapy — Zolgensma (AveXis, Inc.) — was approved to treat children with a rare genetic form of spinal muscular atrophy. These landmark successes fuel intense interest in AAV-based gene therapy to treat genetic and acquired diseases.[2–4]

AAV was first discovered from laboratory adenovirus preparations and humans in the 1960s.[5–7] AAV is a nonpathogenic parvovirus with a non-enveloped capsid of a size of 25 nm, among the smallest viruses. They depend on a helper virus, for example adenovirus, for a productive infection cycle. The AAV genome consists of a linear single-stranded DNA genome of approximately 4.7 or 4.9 kilobases (kb). Two 145-nucleotide palindromic inverted terminal repeats (ITR) flank viral genes including *Rep* (replication), *Cap* (capsid), and the assembly-activation protein (AAP), which are important for some, but not all AAV serotypes.[8–11] The *Rep* gene encodes four regulatory proteins (*Rep78*, *Rep68*, *Rep52*, and *Rep40*) required for AAV genome replication. The *Cap* gene generates three capsid proteins, VP1 (virion protein1), VP2 (virion protein2), and VP3 (virion protein3), which assemble an AAV capsid encapsulating the AAV genome.

Currently, 13 naturally occurring AAV serotypes have been identified with varying tissue tropisms, and at least 11 serotypes are commonly available in the laboratory setting.[12] Serotypes 1, 4, and 7–11 were isolated from nonhuman primates, whereas serotypes 2, 3, 5, and 6 were discovered in humans.[13,14] Because ITRs are the sole requirement for packaging DNA into AAV capsids, AAV genome can be replaced by any gene expression cassette and regulatory elements up to 4.7–4.9 kb. In other words, a recombinant AAV vector (rAAV) consists of no AAV genome except the ITRs and therefore unable to replicate upon administration to the body.

The process of producing rAAV vector, often termed as packaging, typically requires transfection of three plasmids to HEK293 cells: a *cis* plasmid containing the genomic core with ITRs flanking an expression cassette to drive gene of interest (transgene), a *trans* plasmid containing *Rep* and *Cap* genes to generate *Rep* and *Cap* proteins in HEK293 cells but not packaged to AAV capsid, and an adeno-helper to facilitate AAV replication in HEK293 cells.

AAVs have low immunogenicity and can transduce both dividing and nondividing cells.[1] In contrast to frequent genome insertion by retrovirus family,[15] rAAV vectors primarily remain episomal (extrachromosomal) in the nucleus of transduced cells. Random integration of AAV vectors into host DNA is low frequent events[8] although the relatively rare integrations and subsequent toxicity have been observed in mouse models.[16] Hence, AAVs achieve long-term transgene expression with substantially lower risk of genome insertion and associated adverse effects such as carcinogenesis.[17]

Sustained transgene expression by AAVs has been documented in species from mouse to human.[1,18] In animal models, liver, heart, skeletal muscle, eyes, and central nervous system (CNS) have been safely and successfully targeted for gene transfer.[1,19] Yet AAV-mediated gene delivery to adipose tissue has been a challenge largely due to relatively low transduction efficiency and tropism with naturally occurring serotype vectors. In recent years, we have characterized a novel engineered AAV serotype, Rec2, whose efficacy of gene transfer to adipose tissue surpassing all naturally occurring serotype vectors being tested.[20]

Targeting Brain for Obesity Gene Therapy

Obesity is a major risk factor for serious chronic illnesses such as diabetes, cardiovascular disease, depression, stroke, sleep apnea, and some cancers.[21,22] The prevalence of obesity and its comorbidities — metabolic syndrome (or syndrome X) — is rising rapidly worldwide with significant morbidity and mortality and socioeconomic burden.[23,24] United States is severely afflicted by obesity. In 2017–18, the prevalence of obesity in adult was 42.4%, and perhaps more alarming, 18.5% of children and adolescents aged 2–19 years were obese, about 13.7 million.[25] Obesity is a costly disease with the estimated annual medical cost of $147 billion US dollars in 2008.[26]

Life style modifications such as exercise and diet as well as approved drugs have limited efficacy.[27–29] Both randomized and prospective studies reveal that the long-term weight loss with intensive lifestyle intervention in diabetic patients with a body mass index (BMI) of 30 is ~2% at 10 years,[30] and is even less in patients with BMI above 35.[31] Bariatric surgery in extreme circumstances can lead to large and sustained weight loss and has become the most effective treatment for severe obesity at the cost of significant morbidity.[32,33] Patient response to bariatric surgery is highly variable ranging from losing 100% of their excess weight to minimal weight loss.[34] Most weight loss occurs in the 18 months following bariatric surgery, and most patients experience weight regain in the following years.[35,36] There is unmet need to develop safer and more effective therapeutics for obese patients recalcitrant to current treatments.

Direct infusion of a drug into a defined brain region has been considered either because the drug has poor blood–brain barrier permeability (e.g., most neuropeptides and growth factors), or the drug has unwanted systemic or CNS effects outside the target region. Gene therapy provides a significant advantage than infusion of proteins because it provides a potentially long-term and stable delivery method avoiding the need for catheters, pumps, and other hardware. Moreover, the therapeutic vector needs only be given once. The limited experience of stereotactic delivery of AAV vector in the human brain has shown excellent safety and tolerability.[37–40]

There have been several studies targeting the hypothalamus for obesity gene therapy.[41–47] The majority of these studies use viral vectors to overexpress leptin or the leptin receptor in order to overcome the problems of peripheral leptin delivery. However, in diet-induced obesity (DIO) rats, an AAV vector expressing leptin is unable to decrease body weight. The failure is consistent with an obesity-induced leptin resistance at the hypothalamus because leptin gene therapy shows robust effect in animals of normal weight.[48] An alternative therapeutic gene is proopiomelanocortin (POMC). The hypothalamic injection of an AAV vector expressing POMC leads to significant weight loss and improved insulin sensitivity in obese rats.[49,50] However, the same authors report that AAV-POMC predisposes the lean rats to increased weight gain when the animals are switched to high-fat diet.[51] The authors conclude that the hypothalamic overexpression of POMC leads to downregulation of melanocortin-4 receptor (MC4R) and the adaptive response counters the anorexigenic activity.

Why Hypothalamic BDNF?

Obesity is a complex acquired disease with both environmental and genetic factors. In fact, obesity has one of the strongest genetic components among all the chronic disorders of humans. It is estimated that inheritance accounts for 40%–70% of an individual's predisposition to obesity.[52] Although this genetic component stems from a small effect of a large number of genes,[53] there are examples of monogenic obesity caused by defect of a single gene. Prominent examples of monogenic obesity are mutations of genes critical for the leptin-POMC signaling pathway controlling energy balance (**Fig. 4.1**). Genetic studies demonstrate there are only three receptor–ligand pairs that have profound effects on body weight and food intake in mouse and human: leptin and leptin receptor, POMC and MC4R, and brain-derived neurotrophic factor (BDNF) and its receptor TrkB.

BDNF is believed to function downstream of the leptin-POMC signaling pathway.[54–57] In animal studies, MC4R appears to serve

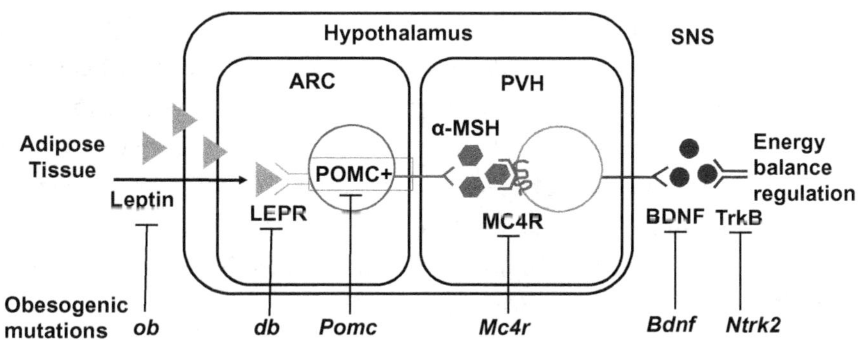

Fig. 4.1. Monogenic obesity is mostly caused by mutations in leptin–melanocortin–BDNF signaling pathway. Peripheral leptin communicates to hypothalamic nuclei to regulate energy balance. Prominent examples of obesogenic mutations in humans can be studied in transgenic mice with equivalent defects.

an intermediary role within the leptin pathway, acting downstream of the leptin receptor and upstream of BDNF signaling. Leptin receptor–deficient *db/db* mice have decreased hypothalamic BDNF expression and their obesity and impaired glucose metabolism are ameliorated by intracerebroventricular administration of BDNF protein.[58,59] MC4R activation induces BDNF expression in the hypothalamus.[54] MC4R knockout mice are hyperphagic, obese, and have decreased hypothalamic BDNF expression.[54] The anorexic effects of MC4R activation can be blocked by administration of an anti-BDNF antibody in the third ventricle[55] and the orexigenic effects of MC4R antagonism are attenuated by BDNF coadministration in the fourth ventricle.[56] These data collectively suggest an important role for BDNF downstream of MC4R within the CNS.

Genetic evidence from animal studies strongly supports the notion that BDNF serves as a final downstream mediator of the leptin-POMC pathway. BDNF heterozygous knockout mice display hyperphagia and obesity.[60,61] Conditional knockout of BDNF in postnatal brain[62] as well as selective deletion of BDNF in the ventromedial and dorsomedial hypothalamus of adult mice also results in hyperphagia and obesity.[63] Moreover, animals that are hypomorphic for TrkB, the high affinity receptor for BDNF, are obese.[54]

Human studies also support the role of BDNF in the regulation of energy balance. Human BDNF haploinsufficiency, either due to heterozygous deletion in patients with WAGR/11p deletion syndrome[64] or disruption of BDNF expression in a child with interstitial 11p inversion,[65] is associated with decreased serum BDNF concentrations, hyperphagia, and obesity. Patients with Prader–Willi syndrome (PWS), a genetic disorder characterized by compulsive eating and obesity, have decreased serum and plasma BDNF concentrations compared with BMI-matched controls.[66] Genome-wide association studies have found that BDNF is 1 of 18 genetic loci associated with BMI.[53,67] A *de novo* mutation affecting human TrkB is associated with severe obesity.[68]

In addition to genetic evidence, pharmacological studies also support BDNF effects on appetite and energy balance. Intracerebroventricular infusion of BDNF protein or direct delivery to the hypothalamus suppresses food intake and induces weight loss.[69,70] Chronic treatment with BDNF protein also alleviates obesity by reducing food intake and increasing energy expenditure in DIO as well as *db/db* mice.[70,71] Investigators at Pfizer undertook preclinical studies of BDNF, the related TrkB ligand neurotrophin-4 (NT4), and a TrkB agonist antibody for the treatment of obesity and associated metabolic conditions. Peripheral administration of BDNF protein or TrkB agonists result in potent weight loss in a variety of models of obesity and diabetes in mice, rats, hamsters, and dogs.[72,73] However, peripheral injection of TrkB ligand NT-4 or a humanized TrkB agonist antibody, TAM-163, lead to a paradoxical increase in food intake and weight gain in lean and obese nonhuman primates.[74,75] On the contrary, central administration of both BDNF and NT-4 significantly reduces food intake in nonhuman primate.[75] The authors suggest that the possible difference in brain neuroanatomy and/or neuronal projections between species may determine the recruitment of different downstream effectors involved in the regulation of energy balance. Nevertheless, these studies do support the notion that it is likely important to deliver BDNF directly into the CNS and ideally into the hypothalamus for therapeutic effects.

When we needed genetic interrogation of the hypothalamic BDNF in mediating EE phenotypes, we generated AAV vector to deliver BDNF gene to the hypothalamus of mice via stereotaxic surgery. Overexpressing BDNF in the hypothalamus led to sustained weight loss and robust reduction of adiposity.[76,77] These data quickly triggered our interest in developing AAV-mediated BDNF gene therapy for obesity and related metabolic syndrome. We also noticed that visceral fat depots were barely palpable in some mice receiving high dose of AAV-BDNF while maintained on normal chow diet. As such, a regulatory strategy is likely necessary to facilitate clinical translation of BDNF gene therapy.

A Physiologically Autoregulatory BDNF Vector

Ideally, the expression of a therapeutic gene can be dialed down and up automatically according to the physiological effects induced by the introduced therapeutic gene. We first thought about a conventional approach: use a promoter that would be turned off by the phenotypic changes brought out by the transgene to drive the transgene expression. Therefore, in order to identify genes that would be suppressed following weight loss, we carried out transcriptome analysis of the hypothalamus samples from mice receiving AAV-BDNF. A little bit surprising, few neuronal genes were downregulated whereas neuropeptide Y (*Npy*) and agouti-related peptide (*Agrp*) were highly upregulated. The stimulation of orexigenic neuropeptides reflects a natural negative feedback to weight loss. We then conducted quantitative real-time polymerase chain reaction (qRT-PCR) to validate the microarray data and found *Agrp* the most robustly upregulated, with 15-fold and 16-fold increases in expression in mice on normal chow and high fat diet (HFD), respectively.[78]

We amplified two human AGRP promoter fragments of different lengths each containing the hypothalamus-specific exon.[79] We coupled the AGRP promoter fragments to a luciferase reporter gene and injected these AGRP promoter–driven reporter vectors into the hypothalamus together with the AAV-BDNF vector to induce weight loss. The 484-bp fragment promoter (referred to AGRP484) showed better inducibility than the 814-bp fragment, displaying 2.66-fold induction of reporter activity when BDNF-overexpressing mice had lost 1.5 g while yellow fluorescent protein (YFP)-expressing control mice gained 1.5 g.

At that time, I was simultaneously working on a loss-of-function study for EE's cancer inhibitory effect. To interfere with the *Bdnf* upregulation by EE, I generated a microRNA against *Bdnf* with high efficacy. Then these pieces fell in place to make a new idea of automatically regulating transgene BDNF expression by mimicking the body's natural feedback mechanism. We constructed a single AAV vector harboring two expression cassettes. One cassette constitutively

Autoregulatory BDNF vector

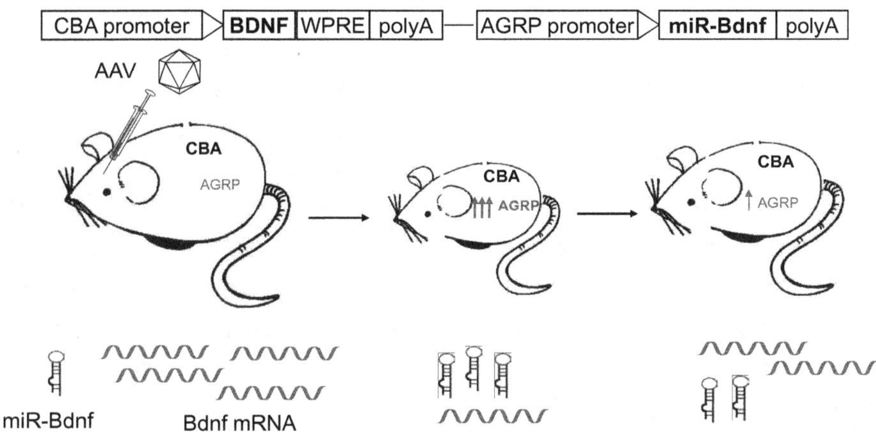

Fig. 4.2. Dual-cassettes design of a physiological autoregulatory gene therapy vector. The therapeutic gene BDNF expression is dialed up and down according to BDNF-induced weight change to achieve a plateau of body weight after significant alleviation of obesity.

expresses BDNF driven by the hybrid cytomegalovirus enhancer/chicken β-actin (CBA) promoter, and the other expresses a microRNA against BDNF driven by the AGRP promoter, which increases activity following weight loss and fat depletion (**Fig. 4.2**). When the vector is administered to an obese individual, the constitutive CBA promoter, much stronger than the AGRP promoter, drives high-level transgene BDNF expression leading to substantial weight loss and reduction of adiposity. Then the weight loss in turn stimulates the AGRP promoter activity as a negative feedback countering the weight loss, whereby producing more microRNA inhibiting the expression of BDNF. Tuning down of BDNF expression automatically can prevent further weight loss. If weight is regained, the stimulation of AGRP promoter will ease and microRNA will decrease accordingly so that BDNF expression will rise to counter the weight gain. Eventually, a plateau of body weight is achieved after significant alleviation of obesity (**Fig. 4.2**).

We carried out a proof-of-concept study using a mouse model of obesity and type 2 diabetes, *db/db* mice, and delayed the intervention until they were extremely obese (~55 g of body weight) and diabetic to investigate the therapeutic efficacy. A high dose was used to assess the autoregulatory efficiency of the dual-cassettes vectors. The *db/db* mice receiving a control YFP virus continued to gain weight. In contrast, mice receiving a nonregulated BDNF vector (the BDNF cassette coupled with microRNA targeting no known genes) lost weight rapidly by 45% in 3 weeks. The precipitous drop of weight showed no sign of stabilization, ultimately requiring euthanasia. The weights of the *db/db* mice receiving the autoregulatory BDNF virus dropped significantly but began to level off and stabilize between 3 and 4 weeks after AAV injection. Weight fluctuated in a narrow range for the entire 11-week duration of the experiment indicating efficient autoregulation of the BDNF transgene expression (**Fig. 4.3**).

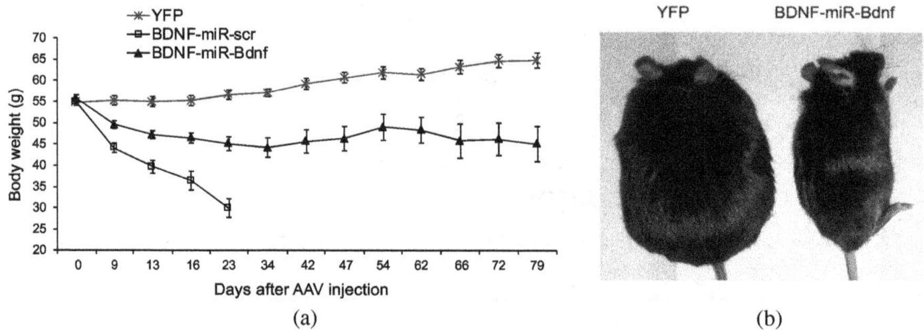

Fig. 4.3. Autoregulatory BDNF vector to treat obese and diabetic *dbldb* mice. AAV vectors were bilaterally injected to the hypothalamus at the dose of 3.4×10^{10} viral genome particles per site. (a) Body weight, $n = 8$ YFP-expressing mice, $n = 7$ BDNF-miR-scr-expressing mice (nonregulated BDNF vector), $n = 9$ BDNF-miR-Bdnf-expressing mice (autoregulatory BDNF vector); $P < 0.0001$ for comparisons between each pair of groups. (b) Mice receiving autoregulatory BDNF vector remained lean 3 months after AAV injection. Reprinted from Cao *et al.* Molecular therapy of obesity and diabetes by a physiological autoregulatory approach. Nat Med 2009, 15, 447–454.

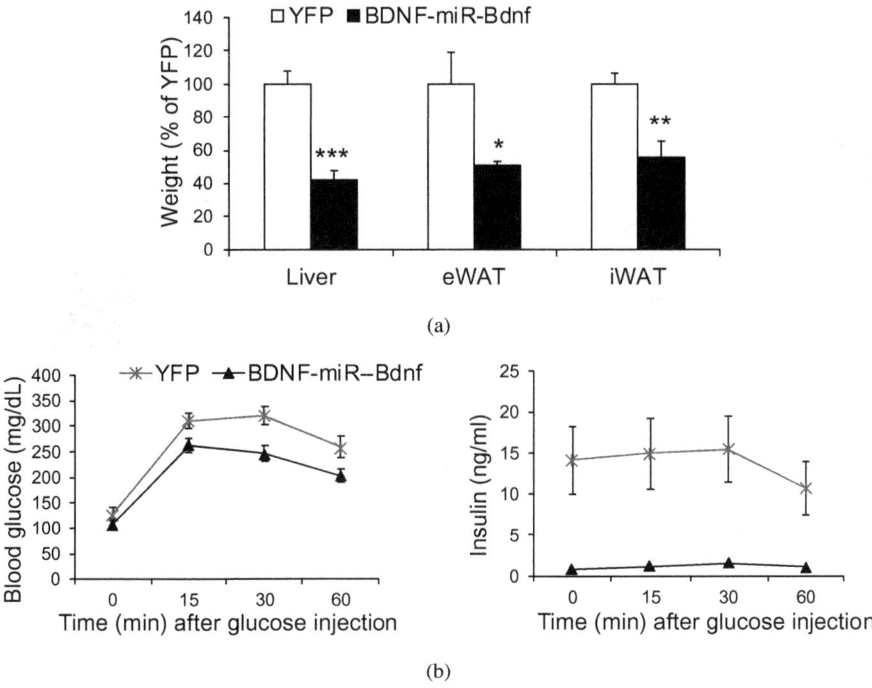

Fig. 4.4. Autoregulatory BDNF gene therapy alleviates obesity and improves glycemic control. (a) Liver, epididymal white adipose tissue (eWAT), and inguinal white adipose tissue (iWAT) mass; n = 8 each group, *P<0.05, **P<0.01, ***P<0.001. (b) Glucose tolerance test on mice after overnight fast; n = 6 YFP-expressing mice, n = 5 BDNF-miR-Bdnf-expressing mice; P<0.05 for glucose concentration and P<0.0001 for insulin concentration. Reprinted from Cao *et al.* Molecular therapy of obesity and diabetes by a physiological autoregulatory approach. Nat Med 2009, 15, 447–454.

Autoregulatory BDNF gene therapy alleviated the obesity (**Fig. 4.4(a)**), vastly improved insulin sensitivity and glucose tolerance (**Fig. 4.4(b)**), and ameliorated the metabolic disturbances in *db/db* mice. BDNF gene therapy reduced food intake compared to YFP controls and increased rectal temperature indicating increased energy expenditure.[78] Autoregulatory vector led to a more controlled BDNF overexpression. Hypothalamic BDNF levels were 2055.6 ± 402.7 pg/mg protein in BDNF-miR-Bdnf (regulated vector) mice, an 85% reduction from the

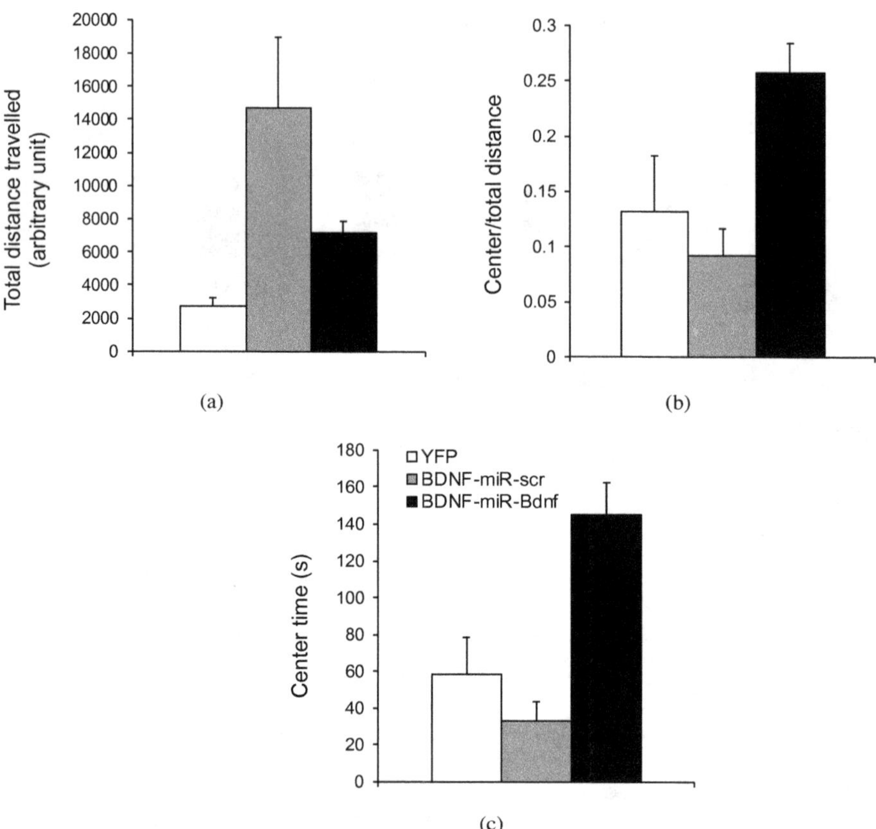

Fig. 4.5. BDNF gene therapy improves mobility and exploration behavior of obese *dbldb* mice. (a) Total distance, $P<0.001$ BDNF-miR-scr and BDNF-miR-Bdnf compared to YFP. (b) Ratio of central to total distance traveled, $P<0.05$ BDNF-miR-Bdnf compared to YFP and BDNF-miR-scr. (c) Center time, $P<0.01$ BDNF-miR-Bdnf compared to YFP and BDNF-miR-scr. $n = 6$ YFP-expressing mice, $n = 5$ BDNF-miR-scr-expressing mice, $n = 9$ BDNF-miR-Bdnf-expressing mice. Reprinted mice. Reprinted from Cao *et al.* Molecular therapy of obesity and diabetes by a physiological autoregulatory approach. Nat Med 2009, 15, 447–454.

13,323.3 ± 3899.8 pg/mg concentration in the BDNF-miR-Scr (non-regulated vector) mice, ($P = 0.023$); and 100.7 ± 13.1 pg/mg protein in the YFP animals. BDNF gene therapy also improved mobility of the extremely obese *db/db* mice and enhanced their physical activity and exploration behavior as shown in an open field test (**Fig. 4.5**).[78]

BDNF-Induced Weight Loss Is Reversible by a Cre-loxP System

In order to provide a further safeguard of BDNF gene therapy and the potential for a clinical rescue procedure, we used the loxP/Cre recombination system to knockout the transgene if the need ever arose because of adverse events.[80] We generated an AAV vector with the BDNF transgene flanked by two *loxP* sites (flox-BDNF), which could be subsequently excised out by a second AAV vector delivering Cre recombinase. The AAV vector encoding a green fluorescent protein (GFP)/Cre fusion protein has been shown to efficiently ablate *loxP* modified genes in the brain including hypothalamus with low toxicity.[81] Bilateral injection of Cre vector alone did not influence body weight, and no toxicity was observed in our study.[78]

To test the efficacy of this rescue approach, we used a DIO model with greater clinical relevance. C57BL/6 mice were fed with the HFD for 10 weeks until their body weight reached 40 g. The flox-BDNF vector was injected into the hypothalamus of the DIO mice with YFP as a control. The flox-BDNF mice started to lose weight 7 days after AAV injection and by 24 days had lost 29.3% of their body weight at which time the YFP control mice had gained 9.0% of their baseline weight (**Fig. 4.7(b)**). Food intake was slightly but significantly reduced in BDNF-treated mice whereas energy expenditure was markedly increased in BDNF mice during both the dark phase and light phase concomitant with higher physical activity particularly in the dark phase (**Fig. 4.6(a), (b)**). Notably, the respiratory exchange ratio (RER), an indicator of the relative contribution of carbohydrates and lipids to overall energy expenditure,[82] was increased in BDNF mice compared to YFP control (**Fig. 4.6(c)**). The higher RER suggests increased carbohydrate oxidation as opposed to lipid oxidation although both groups were fed with HFD, consistent to reduced adiposity and possibly improved fitness[83] after BDNF treatment.

We then randomized flox-BDNF mice to receive a second viral vector injection to the same site as the first surgery, receiving either

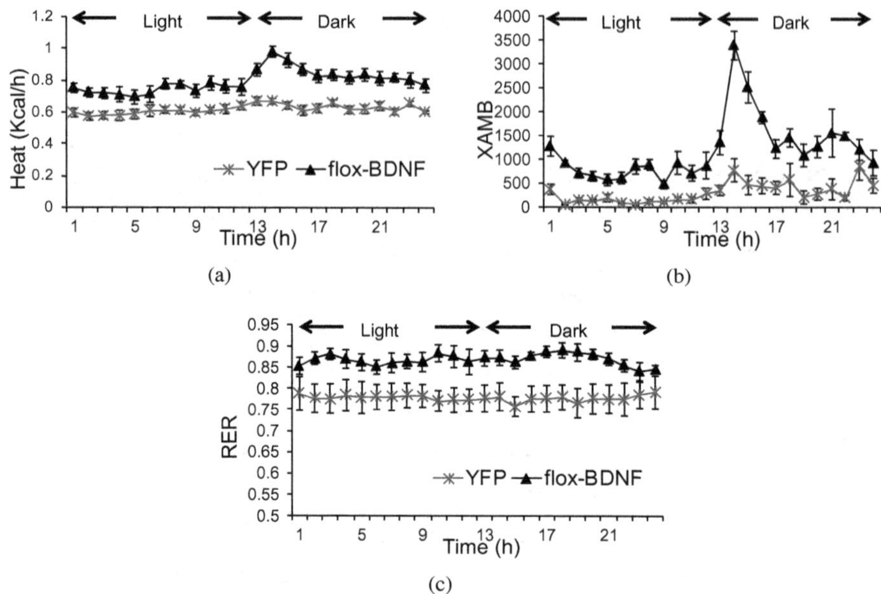

Fig. 4.6. BDNF gene therapy increases energy expenditure in diet-induced obesity. Wild type mice were fed with HFD until their body weight reached 40 g, and then received AAV-flox-BDNF or AAV-YFP control. Energy expenditure was examined by indirect calorimetry during light and dark cycles. (a) Heat. (b) Physical activity. (c) Respiratory exchange ratio (RER). All three parameters were significantly increased in flox-BDNF-expressing mice (n = 6) compared to YFP-expressing mice (n = 5) during both light and dark cycles. Reprinted from Cao *et al.* Molecular therapy of obesity and diabetes by a physiological autoregulatory approach. Nat Med 2009, 15, 447–454.

Cre (fusion with GFP) or empty viral vector (the same expression cassette with no transgene) as a control. All YFP mice received the Cre viral vector in the second surgery (**Fig. 4.7(a)**). Gene expression analysis and immunohistochemistry confirmed ~70% suppression of BDNF mRNA and protein levels by Cre vector injection. After the second surgery, YFP mice continued to gain weight while flox-BDNF mice receiving empty vector in the second surgery continued to lose weight although at a lower rate and eventually became stable. In contrast, flox-BDNF mice receiving Cre virus reversed weight loss, and commenced to regain weight gradually although their weight

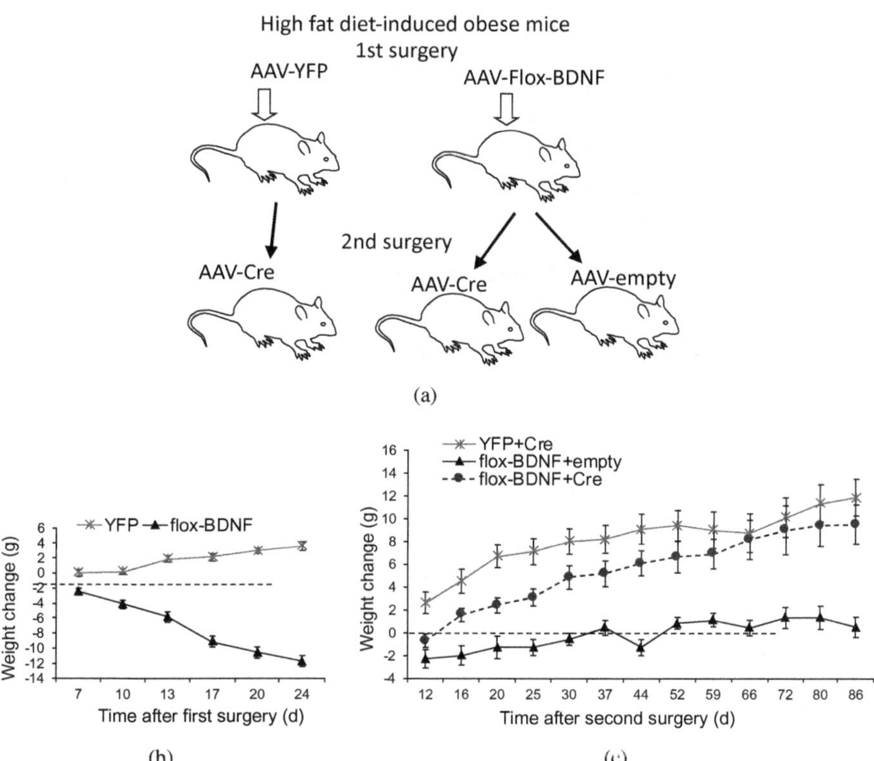

Fig. 4.7. BDNF-induced weight loss is reversible by Cre-loxP-mediated knockout of the transgene. (a) Study design. (b) Weight change after first AAV injection, $n = 10$ YFP-expressing mice and $n = 24$ flox-BDNF-expressing mice, $P<0.01$. (c) Weight change after second AAV injection, $n = 10$ for mice given YFP and Cre, $n = 7$ for mice given flox-BDNF and empty vector, $n = 14$ for mice given flox-BDNF and Cre; $P<0.05$ flox-BDNF+Cre versus flox-BDNF+empty. Reprinted from Cao *et al.* Molecular therapy of obesity and diabetes by a physiological autoregulatory approach. Nat Med 2009, 15, 447–454.

remained significantly lower than the YFP obese mice (**Fig. 4.7(c)**). At the end of the study approximately 4 months after the first surgery, both groups of BDNF mice showed significantly lower BMI than the YFP controls. Because body weight influences bone density, a risk factor for fracture,[84] we measured the bone mineral density of BDNF mice after substantial weight loss and observed no difference in either the whole body skeleton excluding skull or femur only, suggesting a lack of adverse effect on bones following BDNF-induced weight loss in the DIO model.[78]

These data suggest the BDNF-induced weight loss is reversible when the BDNF transgene is excised by the Cre virus. Since the autoregulatory approach is effective, this transgene-excising procedure might be unnecessary. Nevertheless, the rescue strategy can be incorporated to the autoregulatory vector by flanking the entire dual cassettes with *loxP* sites to further enhance safety of BDNF gene therapy.

Advantages of Autoregulatory Vectors

A key advantage of AAV-based gene therapy is its long-term transgene expression, which can last for years in several species and almost for life for rodents. Given the "permanent" nature of AAV-based gene therapy, clinical gene transfer should ideally include some regulatory control of the therapeutic gene expression particularly when constitutive expression of the transgene may be deleterious.[85] Indeed, the inability to regulate or switch off transgene expression is one of the major barriers to clinical application of gene therapy vectors to mediate long-term expression of molecules such as cytokines, neurotrophic, and angiogenic factors.

Several gene regulation technologies based on drug-inducible promoters have been developed. The tetracycline (Tet) regulatory system based on the use of small molecules such as tetracycline or doxycycline is among the most widely used.[86–88] However, the Tet system has concerns including basal leakiness, potential immunogenicity of the foreign proteins, and the need to administer a drug with its own attendant risks. A dimerizer-regulated approach is an alternative. For example, the rapamycin system achieves tight control *in vivo* and is less likely to be immunogenic because the key components of this system originate from human proteins. However, the sequence of the regulatory system is exceeding the packaging capacity of one AAV vector and therefore requires splitting into two separate vectors.[89–91] The use of two separate vectors is inefficient because the two separate AAV vectors must infect the same host cell. Moreover, it is unclear whether the inducer drugs will be appropriate for the clinic given the risk of various potential adverse effects.

To overcome the hurdle, we have designed a built-in autoregulatory system to control therapeutic gene expression mimicking the body's natural feedback systems. We have demonstrated the efficacy of such an approach using BDNF as the therapeutic gene, with weight loss and fat depletion as the physiological readout, and an orexigenic AGRP promoter–driven microRNA cassette as the regulatory agent in various mouse models of obesity[78,92,93] (also see Chapter 7). All components of this system can be packaged into a single rAAV vector for efficient delivery. This autoregulatory approach leads to a sustainable plateau of body weight after substantial weight loss is achieved and prevents some adverse events associated with excessive weight loss caused by unchecked extreme overexpression of BDNF such as compromised immunity and hyperactive behavior. The autoregulatory strategy may represent a significant advance in the area of gene therapy as it can be potentially generalized to other indications in which expression of any given functional transgene is self-regulated by a microRNA driven by promoters activated by the physiological changes caused by the transgene of interest.

Gene Therapy of Melanocortin-4 Receptor Obesity by an Autoregulatory BDNF Vector

Monogenetic obesity is a rare but severe form of the disease. Six forms of human monogenic obesity are linked to inactivating mutations in genes of the leptin–melanocortin pathway (**Fig. 4.1**). Among these, inactivation of MC4R comprises the most common monogenic form of obesity with more than 150 distinct mutations reported.[94]

Dysfunctional mutations in MC4R have been found in approximately 2%–5% of childhood and adult obesity depending on the population background,[95] up to 6% of severe early onset obesity.[96] MC4R variants are found in up to 1% of the general population with a BMI above 30.[97] Due to underdiagnoses, the frequency of MC4R functional mutations could increase to 30% in severely obese children from some populations with high level of consanguinity.[98] In the United States, the two largest population studies have found ~2.5% of Grades 2 and 3 obese patients have a functional MC4R mutation.[99,100] Some researchers believe MC4R obesity is possibly the most common human monogenic disease.[101]

Some evidence suggests that MC4R obese patients respond poorly to current management of obesity. Lifestyle interventions are ineffective in both children and adults with MC4R obesity because functional MC4R may be required for sustained weight loss.[102,103] Bariatric surgery has mixed results and the efficacy may depend on the number of functional MC4R alleles or the specific mutation within the MC4R gene. And some bariatric surgery studies suffer from small sample size of patients.[104–108] Moreover, bariatric surgery has notable disadvantages due to a complication rate of 17%, including nutrient deficiency and postoperative mortality.[109,110]

For two decades, it has been a question whether pharmacological modulation of MC4R is feasible because MC4R is a G-protein-coupled receptor that can bind agonists as well as antagonists, and can couple to multiple classes of G proteins through which stimulating multiple signaling pathways.[94] Moreover, MC4R functions in periphery and brain regions outside the feeding circuitry. Therefore, it is challenging to develop a drug specifically modulating MC4R function in energy homeostasis without unwanted systemic side effects. Indeed, multiple oral small molecules and injectable peptides agonist of MC4R have been produced as therapeutics for treating obesity. Most of these compounds have not yielded promising results in clinical trials such as oral small molecule MK-0493, and peptide agonists LY2112688, MC4-NN-0453, AZD2820.[111] Clinical failure of these MC4R agonist drug candidates has been attributed to: lack of efficacy in humans, significant cardiovascular adverse effects, incidence of nausea and vomiting, and stimulation of sexual arousal. The exception to this disappointment is a cyclic octapeptide setmelanotide (Rhythm Pharmaceuticals), which received FDA approval at the end of 2020 for use in patients with severe obesity caused by genetic defects in POMC, leptin receptor (LEPR), or proprotein convertase subtilisin/kexin type 1 (PCSK1). Setmelanotide activates MC4R signal transduction pathway distinct to alpha-MSH, which differs from other clinically tested MC4R agonists.[111] So far, setmelanotide is approved for severe obesity due to genetic deficiency upstream of MC4R. It remains to be seen whether it is effective for individuals with dysfunctional mutations in MC4R.

Although symptoms manifest in the periphery, the primary defect of MC4R originates within the brain. It makes sense to target brain. Deep brain stimulation (DBS) delivers electrical impulses to specific brain targets to modulate a disturbed neural network[112] and has been approved by FDA for the treatment of advanced Parkinson's disease,[113] dystonia,[114] and essential tremor[115] as well as a number of neurological diseases as humanitarian exemption. DBS is proposed as a potential treatment for obesity.[116,117] A small number of cases provide preliminary evidence for safety and tolerability with mixed and disappointing outcomes.[118] Since available treatment options are ineffective or contraindicated to patients with MC4R deficiency, there is an unmet need for novel therapeutics for MC4R obesity. We propose the autoregulatory BDNF vector may provide a novel gene therapy for MC4R obesity because BDNF acts downstream of MC4R as a final mediator of the leptin–melanocortin pathway.[119]

To test our hypothesis, Jason Siu and colleagues carried out the first gene therapy study on MC4R obesity using heterozygous MC4R-deficient mice (Mc4r$^{loxTB/+}$ mice),[120] which best represent human patient population afflicted with this monogenetic obesity.[101] The

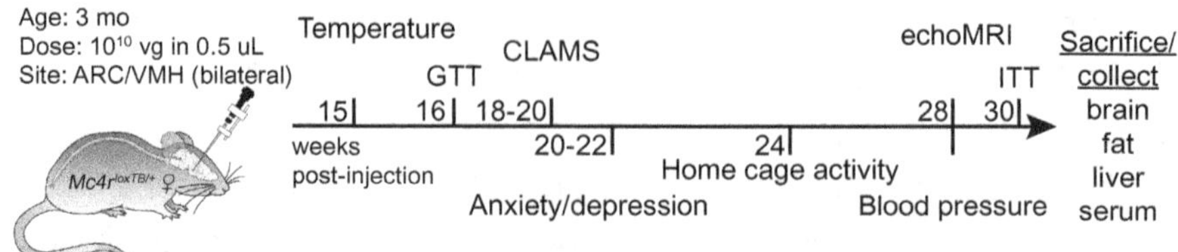

Fig. 4.8. Experimental design. Heterozygous Mc4r-deficient mice were randomized to receive hypothalamic injection of AAV-autoBDNF or AAV-YFP. Parameters above timeline are metabolic assessments; below are safety assessment. GTT, glucose tolerance test; ITT, insulin tolerance test; CLAMS, indirect calorimetry; ARC, arcuate nucleus; VMH, ventral medial hypothalamus. Reprinted from Siu *et al.* Molecular therapy of melanocortin-4-receptor obesity by an autoregulatory BDNF vector. Mol Ther Methods Clin Dev. 2017, 7, 83–95, with permission of American Society of Gene & Cell Therapy.

autoregulatory BDNF vector and YFP control vector are described in previous sections (**Fig. 4.2**). Age-matched 3-month-old male and female heterozygous mice were randomized to two groups, receiving bilateral hypothalamic injections of either the autoregulatory AAV-BDNF (autoBDNF) vector or AAV-YFP vector at equal dose. All mice were maintained on normal chow diet and subjected to a battery of efficacy and safety assessments across the 30-week duration of the study (**Fig. 4.8**).[93]

Mc4r heterozygous mice receiving AAV-YFP gained weight rapidly and developed obesity. In contrast, mice receiving AAV-auto BDNF treatment maintained normal body weight throughout the entire study in both male and female cohorts, indicating complete prevention of obesity by BDNF gene therapy (**Fig. 4.9**).[93] Hyperphagia is the predominant cause of obesity for patients with MC4R deficiency as well as *Mc4r*-deficient mice.[121] BDNF treatment reversed hyperphagia of *Mc4r* heterozygous mice (**Fig. 4.10(a)**). The suppression of food intake was more pronounced than that observed in *db/db* mice, whereas no change or sometimes increased food intake was found in BDNF-treated wild type mice of normal weight. These

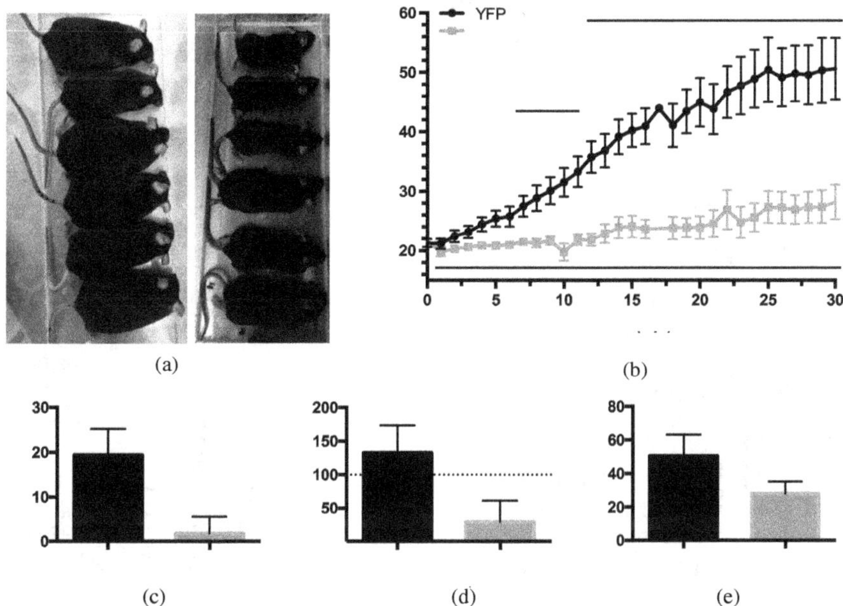

Fig. 4.9. Hypothalamic BDNF gene therapy prevents obesity in Mc4r-deficient mice. (a) Gross images of YFP and autoBDNF mice at 15-week post AAV injection. (b) Body weight of 3-month-old Mc4r heterozygous female mice up to 30 weeks post AAV injection. (c) Weight gain by end of study. (d) Weight gain as a percentage of initial body weight. (e) Final body weight. $n = 7$ for YFP-expressing mice, $n = 6$ for autoBDNF-expressing mice. Error bars, SEM. *$P<0.05$, **$P<0.01$, ***$P<0.001$. Reprinted from Siu *et al.* Molecular therapy of mela nocortin-4-receptor obesity by an autoregulatory BDNF vector. Mol Ther Methods Clin Dev. 2017, 7, 83–95, with permission of American Society of Gene & Cell Therapy.

data appear to indicate *Mc4r*-deficient animals are more sensitive to BDNF treatment.

Weight loss through dieting and exercise may result in a compensatory reduction of basal resting metabolism.[122] BDNF gene therapy elevated basal metabolic rate without significant effect on physical activity in *Mc4r* heterozygous mice (**Fig. 4.10(b)**). The dual actions — suppressing appetite and boosting basal metabolism — of

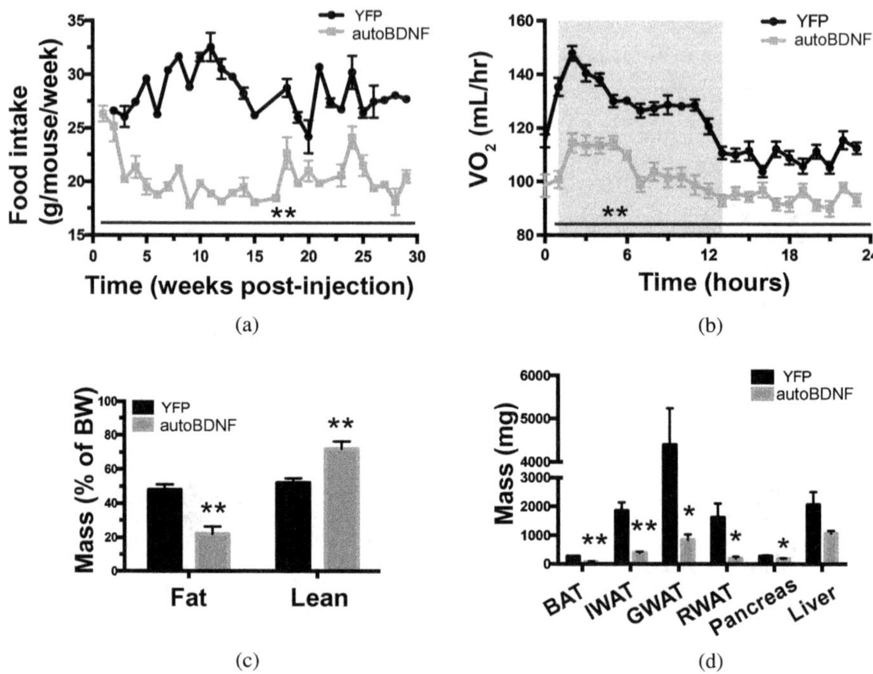

Fig. 4.10. BDNF gene therapy reverses hyperphagia, reduces adiposity, and elevates energy expenditure. (a) Food intake over the duration of the study. (b) Oxygen consumption in metabolic chambers. Shaded area, dark phase. (c) echoMRI analysis of body composition at 28-week post AAV injection. (d) Tissue mass at sacrifice. $n = 7$ for YFP-expressing mice, $n = 6$ for autoBDNF-expressing mice. Error bars, standard error of means (SEM). *$P<0.05$, **$P<0.01$. Reprinted from Siu *et al*. Molecular therapy of melanocortin-4-receptor obesity by an autoregulatory BDNF vector. Mol Ther Methods Clin Dev. 2017, 7, 83–95, with permission of American Society of Gene & Cell Therapy.

BDNF treatment may reset the homeostatic set point for appropriate energy level as to normalized body weight. BDNF treatment reduced adiposity by over 50% and increased the lean mass **(Fig. 4.10(c), (d))**, and alleviated liver steatosis **(Fig. 4.11)**.[93]

Symptoms of *Mc4r* mutant mice include hyperleptinemia, hyperinsulinemia, and slight hyperglycemia. BDNF treatment completely normalized the levels of leptin and insulin. BDNF-treated mice displayed lower fasting blood glucose, ~50% of that in YFP

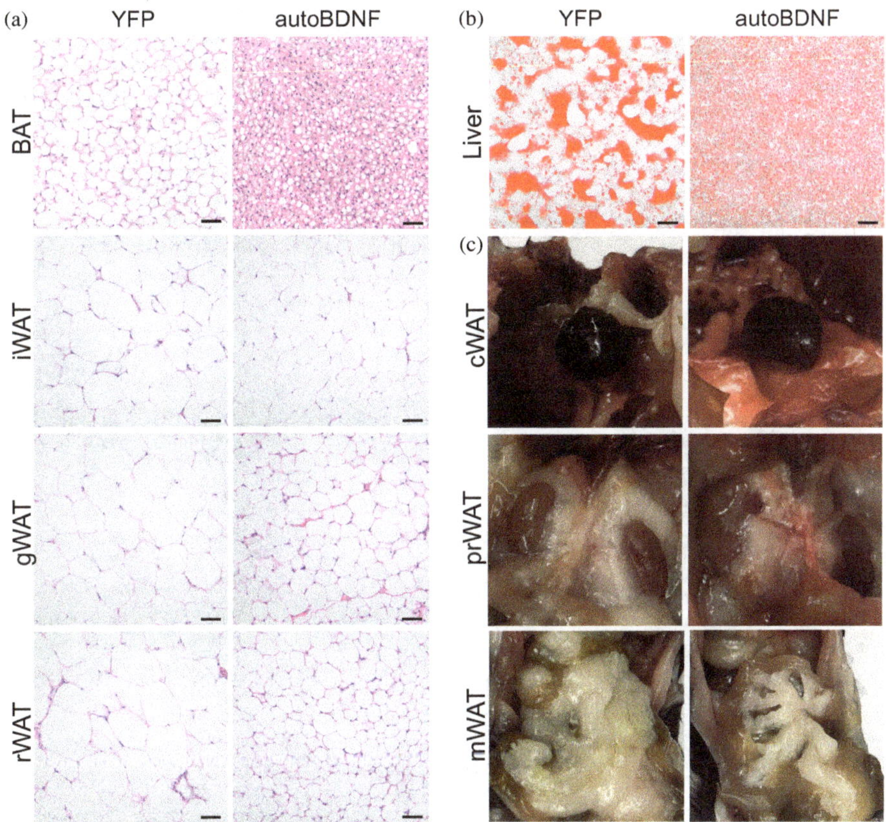

Fig. 4.11. Representative images from YFP-expressing mice and autoBDNF-expressing mice. (a) H&E staining of brown adipose tissue (BAT), inguinal, gonadal, and retroperitoneal white adipose tissue (iWAT, gWAT, rWAT, respectively). (b) Oil red O Staining of liver. (c) Gross images of cardiac, perirenal, and mesenteric white adipose tissue (cWAT, prWAT, mWAT, respectively). Reprinted from Siu *et al.* Molecular therapy of melanocortin-4-receptor obesity by an autoregulatory BDNF vector. Mol Ther Methods Clin Dev. 2017, 7, 83–95, with permission of American Society of Gene & Cell Therapy.

control, and significantly improved glucose tolerance. Moreover, YFP control mice failed to respond to an insulin challenge, an indicator of severe insulin resistance of *Mc4r*-deficient animals. BDNF-treated mice showed substantial improvement in insulin tolerance test (**Fig. 4.12**).[93]

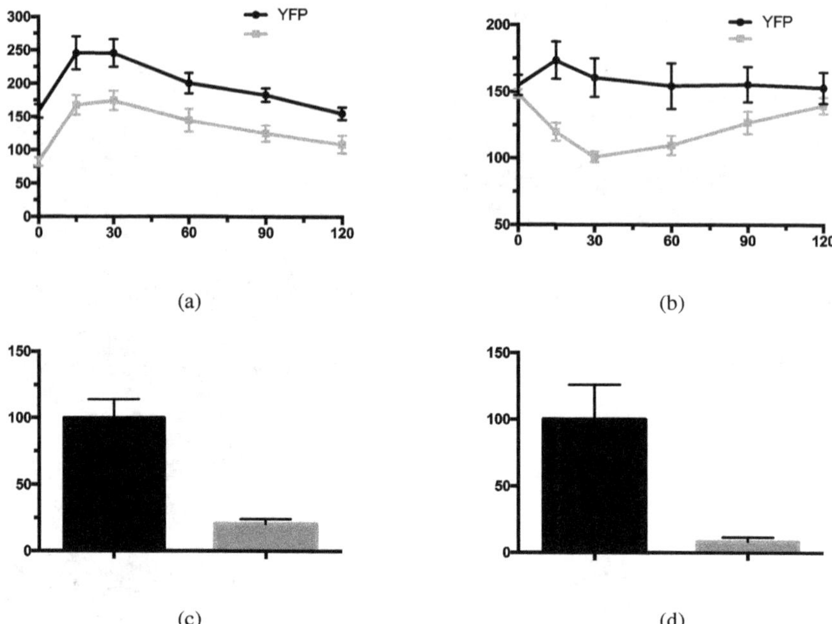

Fig. 4.12. BDNF gene therapy normalizes glycemic control and prevents hyper-leptinemia and insulinemia in Mc4r-deficient mice. (a) Glucose tolerance test. (b) Insulin tolerance test. (c) Serum leptin level. (d) Serum insulin level. $n = 7$ for YFP-expressing mice, $n = 6$ for autoBDNF-expressing mice (a and b); $n = 5$ for YFP-expressing mice, $n = 4$ for autoBDNF-expressing mice (c and d). Error bars, SEM. $*P<0.05$, $**P<0.01$. Reprinted from Siu *et al.* Molecular therapy of melano-cortin-4-receptor obesity by an autoregulatory BDNF vector. Mol Ther Methods Clin Dev. 2017, 7, 83–95, with permission of American Society of Gene & Cell Therapy.

In addition to evaluating the therapeutic efficacy on metabolic outcomes, we aimed to assess the long-term safety of this gene therapy for MC4R obesity in light of the concerns of overexpressing a neurotrophic factor.[123] We performed a series of assays to screen for behavioral alterations. Multiple tests were employed to assess anxiety-like behavior including open field test, cold-induced defe-cation test, elevated T-maze test, and novelty suppressed feeding test. Depression-like behavior was also examined with several tests including tail suspension test, novelty suppressed feeding test, and forced swimming test. All of these behavioral tests demonstrated the absence of adverse behavioral effects in BDNF-treated *Mc4r* heterozygous mice. Moreover, home cage activity was monitored with night vision recordings and no differences were found.[93]

Obese individuals with MC4R deficiency exhibit decreased blood pressure compared to control subject without MC4R mutation.[124,125] BDNF overexpression in the arcuate and ventromedial nucleus of hypothalamus is expected to activate sympathetic nervous system preferentially to the adipose tissue. However, cardiovascular effects should be assessed. Tail cuff manometry showed no significant differences in blood pressure or heart rate between the groups.[93]

The first gene therapy study for MC4R obesity has shown excellent efficacy and safety profile. Hypothalamic BDNF gene therapy using an autoregulatory AAV vector corrects obesity and metabolic syndromes of a clinically relevant animal model of MC4R obesity. Energy balance is reset by suppression of food intake and concomitant increase of basal metabolic rate, with no behavioral or cardiovascular adverse effects.[93] The preclinical evidence suggests an encouraging first step to the long journey toward clinical application. This gene therapy technology has been licensed to Embry that attempts to bring it to clinical trial for patients with MC4R obesity.

Autoregulatory BDNF Gene Therapy for Prader–Willi Syndrome

BDNF gene therapy may be applicable to other diseases with obesity and hyperphagia. PWS is a genetic disorder caused by genetic alterations along chromosome 15q11-13, so called Prader–Willi critical region. Under normal conditions, genes in this region are silenced on maternal chromosome 15 but active on paternal chromosome 15. In PWS patients, this critical region on the paternal chromosome is either missing or inactive. Infants with PWS have trouble feeding and suffer from delay of growth. However, when they get older between ages 2 and 4 years, they become constantly hungry often progressing to severe obesity and diabetes. In addition, PWS patients display intellectual impairment, hypothalamic hypogonadism, behavioral problems, obsessive compulsive behavior, and temper tantrums.[126]

PWS is a rare disease with frequency of 1 in 15,000–25,000 live births. PWS has no cure. Treatment may improve some outcomes if implemented early. Growth hormone therapy[127,128] and experimental drugs[129] may mitigate the impairment of early growth and improve survival. However, up-to-date, effective, and sustained treatments are limited to address the metabolic dysregulations, particularly compulsive eating. Strict supervision of daily food intake may help to prevent rapid weight gain and severe obesity. In order to minimize food stealing and hoarding, parents are recommended to lock all cabinets and refrigerators containing food. Low-calorie diet and regular exercise are essential and must be maintained for the rest of the patient's life, which is extremely difficult to sustain and a huge burden on caregivers. No medications have proven beneficial in managing food-seeking behavior, highlighting the urgent need for new therapeutic strategy.

Patients with PWS have lower serum and plasma BDNF concentrations compared with BMI-matched control subjects.[66] We reason that hypothalamic BDNF gene therapy may mitigate the hyperphagia and obesity of PWS. We are funded by the Foundation for Prader–Willi Research to conduct a preclinical study using a genetic model of PWS. *MAGEL2* is one gene thought to contribute to the metabolic dysregulation observed in PWS.[130] The Magel2[tm1Stw] (hereafter *Magel2*) murine model recapitulates many of the metabolic phenotypes observed in PWS patients. In the hypothalamus, *Magel2* is required for normal leptin signaling in pro-POMC neurons.[131,132] Loss of *Magel2* reduces anorexigenic α-melanocyte-stimulating hormone (α-MSH) axons,[133] while does not influence orexigenic agouti-related peptide (AgRP) fibers.[131,132] Consequently, in the absence of hypothalamic *Magel2*, the satiety response is blunted and feeding continues, leading to systemic metabolic dysregulation.

In a proof-of-concept study, we are applying the autoregulatory BDNF gene therapy, which is effective in DIO and genetic models,[78,93] to a PWS relevant animal model, *Magel2*-null mice. *Magel2*-null mice are obese and have increased circulating levels of leptin, cholesterol, and insulin.[134] Moreover, *Magel2*-null mice display endocrine dysfunctions resembling those found in congenital leptin resistance, including inability to regulate insulin-induced hypoglycemia and mild impairment of glucose tolerance.[135] Although PWS patients display overeating, *Magel2*-null mice have lower food intake as compared to wild type littermates but their food intake is excessive considering lower activity level.[134] With regard to behavior, *Magel2*-null mice exhibit repetitive behaviors,[133] hypoactivity,[133,136] abnormal reactions to novel environments,[133] alterations in exploratory behavior and anxiety,[136] impaired social recognition,[136] and reductions in social novelty seeking behavior.[136] Because *Magel2* is required for normal leptin signaling in POMC neurons[131,132] and BDNF is thought to serve as a final downstream mediator of the leptin–melanocortin pathway, we predict that hypothalamic BDNF gene therapy is likely to ameliorate the metabolic dysfunctions of *Magel2*-null mice. Whether hypothalamic BDNF gene therapy affects some of the behavior deficits is a major objective of this preclinical study. We are excited to complete this study and hope to report the results in 10–12 months.

CRISPR-Based Gene Therapy for Obesity Caused by Haploinsufficiency

Matharu and colleagues recently report a CRISPR-based gene activation approach to amplify the expression of normal endogenous genes in obesity models caused by haploinsufficiency.[137] Haploinsufficiency arises from loss-of-function mutations in one gene copy, often through nonsense or frameshift mutations, or small chromosomal deletions. The gene expression by the intact allele is insufficient to compensate for the loss of lost copy, resulting in reduced expression of the gene product and ultimately leading to pathologic phenotypes.[138] Currently, more than 660 genes are estimated to cause human disease as a result of haploinsufficiency.[137,139,140] What are the therapeutic options for diseases rooted in haploinsufficiency? One is to supply extra copies of the gene through gene therapy. rAAV has become a preferred gene delivery method. However, a crucial hurdle of current rAAV approaches is its 4.7-kb packaging capacity. Considering of regulatory sequences required for stable expression, rAAV is not applicable to genes longer than 3.5 kb. According to Matharu *et al* analysis, 20% of the 660 haploinsufficiency disease-causing genes and 23% of the 3230 genes predicted with heterozygous loss-of-function, harbor coding sequences larger than 3.5 kb. To circumvent this limitation, the authors apply CRISPR-based gene editing to enhance gene expression from the intact allele in animal models of genetic obesity due to haploinsufficiency.

This CRISPR-based gene editing technique uses a nuclease-deficient Cas9 enzyme — dCas9 fused to a protein domain to regulate transcription. Guide RNAs (gRNAs) can recruit these fusion proteins to specific genomic locations that regulate gene expression including promoters and cis-regulatory elements such as enhancers. Depending on the fusion protein domain, the result can be either activation (CRISPRa) or interference (CRISPRi) of transcription.[141] The authors generated CRISPRa system using dCas9 fused to a transcriptional activator, VP64, and target the promoter or hypothalamic specific enhancer of two genes, single-minded 1 (*Sim1*) and *Mc4r*. Haploinsufficiency of either gene causes human obesity, and previous work has established that both SIM1and MC4R regulate energy homeostasis through their expression in the hypothalamus supporting hypothalamus as therapeutic target.[142–144] They packaged the CRISPRa reagents into rAAV and directly delivered into the hypothalamus of heterozygous $Sim1^{+/-}$ mice or $Mc4r^{+/-}$ mice. Postnatal injection of CRISPRa-rAAV upregulated the expression of the existing normal copy of *Sim1* or *Mc4r*, sufficient to rescue the obesity phenotype.[137]

In this study, CRISPRa-rAAV was administered at the age of 4 weeks, prior to the onset of obesity, and the gene therapy prevented obesity due to haploinsufficiency. It remains to be seen whether CRISPRa can rescue the phenotype later in life as many haploinsufficient diseases are likely to be treated only after disease phenotypes are partially or fully developed in patients. Moreover, the success of CRISPRa and CRISPRi technology may hinge on identification and characterization of the cis-regulatory elements that control gene expression. This proof-of-concept study utilized a developmentally stable tissue-specific enhancer. However, it is not clear how often this will be the case for other haploinsufficient genes as many enhancers act at specific developmental stages and dynamically change their tissue specificity.[145] Nevertheless, these exciting advances in CRISPR-based gene therapy of obesity may pave a way to develop novel gene-regulating therapies for wide range of gene dosage-associated diseases.[146]

Targeting Adipose Tissue for Obesity Gene Therapy

Adipose tissue is one of the largest organs of the body and manifests many symptoms of obesity. Yet adipose tissue has been ignored in the field of gene therapy largely due to the relatively poor transduction efficiency and tropism with naturally occurring AAV serotypes.[20,147–149] Research in the past two decades has shown AAV8 outperform other naturally occurring serotypes with regard to adipose tissue gene delivery. However, in order to achieve therapeutic effect, a relative high dose in the order of 10^{11} or 10^{12} viral genome (vg) is required for systemic administration or even intra-adipose injection to mouse.[149–151] Furthermore, AAV8 is the serotype preferable for gene delivery to liver,[19,152] underscoring the challenge of avoiding off-target transduction with AAV8 vectors.

Two approaches have been employed to mitigate off-target effects in liver. One is to add target sequence of microRNA-122 that abundantly expresses in liver and thereby suppressing transgene expression in liver. This approach might cause toxicities at least theoretically, because large amount of microRNA-122 target sequence from AAV vector inside a hepatocyte may compete with endogenous target sequence for microRNA-122. Liver toxicities including hepatic steatosis, hepatitis, or hepatocellular carcinoma have been reported in microRNA-122 knockout mice.[153] Although this risk is very low,[154,155] it remains a safety concern of clinical application of a long-term gene therapy. The other approach is to use an adipose-specific promoter to drive transgene expression. The size limitation of AAV vectors only accommodates a short version of promoter (mini-promoters). These adipose-specific mini-promoters are much less potent than a ubiquitous promoter such as CBA or CAG (CBA fused with rabbit β-globin splice acceptor site), often resulting in weak transgene expression in adipose tissue.[20] As an advancement in the field, our recent studies have characterized an engineered hybrid serotype Rec2 with high efficacy of gene transfer to both brown and white fat via either local or systemic administration,[156–161] opening doors to adipose-oriented gene therapy.

Rec2 Serotype AAV Vector

Modifications of the capsid of AAV, often referred to AAV capsid engineering, have been employed to improve efficiency and tropism of gene delivery.[19] However, scarce efforts have been reported regarding capsid engineering targeting adipose tissue. The During lab attempted to create novel hybrid serotypes more efficiently targeting brain and retina. They generated six engineered serotypes, named Rec1~6, by capsid domain exchange or shuffling among AAV8, and three newer AAV variants isolated from nonhuman primate by Gao lab: cy5 (cynomolgus macaque-variant 5), rh20 (rhesus macaque-variant 20), and rh39 (rhesus macaque-variant 39). *In vivo* studies in mouse and primate demonstrate that these novel serotypes transduce retina tissue no better than AAV2 or AAV5.[162]

Direct Adipose Injection of Rec2

In search of a tool to genetic engineer adult adipose tissue, we assessed several hybrid capsids among this family (Rec1, 2, 3, 4) and compared them with AAV1, AAV8, and AAV9, the naturally occurring serotypes able to transduce adipose tissue. By direct injection to white adipose tissue (WAT), Rec2 vector exhibited widespread transgene expression and highest efficiency among the seven serotypes tested at the dose of 1×10^{10} vg per iWAT pad. Rec2 vector transduced BAT more efficiently than the WAT with a dose at least 5-fold lower than that used in iWAT. We tested the functional efficacy of Rec2-mediated adipose gene transfer using conditional insulin receptor mice (IR^{lox}). Injection of Rec2 vector carrying Cre recombinase (Rec2-Cre) to iWAT (1×10^{10} vg per fat pad) and BAT (2×10^9 vg per fat pad) resulted in 50% reduction of insulin receptor protein level and the ensuring shrink of fat mass, molecular and morphological features consistent with impairment of adipose function. Importantly, intra-adipose injection of Rec2-Cre at these low doses showed minimal effect on insulin receptor in liver and muscle.[163] Since the first publication of Rec2 gene transfer to adipose tissue, other labs have successfully applied Rec2 vectors to genetically manipulate adipose tissues in adult animals.[157–159]

Intravenous Injection of Rec2

We have expanded characterization of the Rec2 serotype and found the bio-distribution of Rec2 dependent on administration route. Intravenous injection of Rec2 via tail vein leads to predominantly liver transduction.[164]

Oral Administration of Rec2

Oral administration results in preferential transduction of BAT with absence of transgene expression in the gastrointestinal track.[165] We were amazed by this surprising finding and carried out experiments to compare six engineered and natural serotypes (Rec1~4, AAV1, AAV8) by oral gavage with a GFP reporter virus at equal dose of 2×10^{10} vg per mouse. Rec2 led to the highest reporter gene expression in BAT.

Next, Wei Huang and colleagues tested approaches to improve selective transduction of BAT. First, lowering the dose of oral administration by 5-fold (5×10^9 vg per mouse) resulted in GFP content in BAT more than 10-fold higher than that in the liver, suggesting decreasing dose favoring BAT transduction over liver. Moreover, large amount of viral vector genome was detected in the BAT 2-week post oral administration of Rec2 (5×10^9 vg per mouse) whereas minimal or negligible copy number was found in liver, heart, stomach, intestine, muscle, and WAT. Second, we incorporated four repeats of the target sequence of microRNA-122 to the AAV transgene expression cassette so that transgene expression would be suppressed by hepatically abundant microRNA-122. When orally administered at high dose (2×10^{10} vg per mouse), the transgene mRNA level in the BAT was 100- to 500-fold higher than that in the liver of the same animal.[165]

Considering the exceptionally efficient transduction of BAT by direct injection, we tested how efficient oral administration compared to direct injection using a Rec2 vector carrying luciferase reporter. Impressively, oral administration of Rec2 vector at the dose of 5×10^9 vg per mouse led to 3-fold higher luciferase reporter activity in BAT than direct injection at the dose of 5×10^8 vg per mouse.[165]

To test whether oral Rec2 vector delivery could augment BAT sufficiently to yield a phenotypic readout, we manipulated VEGF expression in BAT both positively and negatively. Oral administration of Rec2-VEGF to overexpress VEGF in BAT led to enhanced cold response, increased BAT mass, molecular features consistent with elevated angiogenesis and thermogenesis capacity, as well as consequentially reduced WAT mass. Conversely, loss-of-function experiment via Cre-LoxP knockdown (2×10^{10} vg per mouse) resulted in opposing effects including decreased BAT mass, impaired cold response, and increased WAT mass.[165]

This study is the first to demonstrate oral administration of an AAV vector achieves high-level transgene expression in BAT at a dose at least 1~2 orders lower than commonly reported dose of intravenous injection. Feeding a Rec2 vector can genetically manipulate BAT sufficiently to alter BAT functions and the ensuring systemic adaptation. The combined features including high transduction efficiency, low dose, easy and noninvasive administration, selective tropism to BAT, make Rec2 vector a novel and powerful vehicle for both basic research on BAT and potential therapeutic applications boosting BAT for management of obesity and metabolic syndromes.

Up to date, few studies on oral administration of AAV vectors have been reported, and the majority of which focusing on vaccines.[166–169] Oral administration of AAV2 serotype shows limited transduction of the lamina propria and epithelia of gastrointestinal track without notable transduction in other tissues at the dose of 5×10^{11} vg.[170,171] One study shows oral administration of AAV6 vector leads to luciferase reporter activity in the stomach and liver at the dose of 1×10^{11} vg per mouse.[167] None of these publications document adipose tissue transduction.

We are puzzled by the interesting finding that oral administration of Rec2 vector fails to transduce gastrointestinal track but instead transduces distal interscapular BAT. AAV5 transcytosis through gut epithelial cells has been documented.[172] Whether Rec2 is transported in similar fashion is not known. If orally administered Rec2 vectors primarily distribute through blood circulation, they will enter portal vein and reach liver first and thus predominantly transduce liver as seen with intravenous injection. But oral administration of Rec2 preferentially transduces BAT suggesting blood circulation unlikely the major route.

We did a kinetic experiment to track the presence of viral vector DNA in blood and tissues (BAT, liver, thymus, and mesenteric fat) at 10-, 20-, and 30-min post oral gavage of Rec2 vector. Indeed, tail vein injection and oral administration displayed distinct profiles. Oral administration resulted in very limited viral vector presence in the blood, only detectable at 30 min but not 10- and 20-min timepoints. In contrast, viral vector was detected in the thymus 10- and 20-min after the oral administration earlier than the blood. Remarkably, high level of viral vector was detected in the mesenteric fat that is rich in lymph nodes as early as 10 min after oral gavage, and the mesenteric fat viral DNA level gradually declined overtime.[165] Based on available data, we hypothesize that orally administered Rec2 vector might circulate through lymphatic system to transduce BAT. Blood circulation is certainly involved but the lymphatic system might play a major role. Lower dose might favor this lymphatic route further. We are currently attempting to address these fascinating questions whether Rec2 transcytoses to allow systemic delivery and how Rec2 is circulated via blood and/or possibly via lymphatic system.

Intraperitoneal Injection of Rec2

With regard to obesity-associated disease risk, location of adipose tissue matters substantially. Accumulation of subcutaneous fat has neutral or even beneficial effects on metabolism in conditions of energy surplus while excessive visceral adipose tissue (VAT) is strongly associated with adverse metabolic outcomes.[173] Visceral fat or intra-abdominal fat locates within the abdominal cavity surrounding vital organs such as liver, stomach, and intestine. Studies have revealed intrinsic functional differences of adipocytes in different depots, including insulin sensitivity, glucose uptake, rate of lipolysis, and adipokine and cytokine secretion.[174,175] In comparison to subcutaneous fat, VAT is a more active endocrine organ producing a higher proportion of molecules with potentially deleterious health effects. For example, VAT secretes more of pro-inflammatory cytokines that can trigger low-grade chronic inflammation. VAT is implicated in a number of chronic conditions including cardiovascular disease, diabetes, dementia, asthma, and cancers of breast and colon. Thus, management of obesity should aim to VAT first.

Visceral fats are of particular interest to studies on obesity and related metabolic disorders, but they are less accessible to direct injection of viral vectors. Therefore, we attempted intraperitoneal injection and found that Rec2 vector at the dose of 1×10^{10} vg per mouse resulted in robust reporter gene expression (luciferase and GFP) in multiple VAT depots (gonadal, retroperitoneal, and mesenteric fat depots), whereas no reporter activities were detected in small intestine, large intestine, spleen, kidney, testis, BAT, and subcutaneous WAT.[161] Unpublished data show no detectable GFP fluorescence in heart. This data is another example of the interesting characteristic of Rec2 vector whose tissue tropism dependent on administration route. Upon intraperitoneal administration, the majority of Rec2 vectors likely encounter the liver and VAT depots. Due to tropism of Rec2 serotype, both liver and VATs are efficiently transduced, which may limit the quantity of Rec2 vectors entering blood circulation, whereby leading to minimal transduction of subcutaneous WAT and BAT. The preferential modulation of VAT via intraperitoneal administration can be a highly desirable feature because VAT depots are closely associated with risk of metabolic syndromes and heart disease. Furthermore, intraperitoneal administration of Rec2 vector enables genetic manipulation of mesenteric fat that is otherwise difficult to access even via invasive surgical approaches.

In addition to visceral fats, liver was also transduced considerably. To prevent transgene expression in the liver, we developed a novel AAV expression plasmid harboring two expression cassettes: one

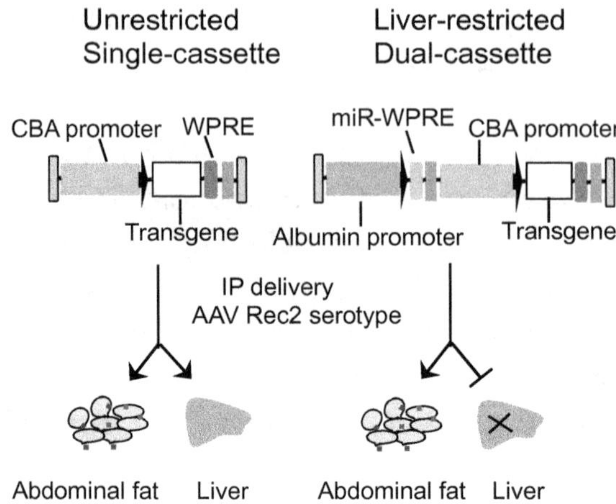

Fig. 4.13.   A novel AAV system for selective transduction of adipose tissue while restricting off-target expression in liver. A single AAV vector harbors two expression cassettes. The liver-restricting cassette interferes with the transgene expression specifically in the liver through a microRNA against WPRE sequence driven by liver-specific album promoter. Upon intraperitoneal administration, the Rec2 serotype AAVs with dual-cassette design lead to selective transduction of visceral fats while severely restricting hepatic transgene expression. Reprinted from Huang *et al.* Targeting visceral fat by intraperitoneal delivery of novel AAV serotype vector restricting off-target transduction in liver. Mol Ther Methods Clin Dev. 2017, 6, 68–78, with permission of American Society of Gene & Cell Therapy.

using the nonselective CBA promoter to drive transgene expression, and the other using the liver-specific proximal albumin promoter to drive a microRNA against woodchuck posttranscriptional regulatory element (WPRE) sequence that only exists in this AAV vector (**Fig. 4.13**). WPRE enhances transgene expression[176,177] and is widely used in AAV expression plasmids. The microRNA targeting WPRE (miR-WPRE) knocked down transgene expression more than 90% *in vitro*. Incorporation of the liver-restricting cassette does not interfere with the transgene expression in the adipose tissue but suppresses transgene expression specifically in the liver. This dual-cassette vector (named AS/Rec2) achieved highly selective transduction of visceral fats while severely restricting hepatic transgene expression in the range from 1×10^{10} to 4×10^{10} vg/mouse even though large amount of viral DNA was detected in liver.[161] Efficacy of the dual-cassette vector design has been confirmed in later *in vivo* studies by our lab[160,178,179] and collaborators (personal communications).

Visceral Fat-Oriented Gene Therapy of Congenital Leptin Deficiency

Leptin, an adipocyte-derived hormone, plays a critical role in energy homeostasis. Congenital leptin deficiencies in humans cause severe obesity, hyperphagia, and hyperinsulinemia.[180] Leptin replacement therapy is necessary in patients with homozygous mutations in leptin or acquired leptin deficiency derived from congenital or acquired lipodystrophy.[181–183] Treatment with recombinant leptin protein through subcutaneous injection produces short-lasting effects, and therefore requires repetitive doses. And the supra-physiological increase in circulating leptin level following regular injection is associated with considerable side effects.[184] Given the requirement of lifelong leptin replacement, gene therapies with AAV vectors have been attempted in an animal model best recapitulating human congenital leptin deficiency. The *ob/ob* mouse, a homozygous mutant in leptin gene (*Lep* or *ob* gene), rapidly develops severe obesity and metabolic syndromes.[185,186] Moreover, the leptin-deficient *ob/ob* mice display abnormalities in almost all physiologic systems.[187,188] AAV-mediated intramuscular leptin gene transfer (1 × 10^{11} vg per injection) alleviates obesity and diabetes.[189] The Reilly group reports a gene therapy to reintroduce the leptin gene in its native tissue[150] by combined use of adipose-specific mini promoter and microRNA-122-targeting sequence. Intravenous injection of AAV8-based adipose-targeting vector to *ob/ob* mice at the dose of 1 × 10^{12} vg per mouse, results in peak leptin level approximately 7% of circulating leptin level in the age-matched wild type mice and partially ameliorates the metabolic syndromes.[150] Of note, the dose for adipose-targeting vector is 10-fold higher than that for muscle-directed gene transfer in this study whereas the therapeutic outcomes are relatively moderate.[150]

Wei Huang used the same *ob/ob* mouse model to assess the therapeutic potential of our novel adipose-targeting Rec2 vector system.[161] Intraperitoneal injection of the dual-cassette Rec2 vector carrying leptin gene (AS/Rec2-leptin) at the dose of 4×10^{10} vg per mouse, 25-fold lower than the reported dose in the abovementioned study,[150] normalized leptin level to the age-matched wild type mice (**Fig. 4.14(a)**). AS/Rec2-leptin treatment completely prevented excessive weight gain and normalized body weight of *ob/ob* mice to that of wild type mice by 4-week post AAV injection, which sustained throughout the entire 9-week duration of the study (**Fig. 4.14(b), (c)**). Mice receiving AS/Rec2-leptin showed a sharp drop of food intake as early as 1-week post AAV injection and the reversal of hyperphagia was maintained similarly to the weight loss (**Fig. 4.14(d)**).

In addition, AS/Rec2-leptin treatment corrected the abnormally low body temperature of *ob/ob* mice and their impaired thermogenesis response to fast. Adiposity was decreased by 65% in mice receiving AS/Rec2-leptin while lean mass increased by 75% (**Fig. 4.14(e)**). AS/Rec2-leptin treatment completely reversed hyperinsulinemia and impaired glucose tolerance, and robustly corrected low energy expenditure. At the end of the study, visceral fat of AS/Rec2-leptin-treated mice was reduced by 82.5% compared to AS/Rec2-GFP control mice when calibrated to body weight and the fatty liver was completed reversed.[161]

Taken together, this proof-of-concept study suggests a cure for congenital leptin deficiency in animal model.[161] A single intraperitoneal injection of AS/Rec2-leptin at a low dose is sufficient to normalize leptin level and reverse metabolic symptoms including obesity, hyperphagia, hyperinsulinemia, impaired glycemic control, low metabolic rate, impaired thermogenesis, and low physical activity close to the age-matched wild type animals, indicating advances compared to the limited efficacy with previously reported AAV system.[150]

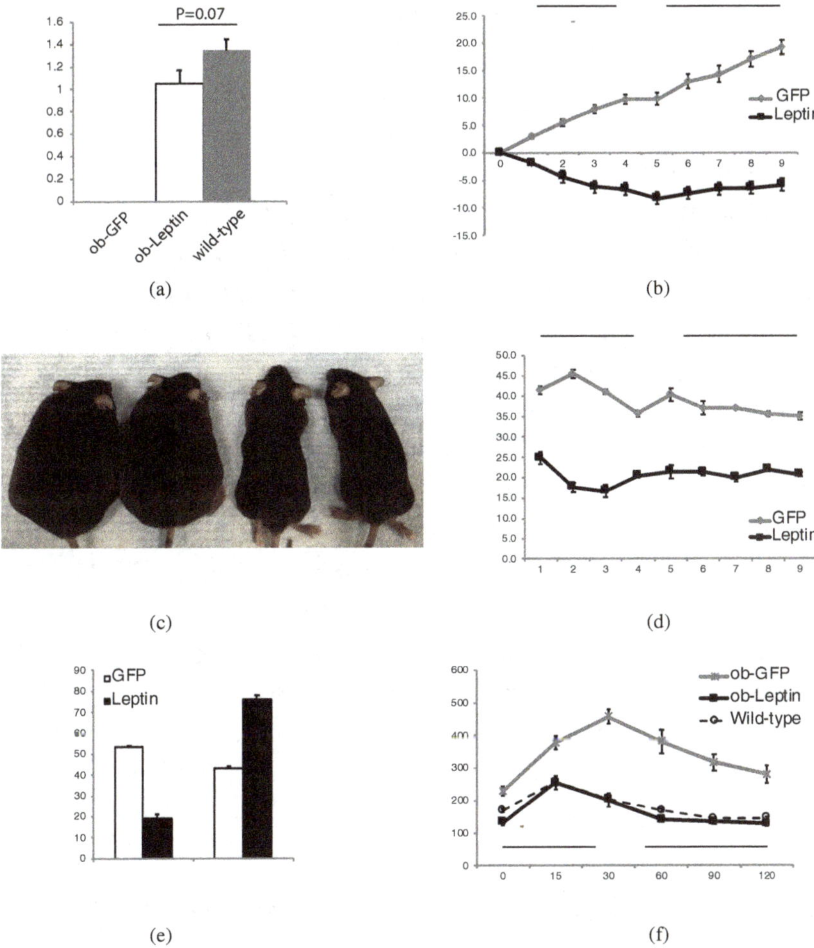

Fig. 4.14. Visceral fat-directed gene therapy rescues leptin deficiency in *oblob* mice. Mice were randomized to receive a single dose of AS/Rec2-Leptin or AS/Rec2-GFP (4 × 10^{10} vg per mouse) by intraperitoneal injection. (a) Serum leptin level 4 weeks after AAV injection. Leptin undetectable in *oblob* mice treated with AS/Rec2-GFP. (b) Weight gain. (c) Representative picture 9 weeks after AAV injection. (d) Cumulative food intake. (e) echoMRI analysis of body composition 4 weeks after AAV injection. (f) Glucose tolerance test 4 weeks after AAV injection. $n = 6$ for AS/Rec2-GFP, $n = 6$ for AS/Rec2-Leptin, $n = 6$–8 for age-matched wild type mice. Error bars, SEM. ***$P<0.001$. Reprinted from Huang *et al*. Targeting visceral fat by intraperitoneal delivery of novel AAV serotype vector restricting off-target transduction in liver. Mol Ther Methods Clin Dev. 2017, 6 ,68–78, with permission of American Society of Gene & Cell Therapy.

Both animal and human studies have demonstrated that restoring circulating leptin level to approximately 10% of normal level is sufficient to alleviate metabolic symptoms caused by congenital leptin deficiency.[150,190] Accordingly, the dose of AS/Rec2-leptin could likely be lowered further to 1×10^{10} vg per mouse, a dose based on body mass close to the dose of 1×10^{12} vg per kg for alipogene tiparvovec (Glybeta), the first gene therapy product approved in Europe, that has been documented to be safe and effective in patients.[191] The encouraging preclinical data suggest the AS/Rec2-leptin worthy of further assessment of translational potential.

Clinical studies have shown that AAV-based systemic gene therapy of genetic deficiencies, such as factor VIII, factor IX hemophilia, and LPL deficiencies, are able to profoundly rescue physiologic aberrancies albeit achieving small corrections of physiological levels in the range from 5% to 10% of normal levels.[192–194] In light of adipose tissue as a secretory organ, the terminally differentiated and nondividing adipocytes can be used as a "factory" to produce therapeutic molecules beyond replacing a defective gene in adipose tissue.[180,195,196] We have applied the highly effective adipose-targeting Rec2 vector system in gene therapy of DIO [197] as well as cancer immune therapy[179] (see Chapter 6).

Visceral Fat-Directed FGF21 Gene Therapy

Fibroblast growth factor 21 (FGF21) is a peptide hormone that exerts its biological effects by binding to ubiquitous FGF receptors (FGFRs) in complex with a co-receptor the transmembrane protein β-Klotho (KLB) that is restricted to adipose tissue, liver, and particular regions of brain.[198,199] FGF21 is primarily produced by the liver in response to metabolic stress such as fasting and a ketogenic diet. With regard to metabolic regulation, adipose tissue is the main target of FGF21 action[200–204] including stimulation of insulin-independent glucose uptake,[205] modulation of lipolysis,[202] mitochondrial activity,[206] and adaptive thermogenesis.[207] Moreover, the antidiabetic actions of FGF21 are thought to occur primarily within WAT.[200,201]

FGF21 is increasingly recognized as a potential therapeutic agent for type 2 diabetes, nonalcoholic fatty liver disease, and other metabolic complications, attracting intensive drug development investigations.[208] Exogenous administration of recombinant FGF21 protein has been shown to improve metabolic health in various animal models.[205,209,210] But the use of native FGF21 peptide has a substantial shortcoming due to the short half-life and biophysical deficiencies.[211] To overcome the hurdle, FGF21 analogs and mimetics have been developed with promising improvement in animal studies, and are under clinical investigations.[212] Despite of improvement in long-lasting FGF21 analogs, the use of FGF21 peptide drugs may still require repeated administrations to achieve sustained clinical benefit, raising concerns about immunological reactions associated with exogenous protein administration, patient comfort, and treatment noncompliance.[213–215]

AAV-mediated FGF21 gene therapy has been investigated to treat obesity and insulin resistance in mouse models[152,216] mostly targeting the liver. Nicholas Queen and others of our lab recently report a VAT-directed FGF21 gene therapy in obese and insulin-resistant BTBR mice.[197] This gene therapy combines an adipose-selective dual-cassette vector and the VAT preferential tropism of Rec2 serotype with the noninvasive intraperitoneal administration (**Fig. 4.15**). Under HFD condition, a single intraperitoneal injection of AS/Rec2-FGF21 (2×10^{10} vg per mouse) led to sustained metabolic benefits including improved insulin sensitivity and glycemic control, reduced whole-body adiposity, and alleviation of hepatic steatosis compared to mice receiving a vector carrying no transgene. Notably, AS/Rec2-FGF21 mice had higher oxygen consumption and increased food intake calibrated to body weight. These data indicate the reduction of adiposity is caused primarily by elevation of energy expenditure rather than appetite suppression. At the end

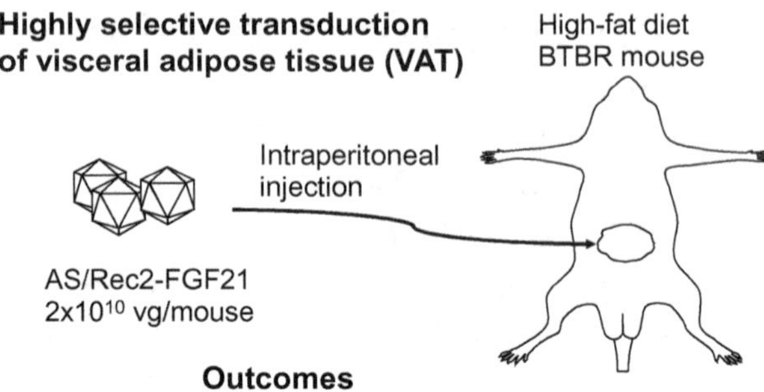

Outcomes
- VAT overexpressing FGF21
- Increasing circulating FGF21 level
- Enhancing insulin sensitivity
- Improving glycemic control
- Increasing anti-inflammatory M2 macrophage in VAT
- Reducing adiposity
- Suppressing hepatic steatosis
- Decreasing inflammatory cytokines

Fig. 4.15. Visceral fat-directed FGF21 gene therapy improves metabolic and immune health. Adapted from Queen *et al.* Visceral adipose tissue-directed FGF21 gene therapy improves metabolic and immune health in BTBR mice. Mol Ther Methods Clin Dev 2020, 20, 409–422, with permission of American Society of Gene & Cell Therapy.

of the 21-week study, high level FGF21 expression was observed in VAT but not liver associated with a 2-fold increase in circulating FGF21 level. FGF21 gene therapy led to a favorable adipokine profile — decreasing serum leptin level by approximately 70% while significantly increasing high-molecular weight adiponectin that is an advanced biomarker of metabolic and cardiac health.[197]

Chronic low-grade inflammation is thought to link obesity to various metabolic disorders and other chronic illnesses. Hence, we examined several pro-inflammatory cytokines and chemokines in serum.[197] We observed a strong trend of reduction of Serum amyloid A (SAA) in the Rec2-FGF21 group as compared to controls. Plasminogen activator inhibitor-1 (PAI-1) is implicated in fibrinolysis whose elevation contributing to vascular disease and inflammation in obese states.[217,218] PAI-1 levels were significantly reduced by ~45%

in the AS/Rec2-FGF21 group consistent with improved metabolic function and reduced inflammation. Serum C-C motif chemokine ligand 2 (CCL2) levels were reduced by ~60% in the AS/Rec2-FGF21 group also indicative of decreased inflammation and improved insulin sensitivity.[219]

Gene expression profiling of the VAT found downregulation of *Pai1* consistent with serum observation. Two markers of inflammation involved in the NLRP3 (NLR family pyrin domain containing 3) inflammasome complex, *Casp1* (encoding caspase-1) and *Pycard* (encoding apoptosis-associated speck-like protein containing a CARD) were also downregulated in AS/Rec2-FGF21–treated mice.[197]

Next, we examined immune populations residing in the VAT.[197] Adipose tissue macrophages (ATMs) are the largest immune population in adipose tissue. In lean animals, ATMs are primarily M2-polarized (defined as CD11c−, CD206+), protecting adipocytes from inflammation. In contrast, under obese conditions, ATMs accumulate in large numbers in VAT and exhibit a pro-inflammatory M1 polarization (defined as CD11c+, CD206−), contributing to insulin resistance.[220] Flow cytometry showed distinct changes in ATM polarization within the VAT treated with AS/Rec2-FGF21 (**Fig. 4.16(a)**). Although the frequency of total ATMs (**Fig. 4.16(b)**) or M1-polarized ATMs (**Fig. 4.16(c)**) was not different between the two groups, a significant proportional increase in M2 polarization (**Fig. 4.16(d)**) was observed and was accompanied by a significant proportional decrease in double-positive (defined as CD11c+, CD206+) ATMs (**Fig. 4.16(e)**). Of interest, the double-positive ATMs have been identified as sources of pro-inflammatory cytokines and drivers of insulin resistance.[221]

Previous work from Bosch group found that FGF21 gene therapy reduced immunostaining of a macrophage marker, Mac2, and expression of F4/80.[152] Our work expanded to a more comprehensive immune profiling including ATMs polarization, T cell subsets, and natural killer T cells. AS/Rec2-FGF21 treatment resulted in a favorable ATM polarization in VAT associated with suppression of

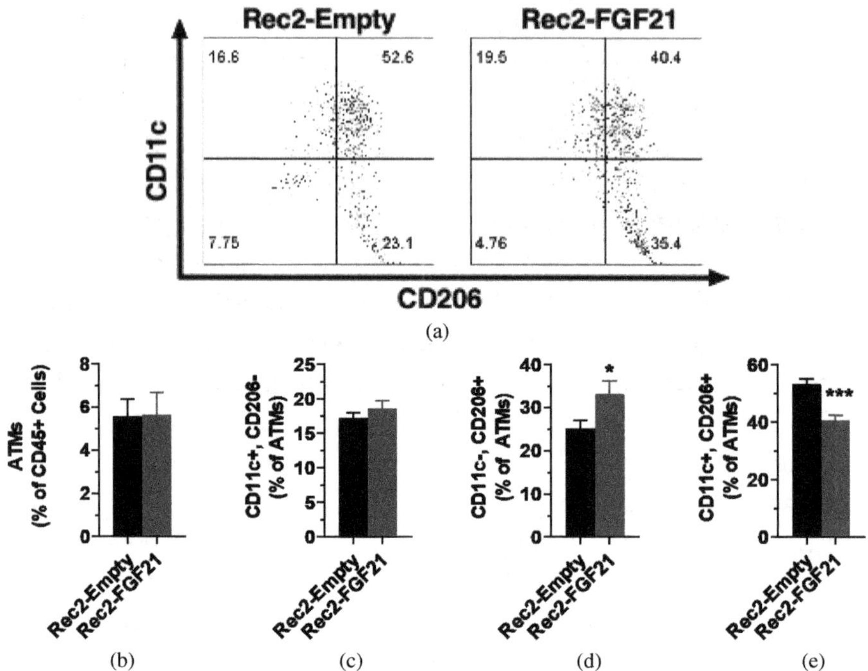

Fig. 4.16. VAT-directed FGF21 gene therapy reduces adipose tissue macrophage (ATM) inflammation. (a) Representative FACS plot of ATMs in gWAT. (b) ATMs as a percentage of immune cells. (c) Frequency of CD11c+, CD206– M1 ATMs. (d) Frequency of CD11c–, CD206+ M2 ATMs. (e) Frequency of CD11c+, CD206+ double-positive ATMs. n = 5 for Rec2-Empty, n = 7 for Rec2-FGF21. Error bars, SEM. *$P<0.05$, ***$P<0.001$. Reprinted from Queen *et al.* Visceral adipose tissue-directed FGF21 gene therapy improves metabolic and immune health in BTBR mice. Mol Ther Methods Clin Dev 2020, 20, 409–422, with permission of American Society of Gene & Cell Therapy.

gene expression of pro-inflammatory cytokines and inflammasome components in VAT adipocytes, all indicating reduced local inflammation in VAT under obesogenic conditions.[197] The alleviation of VAT inflammation is sufficient to lessen systemic chronic inflammation that is implicated in a wide variety of chronic diseases beyond obesity and type 2 diabetes.

In addition to obesity, diabetes, and nonalcoholic steatohepatitis individuals,[222] aging is considered as an indication for FGF21-related therapeutics. Davidsohn and colleagues recently report a combination gene therapy based on three longevity associated genes (FGF21, β-Klotho, soluble form of transforming growth factor-β receptor 2) to treat multiple age-related diseases.[216] Adipose tissue dysfunction is considered a key driver of systemic aging by causing a systemic pro-inflammatory state and multi-organ dysfunction. The age-related pathophysiology often mirrors the pathologies associated with obesity.[223] Consequently, we are compelled to ask whether a VAT-directed FGF21 gene therapy could benefit healthy aging. A long-term study is underway to examine the effects on health span and life span in middle-aged mice treated with a single dose of AS/Rec2-FGF21.

Summary

This chapter focuses on AAV-based gene therapy approaches for obesity and associated metabolic disorders targeting either the CNS or the adipose tissue. One example of the hypothalamus-directed gene therapy is AAV-mediated gene transfer of BDNF, which has been shown to be highly effective in animal models of both diet-induced and genetic obesity. The development of an autoregulatory AAV system is expected to improve the safety and translatability of BDNF gene therapy. The entire system can be packaged into a single rAAV vector allowing efficient delivery. This autoregulatory approach mimics the body's natural feedback systems to achieve self-regulation of the level of therapeutic gene expression according to its therapeutic outcomes. In several mouse models of obesity, AAV-mediated autoregulatory BDNF gene therapy leads to a sustainable plateau of body weight after substantial weight loss is achieved and minimizes adverse events associated with extreme weight loss. Future research will further assess the translational potential of the BDNF gene therapy for genetic forms of obesity.

As one of the largest organs, adipose tissues play important roles in physiology and pathologies of multiple diseases not limited to obesity. Yet, adipose tissues have been ignored as a target for gene therapy while far more investigations focus on liver and muscle as peripheral gene delivery targets, largely due to lack of efficient gene delivery vehicles to adipose tissue. In a review article,[20] we summarize recent progress in developing AAV systems with improved selectivity and efficiency for adipose tissue. These strategies include generating adipo-tropic serotypes and engineering transgene expression cassettes. An engineered hybrid serotype Rec2 displays high transduction efficacy to adipose tissue superior than naturally occurring serotypes. An interesting feature of Rec2 serotype is that its tissue tropism depends on administration route: intravenous injection predominantly transducing liver; oral administration favoring distal BAT; intraperitoneal injection transducing all visceral fat depots and liver. Incorporating a regulatory cassette can severely restricts transgene expression in liver while maintains high level transgene expression in visceral adipose depots. These promising developments are expected to stimulate interest in research of adipose-oriented gene therapy not only for obesity and metabolic disorders but also for other indications that may benefits from continuous secretion of therapeutic molecules.

Adipose-oriented gene therapy is in the infancy. As the vast majority of peripheral gene therapies target liver or muscle, the advantages and disadvantages of such approaches are well characterized.[224] In contrast, the strengths and shortcomings of adipose tissue as a targeting tissue remain largely unknown. Currently, scarce or almost no data are available regarding long-term transgene expression, immune responses to either AAV capsids or transgene expressed in adipocytes, genome insertion risk, dynamic transgene expression in adipocytes during drastic change in response to nutritional demands and environmental cues, and other adverse effects. More efforts are needed to fill these gaps and address the many challenges in order to develop optimal AAV vector tailored to adipose tissue and feasible to clinical applications.[20]

References

1. Mingozzi F, High KA. (2011) Therapeutic in vivo gene transfer for genetic disease using AAV: Progress and challenges. *Nat Rev Genet* **12**:341–355.
2. Domenger C, Grimm D. (2019) Next-generation AAV vectors — do not judge a virus (only) by its cover. *Hum Mol Genet* **28**:R3–R14.
3. Keeler AM, Flotte TR. (2019) Recombinant adeno-associated virus gene therapy in light of luxturna (and zolgensma and glybera): Where are we, and how did we get here? *Annu Rev Virol* **6**: 601–621.
4. Gruntman AM, Flotte TR. (2018) The rapidly evolving state of gene therapy. *FASEB J* **32**:1733–1740.
5. Atchison RW, Casto BC, Hammon WM. (1965) Adenovirus-associated defective virus particles. *Science* **149**:754–756.
6. Hoggan MD, Blacklow NR, Rowe WP. (1966) Studies of small DNA viruses found in various adenovirus preparations: Physical, biological, and immunological characteristics. *Proc Natl Acad Sci U S A* **55**:1467–1474.
7. Blacklow NR, Hoggan MD, Rowe WP. (1967) Isolation of adenovirus-associated viruses from man. *Proc Natl Acad Sci U S A* **58**:1410–1415.
8. Colella P, Ronzitti G, Mingozzi F. (2018) Emerging issues in AAV-mediated in vivo gene therapy. *Mol Ther Methods Clin Dev* **8**:87–104.
9. Sonntag F, Köther K, Schmidt K, *et al.* (2011) The assembly-activating protein promotes capsid assembly of different adeno-associated virus serotypes. *J Virol* **85**:12686–12697.
10. King JA, Dubielzig R, Grimm D, Kleinschmidt JA. (2001) DNA helicase-mediated packaging of adeno-associated virus type 2 genomes into preformed capsids. *EMBO J* **20**:3282–3291.
11. Surosky RT, Urabe M, Godwin SG, *et al.* (1997) Adeno-associated virus Rep proteins target DNA sequences to a unique locus in the human genome. *J Virol* **71**:7951–7959.
12. Pipe S, Leebeek FWG, Ferreira V, *et al.* (2019) Clinical considerations for capsid choice in the development of liver-targeted AAV-based gene transfer. *Mol Ther Methods Clin Dev* **15**:170–178.

13. Gao GP, Alvira MR, Wang L, *et al.* (2002) Novel adeno-associated viruses from rhesus monkeys as vectors for human gene therapy. *Proc Natl Acad Sci U S A* **99**:11854–11859.

14. Gao G, Vandenberghe LH, Alvira MR, *et al.* (2004) Clades of Adeno-associated viruses are widely disseminated in human tissues. *J Virol* **78**:6381–6388.

15. Kvaratskhelia M, Sharma A, Larue RC, *et al.* (2014) Molecular mechanisms of retroviral integration site selection. *Nucleic Acids Res* **42**:10209–10225.

16. Chandler RJ, LaFave MC, Varshney GK, *et al.* (2015) Vector design influences hepatic genotoxicity after adeno-associated virus gene therapy. *J Clin Invest* **125**:870–880.

17. von Kalle C, Deichmann A, Schmidt M. (2014) Vector integration and tumorigenesis. *Hum Gene Ther* **25**:475–481.

18. Samulski RJ, Muzyczka N. (2014) AAV-mediated gene therapy for research and therapeutic purposes. *Annu Rev Virol* **1**:427–451.

19. Wang D, Tai PWL, Gao G. (2019) Adeno-associated virus vector as a platform for gene therapy delivery. *Nat Rev Drug Discov* **18**:358–378.

20. Bates R, Huang W, Cao L. (2020) Adipose tissue: An emerging target for Adeno-associated viral vectors. *Mol Ther Methods Clin Dev* **19**:236–249.

21. Bhaskaran K, Douglas I, Forbes H, *et al.* (2014) Body-mass index and risk of 22 specific cancers: A population-based cohort study of 5.24 million UK adults. *Lancet* **384**:755–765.

22. Luppino FS, de Wit LM, Bouvy PF, *et al.* (2010) Overweight, obesity, and depression: A systematic review and meta-analysis of longitudinal studies. *Arch Gen Psychiatry* **67**:220–229.

23. Anghel SI, Wahli W. (2007) Fat poetry: A kingdom for PPARgamma. *Cell Res* **17**:486–511.

24. TOE Panel. (2013) *Managing Overweight and Obesity in Adults: Systematic Evidence Review from the Obesity Expert Panel.* National Heart, Lung, and Blood Institute, Bethesda, MD.

25. Hales CM, Fryar CD, Ogden CL. (2017) *Prevalence of Obesity Among Adults and Youth: United States, 2015-2016.* NCHS data brief. National Center for Health Statistics, Hyattsville, MD.

26. Finkelstein EA, Trogdon JG, Cohen JW, Dietz W. (2009) Annual medical spending attributable to obesity: Payer-and service-specific estimates. *Health Aff (Millwood)* **28**:w822–831.

27. Wadden TA, Butryn ML, Hong PS, Tsai AG. (2014) Behavioral treatment of obesity in patients encountered in primary care settings: A systematic review. *JAMA* **312**:1779–1791.

28. Kushner RF, Ryan DH. (2014) Assessment and lifestyle management of patients with obesity: Clinical recommendations from systematic reviews. *JAMA* **312**:943–952.

29. Yanovski SZ, Yanovski JA. (2014) Long-term drug treatment for obesity: A systematic and clinical review. *JAMA* **311**:74–86.

30. Knowler WC, Fowler SE, Hamman RF, *et al.* (2009) 10-year follow-up of diabetes incidence and weight loss in the Diabetes Prevention Program Outcomes Study. *Lancet* **374**:1677–1686.

31. Sjostrom L, Narbro K, Sjöström CD, *et al.* (2007) Effects of bariatric surgery on mortality in Swedish obese subjects. *N Engl J Med* **357**:741–752.

32. Courcoulas AP, Yanovski SZ, Bonds D, *et al.* (2014) Long-term outcomes of bariatric surgery: A National Institutes of Health symposium. *JAMA Surg* **149**:1323–1329.

33. Puzziferri N, Roshek TB, 3rd, Mayo HG, *et al.* (2014) Long-term follow-up after bariatric surgery: A systematic review. *JAMA* **312**:934–942.

34. Puzziferri N, Nakonezny PA, Livingston EH, *et al.* (2008) Variations of weight loss following gastric bypass and gastric band. *Ann Surg* **248**:233–242.

35. Courcoulas AP, Christian NJ, Belle SH, *et al.* (2013) Weight change and health outcomes at 3 years after bariatric surgery among individuals with severe obesity. *JAMA* **310**:2416–2425.

36. Arterburn D, Wellman R, Emiliano A, *et al.* (2018) Comparative effectiveness and safety of bariatric procedures for weight loss: A PCORnet Cohort Study. *Ann Intern Med* **169**:741–750.

37. McPhee SW, Janson CG, Li C, *et al.* (2006) Immune responses to AAV in a phase I study for Canavan disease. *J Gene Med* **8**:577–588.

38. Worgall S, Sondhi D, Hackett NR, *et al.* (2008) Treatment of late infantile neuronal ceroid lipofuscinosis by CNS administration of a

serotype 2 adeno-associated virus expressing CLN2 cDNA. *Hum Gene Ther* **19**:463–474.

39. Marks WJ, Jr., Ostrem JL, Verhagen L, *et al.* (2008) Safety and tolerability of intraputaminal delivery of CERE-120 (adeno-associated virus serotype 2-neurturin) to patients with idiopathic Parkinson's disease: An open-label, phase I trial. *Lancet Neurol* **7**:400–408.

40. Kaplitt MG, Feigin A, Tang C, *et al.* (2007) Safety and tolerability of gene therapy with an adeno-associated virus (AAV) borne GAD gene for Parkinson's disease: An open label, phase I trial. *Lancet* **369**:2097–2105.

41. Beretta E, Dube MG, Kalra PS, Kalra SP. (2002) Long-term suppression of weight gain, adiposity, and serum insulin by central leptin gene therapy in prepubertal rats: Effects on serum ghrelin and appetite-regulating genes. *Pediatr Res* **52**:189–198.

42. Boghossian S, Ueno N, Dube MG, *et al.* (2007). Leptin gene transfer in the hypothalamus enhances longevity in adult monogenic mutant mice in the absence of circulating leptin. *Neurobiol Aging* **28**:1594–1604

43. Couturier C, Sarkis C, Séron K, *et al.* (2007) Silencing of OB-RGRP in mouse hypothalamic arcuate nucleus increases leptin receptor signaling and prevents diet-induced obesity. *Proc Natl Acad Sci USA* **104**:19476–19481.

44. Keen-Rhinehart E, Kalra SP, Kalra PS. (2005) AAV-mediated leptin receptor installation improves energy balance and the reproductive status of obese female Koletsky rats. *Peptides* **26**:2567–2578.

45. Lundberg C, Jungles SJ, Mulligan RC. (2001) Direct delivery of leptin to the hypothalamus using recombinant adeno-associated virus vectors results in increased therapeutic efficacy. *Nat Biotechnol* **19**:169–172.

46. Morton GJ, Niswender KD, Rhodes CJ, *et al.* (2003) Arcuate nucleus-specific leptin receptor gene therapy attenuates the obesity phenotype of Koletsky (fa(k)/fa(k)) rats. *Endocrinology* **144**:2016–2024.

47. Dhillon H, Kalra SP, Prima V, *et al.* (2001) Central leptin gene therapy suppresses body weight gain, adiposity and serum insulin without affecting food consumption in normal rats: A long-term study. *Regul Pept* **99**:69–77.

48. Wilsey J, Zolotukhin S, Prima V, Scarpace PJ. (2003) Central leptin gene therapy fails to overcome leptin resistance associated with diet-induced obesity. *Am J Physiol Regul Integr Comp Physiol* **285**:R1011–1020.

49. Li G, Mobbs CV, Scarpace PJ. (2003) Central pro-opiomelanocortin gene delivery results in hypophagia, reduced visceral adiposity, and improved insulin sensitivity in genetically obese Zucker rats. *Diabetes* **52**:1951–1957.

50. Li G, Zhang Y, Wilsey JT, Scarpace PJ. (2005) Hypothalamic pro-opiomelanocortin gene delivery ameliorates obesity and glucose intolerance in aged rats. *Diabetologia* **48**:2376–2385.

51. Li G, Zhang Y, Cheng KY, Scarpace PJ. (2007). Lean rats with hypothalamic pro-opiomelanocortin overexpression exhibit greater diet-induced obesity and impaired central melanocortin responsiveness. *Diabetologia* **50**:1490–1499.

52. Herrera BM, Lindgren CM. (2010) The genetics of obesity. *Curr Diab Rep* **10**:498–505.

53. Speliotes EK, Willer CJ, Berndt SI, *et al.* (2010) Association analyses of 249,796 individuals reveal 18 new loci associated with body mass index. *Nat Genet* **42**:937–948.

54. Xu B, Goulding EH, Zang K, *et al.* (2003) Brain-derived neurotrophic factor regulates energy balance downstream of melanocortin-4 receptor. *Nat Neurosci* **6**:736–742.

55. Nicholson JR, Peter JC, Lecourt AC, *et al.* (2007) Melanocortin-4 receptor activation stimulates hypothalamic brain-derived neurotrophic factor release to regulate food intake, body temperature and cardiovascular function. *J Neuroendocrinol* **19**:974–982.

56. Bariohay B, Roux J, Tardivel C, *et al.* (2009) Brain-derived neurotrophic factor/tropomyosin-related kinase receptor type B signaling is a downstream effector of the brainstem melanocortin system in food intake control. *Endocrinology* **150**:2646–2653.

57. Caruso C, Carniglia L, Durand D, *et al.* (2013) Astrocytes: New targets of melanocortin 4 receptor actions. *J Mol Endocrinol* **51**:R33–50.

58. Stranahan AM, Arumugam TV, Mattson MP. (2011) Lowering corticosterone levels reinstates hippocampal brain-derived neurotropic factor and Trkb expression without influencing deficits in

hypothalamic brain-derived neurotropic factor expression in leptin receptor-deficient mice. *Neuroendocrinology* **93**:58–64.

59. Nakagawa T, Ono-Kishino M, Sugaru E, *et al.* (2002) Brain-derived neurotrophic factor (BDNF) regulates glucose and energy metabolism in diabetic mice. *Diabetes Metab Res Rev* **18**:185–191.

60. Kernie SG, Liebl DJ, Parada LF. (2000) BDNF regulates eating behavior and locomotor activity in mice. *EMBO J* **19**:1290–1300.

61. Lyons WE, Mamounas LA, Ricaurte GA, *et al.* (1999) Brain-derived neurotrophic factor-deficient mice develop aggressiveness and hyperphagia in conjunction with brain serotonergic abnormalities. *Proc Natl Acad Sci U S A* **96**:15239–15244.

62. Rios M, Fan G, Fekete C, *et al.* (2001) Conditional deletion of brain-derived neurotrophic factor in the postnatal brain leads to obesity and hyperactivity. *Mol Endocrinol* **15**:1748–1757.

63. Unger TJ, Calderon GA, Bradley LC, *et al.* (2007) Selective deletion of Bdnf in the ventromedial and dorsomedial hypothalamus of adult mice results in hyperphagic behavior and obesity. *J Neurosci* **27**:14265–14274.

64. Han JC, Liu Q-R, Jones MP, *et al.* (2008) Brain-derived neurotrophic factor and obesity in the WAGR syndrome. *N Engl J Med* **359**:918–927.

65. Gray J, Yeo GSH, Cox JJ, *et al.* (2006) Hyperphagia, severe obesity, impaired cognitive function, and hyperactivity associated with functional loss of one copy of the brain-derived neurotrophic factor (BDNF) gene. *Diabetes* **55**:3366–3371.

66. Han JC, Muehlbauer MJ, Cui HN, *et al.* (2010) Lower brain-derived neurotrophic factor in patients with prader-willi syndrome compared to obese and lean control subjects. *J Clin Endocrinol Metab* **95**:3532–3536.

67. Jiao H, Arner P, Hoffstedt J, *et al.* (2011) Genome wide association study identifies KCNMA1 contributing to human obesity. *BMC Med Genomics* **4**:51.

68. Yeo GS, Hung C-CC, Rochford J, *et al.* (2004) A de novo mutation affecting human TrkB associated with severe obesity and developmental delay. *Nat Neurosci* **7**:1187–1189.

69. Pelleymounter MA, Cullen MJ, Wellman CL. (1995) Characteristics of BDNF-induced weight loss. *Exp Neurol* **131**:229–238.

70. Nakagawa T, Tsuchida A, Itakura Y, *et al.* (2000) Brain-derived neurotrophic factor regulates glucose metabolism by modulating energy balance in diabetic mice. *Diabetes* **49**:436–444.

71. Tonra JR, Ono M, Liu X, *et al.* (1999) Brain-derived neurotrophic factor improves blood glucose control and alleviates fasting hyperglycemia in C57BLKS-Lepr(db)/lepr(db) mice. *Diabetes* **48**:588–594.

72. Nakagawa T, Ogawa Y, Ebihara K, *et al.* (2003) Anti-obesity and anti-diabetic effects of brain-derived neurotrophic factor in rodent models of leptin resistance. *Int J Obes Relat Metab Disord* **27**:557–565.

73. Tsao D, Thomsen HK, Chou J, *et al.* (2008) TrkB agonists ameliorate obesity and associated metabolic conditions in mice. *Endocrinology* **149**:1038–1048.

74. Lin JC, Tsao D, Barras R, *et al.* (2008) Appetite enhancement and weight gain by peripheral administration of TrkB agonists in non-human primates. *PLoS One* **3**:e1900.

75. Perreault M, Feng G, Will S, *et al.* (2013) Activation of TrkB with TAM-163 results in opposite effects on body weight in rodents and non-human primates. *PLoS One* **8**:e62616.

76. Cao L, Liu X, Lin E-JD, *et al.* (2010) Environmental and genetic activation of a brain-adipocyte BDNF/leptin axis causes cancer remission and inhibition. *Cell* **142**:52–64.

77. Cao L, Choi EY, Liu X, *et al.* (2011) White to brown fat phenotypic switch induced by genetic and environmental activation of a hypothalamic-adipocyte axis. *Cell Metab* **14**:324–338.

78. Cao L, Lin E-JD, Cahill MC, *et al.* (2009) Molecular therapy of obesity and diabetes by a physiological autoregulatory approach. *Nat Med* **15**:447–454.

79. Brown AM, Mayfield DK, Volaufova J, Argyropoulos G. (2001) The gene structure and minimal promoter of the human agouti related protein. *Gene* **277**:231–238.

80. Li XG, Okada T, Kodera M, *et al.* (2006) Viral-mediated temporally controlled dopamine production in a rat model of Parkinson disease. *Mol Ther* **13**:160–166.

81. Kaspar BK, Vissel B, Bengoechea T, *et al.* (2002) Adeno-associated virus effectively mediates conditional gene modification in the brain. *Proc Natl Acad Sci U S A* **99**:2320–2325.

82. Simonson DC, DeFronzo RA. (1990) Indirect calorimetry: Methodological and interpretative problems. *Am J Physiol* **258**:E399–412.

83. Ramos-Jimenez A, Hernández-Torres RP, Torres-Durán PV, *et al.* (2008) The respiratory exchange ratio is associated with fitness indicators both in trained and untrained men: A possible application for people with reduced exercise tolerance. *Clin Med Circ Respirat Pulm Med* **2**:1–9.

84. Reid IR. (2008) Relationships between fat and bone. *Osteoporos Int* **19**:595–606.

85. Le Bec C, Douar AM. (2006) Gene therapy progress and prospects– vectorology: Design and production of expression cassettes in AAV vectors. *Gene Ther* **13**:805–813.

86. Stieger K, Le Meur G, Lasne F, *et al.* (2006) Long-term doxycycline-regulated transgene expression in the retina of nonhuman primates following subretinal injection of recombinant AAV vectors. *Mol Ther* **13**:967–975.

87. Jiang L, Rampalli S, George D, *et al.* (2004) Tight regulation from a single tet-off rAAV vector as demonstrated by flow cytometry and quantitative, real-time PCR. *Gene Ther* **11**:1057–1067.

88. Sohn J, Takahashi M, Okamoto S, *et al.* (2017) A single vector platform for high-level gene transduction of central neurons: Adeno-associated virus vector equipped with the Tet-Off system. *PLoS One* **12**:e0169611.

89. Nguyen M, Huan-Tu G, Gonzalez-Edick M, *et al.* (2007) Rapamycin-regulated control of antiangiogenic tumor therapy following rAAV-mediated gene transfer. *Mol Ther* **15**:912–920.

90. Ye X, Rivera VM, Zoltick P, *et al.* (1999) Regulated delivery of therapeutic proteins after in vivo somatic cell gene transfer. *Science (New York, N.Y)* **283**:88–91.

91. Lebherz C, Auricchio A, Maguire AM, *et al.* (2005) Long-term inducible gene expression in the eye via adeno-associated virus gene transfer in nonhuman primates. *Hum Gene Ther* **16**:178–186.

92. McMurphy T, Huang W, Liu X, *et al.* (2019) Hypothalamic gene transfer of BDNF promotes healthy aging in mice. *Aging Cell* **18**:e12846.

93. Siu JJ, Queen NJ, Liu X, *et al.* (2017) Molecular therapy of melanocortin-4-receptor obesity by an autoregulatory BDNF vector. *Mol Ther Methods Clin Dev* **7**:83–95.

94. Tao YX. (2010) The melanocortin-4 receptor: Physiology, pharmacology, and pathophysiology. *Endocr Rev* **31**:506–543.

95. Kuhnen P, Krude H, Biebermann H. (2019) Melanocortin-4 receptor signalling: Importance for weight regulation and obesity treatment. *Trends Mol Med* **25**:136–148.

96. Farooqi IS, Keogh JM, Yeo GSH, *et al.* (2003) Clinical spectrum of obesity and mutations in the melanocortin 4 receptor gene. *N Engl J Med* **348**:1085–1095.

97. Alharbi KK, Spanakis E, Tan K, *et al.* (2007) Prevalence and functionality of paucimorphic and private MC4R mutations in a large, unselected European British population, scanned by meltMADGE. *Hum Mutat* **28**:294–302.

98. Saeed S, Bonnefond A, Manzoor J, *et al.* (2015) Genetic variants in LEP, LEPR, and MC4R explain 30% of severe obesity in children from a consanguineous population. *Obesity (Silver Spring)* **23**:1687–1695.

99. Calton MA, Ersoy BA, Zhang S, *et al.* (2009) Association of functionally significant Melanocortin-4 but not Melanocortin-3 receptor mutations with severe adult obesity in a large North American case-control study. *Hum Mol Genet* **18**:1140–1147.

100. Lubrano-Berthelier C, Dubern B, Lacorte J-M, *et al.* (2006) Melanocortin 4 receptor mutations in a large cohort of severely obese adults: Prevalence, functional classification, genotype-phenotype relationship, and lack of association with binge eating. *J Clin Endocrinol Metab* **91**:1811–1818.

101. Farooqi S, O'Rahilly S. (2006) Genetics of obesity in humans. *Endocr Rev* **27**:710–718.

102. Reinehr T, Hebebrand J, Friedel S, *et al.* (2009) Lifestyle intervention in obese children with variations in the melanocortin 4 receptor gene. *Obesity (Silver Spring)* **17**:382–389.

103. Hatoum IJ, Stylopoulos N, Vanhoose AM, *et al.* (2012) Melano-cortin-4 receptor signaling is required for weight loss after gastric bypass surgery. *J Clin Endocrinol Metab* **97**:E1023–1031.
104. Aslan IR, Ranadive SA, Ersoy BA, *et al.* (2011) Bariatric surgery in a patient with complete MC4R deficiency. *Int J Obes (Lond)* **35**:457–461.
105. Aslan IR, Campos GM, Calton MA, *et al.* (2011) Weight loss after Roux-en-Y gastric bypass in obese patients heterozygous for MC4R mutations. *Obes Surg* **21**:930–934.
106. Potoczna N, Branson R, Kral JG, *et al.* (2004) Gene variants and binge eating as predictors of comorbidity and outcome of treatment in severe obesity. *J Gastrointest Surg* **8**:971–981; discussion 981–972.
107. Censani M, Conroy R, Deng L, *et al.* (2014) Weight loss after bariatric surgery in morbidly obese adolescents with MC4R mutations. *Obesity (Silver Spring)* **22**:225–231.
108. Elkhenini HF, New JP, Syed AA. (2014) Five-year outcome of bariatric surgery in a patient with melanocortin-4 receptor mutation. *Clin Obes* **4**:121–124.
109. Chang SH, Stoll CRT, Song J, *et al.* (2014) The effectiveness and risks of bariatric surgery: An updated systematic review and meta-analysis, 2003-2012. *JAMA Surg* **149**:275–287.
110. Becker DA, Balcer LJ, Galetta SL. (2012) The neurological complications of nutritional deficiency following bariatric surgery. *J Obes* **2012**:608534.
111. Yeo GSH, Chao DHM, Siegert A-M, *et al.* (2021) The melanocortin pathway and energy homeostasis: From discovery to obesity therapy. *Mol Metab* **48**:101206.
112. Benabid AL, Pollak P, Louveau A, *et al.* (1987) Combined (thalamotomy and stimulation) stereotactic surgery of the VIM thalamic nucleus for bilateral Parkinson disease. *Appl Neurophysiol* **50**:344–346.
113. Odekerken VJ, van Laar T, Staal MJ, *et al.* (2013) Subthalamic nucleus versus globus pallidus bilateral deep brain stimulation for advanced Parkinson's disease (NSTAPS study): A randomised controlled trial. *Lancet Neurol* **12**:37–44.

114. Meoni S, Fraix V, Castrioto A, *et al.* (2017) Pallidal deep brain stimulation for dystonia: A long term study. *J Neurol Neurosurg Psychiatry* **88**:960–967.

115. Barbe MT, Reker P, Hamacher S, *et al.* (2018) DBS of the PSA and the VIM in essential tremor: A randomized, double-blind, crossover trial. *Neurology* **91**:e543–e550.

116. Rezai AR, Machado AG, Deogaonkar M, *et al.* (2008) Surgery for movement disorders. *Neurosurgery* **62 Suppl** **2**:809–838; discussion 838–809.

117. Taghva A, Corrigan JD, Rezai AR. (2012) Obesity and brain addiction circuitry: Implications for deep brain stimulation. *Neurosurgery* **71**:224–238.

118. Formolo DA, Gaspar JM, Melo HM, *et al.* (2019) Deep brain stimulation for obesity: A review and future directions. *Front Neurosci* **13**:323.

119. Flier JS. (2004) Obesity wars: Molecular progress confronts an expanding epidemic. *Cell* **116**:337–350.

120. Balthasar N, Dalgaard LT, Lee CE, *et al.* (2005) Divergence of melanocortin pathways in the control of food intake and energy expenditure. *Cell* **123**:493–505.

121. Farooqi IS, Yeo GSH, Keogh JM, *et al.* (2000) Dominant and recessive inheritance of morbid obesity associated with melanocortin 4 receptor deficiency. *J Clin Invest* **106**:271–279.

122. Fothergill E, Guo J, Howard L, *et al.* (2016) Persistent metabolic adaptation 6 years after "The Biggest Loser" competition. *Obesity (Silver Spring)* **24**:1612–1619.

123. Thoenen H, Sendtner M. (2002) Neurotrophins: From enthusiastic expectations through sobering experiences to rational therapeutic approaches. *Nat Neurosci* **5 Suppl**: 1046–1050.

124. Tallam LS, Stec DE, Willis MA, *et al.* (2005) Melanocortin-4 receptor-deficient mice are not hypertensive or salt-sensitive despite obesity, hyperinsulinemia, and hyperleptinemia. *Hypertension* **46**:326–332.

125. Greenfield JR, Miller JW, Keogh JM, *et al.* (2009) Modulation of blood pressure by central melanocortinergic pathways. *N Engl J Med* **360**:44–52.

126. Elena G, Bruna C, Benedetta M, *et al.* (2012) Prader-willi syndrome: Clinical aspects. *J Obes* **2012**:13.

127. Burman P, Ritzen EM, Lindgren AC. (2001) Endocrine dysfunction in Prader-Willi syndrome: A review with special reference to GH. *Endocr Rev* **22**:787–799.

128. Carrel AL, Myers SE, Whitman BY, Allen DB. (2002) Benefits of long-term GH therapy in Prader-Willi syndrome: A 4-year study. *J Clin Endocrinol Metab* **87**:1581–1585.

129. Kim Y, Lee H-M, Xiong Y, *et al.* (2017) Targeting the histone methyl-transferase G9a activates imprinted genes and improves survival of a mouse model of Prader-Willi syndrome. *Nat Med* **23**:213–222.

130. Schaaf CP, Gonzalez-Garay ML, Xia F, *et al.* (2013) Truncating mutations of MAGEL2 cause Prader-Willi phenotypes and autism. *Nat Genet* **45**:1405.

131. Maillard J, Park S, Croizier S, *et al.* (2016) Loss of Magel2 impairs the development of hypothalamic Anorexigenic circuits. *Hum Mol Genet* **25**:3208–3215.

132. Oncul M, Dilsiz P, Ates Oz E, *et al.* (2018) Impaired melanocortin pathway function in Prader-Willi syndrome gene-Magel2 deficient mice. *Hum Mol Genet* **27**:3129–3136.

133. Mercer RE, Kwolek EM, Bischof JM, *et al.* (2009) Regionally reduced brain volume, altered serotonin neurochemistry, and abnormal behavior in mice null for the circadian rhythm output gene Magel2. *Am J Med Genet B Neuropsychiatr Genet* **150b**: 1085–1099.

134. Bischof JM, Stewart CL, Wevrick R. (2007) Inactivation of the mouse Magel2 gene results in growth abnormalities similar to Prader-Willi syndrome. *Hum Mol Genet* **16**:2713–2719.

135. Tennese AA, Wevrick R. (2011) Impaired hypothalamic regulation of endocrine function and delayed counterregulatory response to hypoglycemia in Magel2-null mice. *Endocrinology* **152**:967–978.

136. Fountain MD, Tao H, Chen CA, *et al.* (2017) Magel2 knockout mice manifest altered social phenotypes and a deficit in preference for social novelty. *Genes Brain Behav* **16**:592–600.

137. Matharu N, Rattanasopha S, Tamura S, *et al.* (2019) CRISPR-mediated activation of a promoter or enhancer rescues obesity caused by haploinsufficiency. *Science* **363**:eaau0629.

138. Huang N, Lee I, Marcotte EM, Hurles ME. (2010) Characterising and predicting haploinsufficiency in the human genome. *PLoS Genet* **6**:e1001154.

139. Dang VT, Kassahn KS, Marcos AE, Ragan MA. (2008) Identification of human haploinsufficient genes and their genomic proximity to segmental duplications. *Eur J Hum Genet* **16**:1350–1357.

140. Landrum MJ, Lee JM, Benson M, *et al.* (2016) ClinVar: Public archive of interpretations of clinically relevant variants. *Nucleic Acids Res* **44**:D862–868.

141. Lau CH, Suh Y. (2018) In vivo epigenome editing and transcriptional modulation using CRISPR technology. *Transgenic Res* **27**:489–509.

142. Krashes MJ, Lowell BB, Garfield AS. (2016) Melanocortin-4 receptor-regulated energy homeostasis. *Nat Neurosci* **19**:206–219.

143. Ramachandrappa S, Raimondo A, Cali AMG, *et al.* (2013) Rare variants in single-minded 1 (SIM1) are associated with severe obesity. *J Clin Invest* **123**:3042–3050.

144. Michaud JL, Boucher F, Melnyk A, *et al.* (2001) Sim1 haploinsufficiency causes hyperphagia, obesity and reduction of the paraventricular nucleus of the hypothalamus. *Hum Mol Genet* **10**:1465–1473.

145. Nord AS, Blow MJ, Attanasio C, *et al.* (2013) Rapid and pervasive changes in genome-wide enhancer usage during mammalian development. *Cell* **155**:1521–1531.

146. Montefiori LE, Nobrega MA. (2019) Gene therapy for pathologic gene expression. *Science* **363**:231–232.

147. Mizukami H, Mimuro J, Ogura T, *et al.* (2006) Adipose tissue as a novel target for in vivo gene transfer by adeno-associated viral vectors. *Hum Gene Ther* **17**:921–928.

148. Zhang FL, Jia SQ, Zheng SP, Ding W. (2011) Celastrol enhances AAV1-mediated gene expression in mice adipose tissues. *Gene Ther* **18**:128–134.

149. Jimenez V, Muñoz S, Casana E, *et al.* (2013) In vivo adeno-associated viral vector-mediated genetic engineering of white and brown adipose tissue in adult mice. *Diabetes* **62**:4012–4022.

150. O'Neill SM, Hinkle C, Chen S-J, *et al.* (2014) Targeting adipose tissue via systemic gene therapy. *Gene Ther* **21**:653–661.

151. Jimenez V, Jambrina C, Casana E, *et al.* (2018) FGF21 gene therapy as treatment for obesity and insulin resistance. *EMBO Mol Med* **10**:e8791.

152. Li C, Samulski RJ. (2020) Engineering adeno-associated virus vectors for gene therapy. *Nat Rev Genet* **21**:255–272.

153. Wen J, Friedman JR. (2012) miR-122 regulates hepatic lipid metabolism and tumor suppression. *J Clin Invest* **122**:2773–2776.

154. Geisler A, Jungmann A, Kurreck J, *et al.* (2011) microRNA122-regulated transgene expression increases specificity of cardiac gene transfer upon intravenous delivery of AAV9 vectors. *Gene Ther* **18**:199–209.

155. Esau C, Davis S, Murray SF, *et al.* (2006) miR-122 regulation of lipid metabolism revealed by in vivo antisense targeting. *Cell Metab* **3**:87–98.

156. Liu X, McMurphy T, Xiao R, *et al.* (2014) Hypothalamic gene transfer of BDNF inhibits breast cancer progression and metastasis in middle age obese mice. *Mol Ther* **22**:1275–1284.

157. Zhu Y, Gao Y, Tao C, *et al.* (2016) Connexin 43 mediates white adiposetTissue beiging by facilitating the propagation of sympathetic neuronal signals. *Cell Metab* **24**:420–433.

158. Ng R, Hussain NA, Zhang Q, *et al.* (2017) miRNA-32 drives brown fat thermogenesis and trans-activates subcutaneous white fat browning in mice. *Cell Rep* **19**:1229–1246.

159. Zhang Y, Xie L, Gunasekar SK, *et al.* (2017) SWELL1 is a regulator of adipocyte size, insulin signalling and glucose homeostasis. *Nat Cell Biol* **19**:504–517.

160. Huang W, Queen NJ, McMurphy TB, *et al.* (2019) Adipose PTEN regulates adult adipose tissue homeostasis and redistribution via a PTEN-leptin-sympathetic loop. *Mol Metab* **30**:48–60.

161. Huang W, Liu X, Queen NJ, Cao L. (2017) Targeting visceral fat by intraperitoneal delivery of novel AAV serotype vector restricting off-target transduction in liver. *Mol Ther Methods Clin Dev* **6**:68–78.

162. Charbel Issa P, De Silva SR, Lipinski DM, *et al.* (2013) Assessment of tropism and effectiveness of new primate-derived hybrid recombinant AAV serotypes in the mouse and primate retina. *PLoS One* **8**:e60361.

163. Liu X, Magee D, Wang C, *et al.* (2014) Adipose tissue insulin receptor knockdown via a new primate-derived hybrid recombinant AAV serotype. *Mol Ther Methods Clin Dev* **1**:8.

164. McMurphy TB, Huang W, Xiao R, *et al.* (2017) Hepatic expression of adenovirus 36 E4ORF1 improves glycemic control and promotes glucose metabolism through AKT activation. *Diabetes* **66**:358–371.

165. Huang W, McMurphy T, Liu X, *et al.* (2016) Genetic manipulation of brown fat via oral administration of an engineered recombinant Adeno-associated viral serotype vector. *Mol Ther* **24**:1062–1069.

166. During MJ, Liu X, Huang W, *et al.* (2015) Adipose VEGF links the white-to-brown fat switch with environmental, genetic, and pharmacological stimuli in male mice. *Endocrinology* **156**:2059–2073.

167. Steel JC, Pasquale GD, Ramlogan CA, *et al.* (2013) Oral vaccination with adeno-associated virus vectors expressing the Neu oncogene inhibits the growth of murine breast cancer. *Mol Ther* **21**:680–687.

168. Xin KQ, Ooki T, Mizukami H, *et al.* (2002) Oral administration of recombinant adeno-associated virus elicits human immunodeficiency virus-specific immune responses. *Hum Gene Ther* **13**:1571–1581.

169. Mouri A, Noda Y, Hara H, *et al.* (2007) Oral vaccination with a viral vector containing Abeta cDNA attenuates age-related Abeta accumulation and memory deficits without causing inflammation in a mouse Alzheimer model. *FASEB J* **21**:2135–2148.

170. During MJ, Symes CW, Lawlor PA, *et al.* (2000) An oral vaccine against NMDAR1 with efficacy in experimental stroke and epilepsy. *Science* **287**:1453–1460.

171. Hao ZM, Cai M, Lv YF, *et al.* (2012) Oral administration of recombinant adeno-associated virus-mediated bone morphogenetic protein-7 suppresses CCl(4)-induced hepatic fibrosis in mice. *Mol Ther* **20**:2043–2051.

172. Di Pasquale G, Chiorini JA. (2006) AAV transcytosis through barrier epithelia and endothelium. *Mol Ther* **13**:506–516.

173. Chau YY, Bandiera R, Serrels A, *et al.* (2014) Visceral and subcutaneous fat have different origins and evidence supports a mesothelial source. *Nat Cell Biol* **16**:367–375.

174. Lafontan M, Berlan M. (2003) Do regional differences in adipocyte biology provide new pathophysiological insights? *Trends Pharmacol Sci* **24**:276–283.

175. Ibrahim MM. (2010) Subcutaneous and visceral adipose tissue: Structural and functional differences. *Obes Rev* **11**:11–18.

176. Zufferey R, Donello JE, Trono D, Hope TJ. (1999) Woodchuck hepatitis virus posttranscriptional regulatory element enhances expression of transgenes delivered by retroviral vectors. *J Virol* **73**: 2886–2892.

177. Loeb JE, Cordier WS, Harris ME, *et al.* (1999) Enhanced expression of transgenes from adeno-associated virus vectors with the woodchuck hepatitis virus posttranscriptional regulatory element: Implications for gene therapy. *Hum Gene Ther* **10**:2295–2305.

178. Queen NJ, Boardman AA, Patel RS, *et al.* (2020) Environmental enrichment improves metabolic and behavioral health in the BTBR mouse model of autism. *Psychoneuroendocrinology* **111**:104476.

179. Xiao R, Mansour AG, Huang W, *et al.* (2019) Adipocytes: A novel target for IL-15/IL-15Ralpha cancer gene therapy. *Mol Ther* **27**:922–932.

180. Montague CT, Farooqi IS, Whitehead JP, *et al.* (1997) Congenital leptin deficiency is associated with severe early-onset obesity in humans. *Nature* **387**:903–908.

181. Farooqi IS, Matarese G, Lord GM, *et al.* (2002) Beneficial effects of leptin on obesity, T cell hyporesponsiveness, and neuroendocrine/metabolic dysfunction of human congenital leptin deficiency. *J Clin Invest* **110**:1093–1103.

182. Gibson WT, Farooqi IS, Moreau M, *et al.* (2004) Congenital leptin deficiency due to homozygosity for the Delta133G mutation: Report of another case and evaluation of response to four years of leptin therapy. *J Clin Endocrinol Metab* **89**:4821–4826.

183. Oral EA, Simha V, Ruiz E, *et al.* (2002) Leptin-replacement therapy for lipodystrophy. *N Engl J Med* **346**:570–578.

184. Baldo BA. (2014) Side effects of cytokines approved for therapy. *Drug Saf* **37**:921–943.

185. Maffei M, Halaas J, Ravussin E, *et al.* (1995) Leptin levels in human and rodent: Measurement of plasma leptin and ob RNA in obese and weight-reduced subjects. *Nat Med* **1**:1155–1161.

186. Ingalls AM, Dickie MM, Snell GD. (1950) Obese, a new mutation in the house mouse. *J Hered* **41**:317–318.

187. Bray GA. (1991) Obesity, a disorder of nutrient partitioning: The MONA LISA hypothesis. *J Nutr* **121**:1146–1162.

188. Friedman J. (2016) The long road to leptin. *J Clin Invest* **126**:4727–4734.

189. Murphy JE, Zhou S, Giese K, *et al.* (1997) Long-term correction of obesity and diabetes in genetically obese mice by a single intramuscular injection of recombinant adeno-associated virus encoding mouse leptin. *Proc Natl Acad Sci U S A* **94**:13921–13926.

190. Farooqi IS, Jebb SA, Langmack G, *et al.* (1999) Effects of recombinant leptin therapy in a child with congenital leptin deficiency. *N Engl J Med* **341**:879–884.

191. Gaudet D, Méthot J, Déry S, *et al.* (2013) Efficacy and long-term safety of alipogene tiparvovec (AAV1-LPLS447X) gene therapy for lipoprotein lipase deficiency: An open-label trial. *Gene Ther* **20**:361–369.

192. Peyvandi F, Palla R, Menegatti M, *et al.* (2012) Coagulation factor activity and clinical bleeding severity in rare bleeding disorders: Results from the European Network of Rare Bleeding Disorders. *J Thromb Haemost* **10**:615–621.

193. Arruda VR, Stedman HH, Nichols TC, *et al.* (2005) Regional intravascular delivery of AAV-2-F.IX to skeletal muscle achieves long-term correction of hemophilia B in a large animal model. *Blood* **105**:3458–3464.

194. Yla-Herttuala S. (2012) Endgame: Glybera finally recommended for approval as the first gene therapy drug in the European union. *Mol Ther* **20**:1831–1832.

195. Agostini M, Schoenmakers E, Mitchell C, *et al.* (2006) Non-DNA binding, dominant-negative, human PPARgamma mutations cause lipodystrophic insulin resistance. *Cell Metab* **4**:303–311.

196. Cortes VA, Curtis DE, Sukumaran S, *et al.* (2009) Molecular mechanisms of hepatic steatosis and insulin resistance in the AGPAT2-deficient mouse model of congenital generalized lipodystrophy. *Cell Metab* **9**:165–176.

197. Queen NJ, Bates R, Huang W, *et al.* (2021) Visceral adipose tissue-directed FGF21 gene therapy improves metabolic and immune health in BTBR mice. *Mol Ther Methods Clin Dev* **20**:409–422.

198. Ogawa Y, Kurosu H, Yamamoto M, *et al.* (2007) BetaKlotho is required for metabolic activity of fibroblast growth factor 21. *Proc Natl Acad Sci USA* **104**:7432–7437.

199. Bookout AL, de Groot MHM, Owen BM, *et al.* (2013) FGF21 regulates metabolism and circadian behavior by acting on the nervous system. *Nat Med* **19**:1147–1152.

200. Véniant MM, Hale C, Helmering J, *et al.* (2012) FGF21 promotes metabolic homeostasis via white adipose and leptin in mice. *PLoS One* **7**:e40164.

201. Lin Z, Tian H, Lam KSL, *et al.* (2013) Adiponectin mediates the metabolic effects of FGF21 on glucose homeostasis and insulin sensitivity in mice. *Cell Metab* **17**:779–789.

202. Chen W, Hoo RL-C, Konishi M, *et al.* (2011) Growth hormone induces hepatic production of fibroblast growth factor 21 through a mechanism dependent on lipolysis in adipocytes. *J Biol Chem* **286**:34559–34566.

203. Ding X, Boney-Montoya J, Owen BM, *et al.* (2012). βKlotho is required for fibroblast growth factor 21 effects on growth and metabolism. *Cell Metab* **16**:387–393.

204. Adams AC, Yang C, Coskun T, *et al.* (2013) The breadth of FGF21's metabolic actions are governed by FGFR1 in adipose tissue. *Mol Metab* **2**:31–37.

205. Kharitonenkov A, Shiyanova TL, Koester A, *et al.* (2005) FGF-21 as a novel metabolic regulator. *J Clin Invest* **115**:1627–1635.

206. Chau MDL, Gao J, Yang Q, *et al.* (2010) Fibroblast growth factor 21 regulates energy metabolism by activating the AMPK–SIRT1–PGC-1α pathway. **107**:12553–12558.

207. Fisher FM, Kleiner S, Douris N, *et al.* (2012) FGF21 regulates PGC-1α and browning of white adipose tissues in adaptive thermogenesis. *Genes Dev* **26**:271–281.

208. Fisher FM, Maratos-Flier E. (2016) Understanding the physiology of FGF21. *Annu Rev Physiol* **78**:223–241.

209. Coskun T, Bina HA, Schneider MA, *et al.* (2008) Fibroblast growth factor 21 corrects obesity in mice. *Endocrinology* **149**:6018–6027.

210. Berglund ED, Li CY, Bina HA, *et al.* (2009) Fibroblast growth factor 21 controls glycemia via regulation of hepatic glucose flux and insulin sensitivity. *Endocrinology* **150**:4084–4093.

211. Kharitonenkov A, Adams AC. (2014) Inventing new medicines: The FGF21 story. *Mol Metab* **3**:221–229.

212. Zarei M, Pizarro-Delgado J, Barroso E, *et al.* (2020) Targeting FGF21 for the treatment of nonalcoholic steatohepatitis. *Trends Pharmacol Sci* **41**:199–208.

213. Gaich G, Chien JY, Fu H, *et al.* (2013) The effects of LY2405319, an FGF21 analog, in obese human subjects with type 2 diabetes. *Cell Metab* **18**:333–340.

214. Talukdar S, Zhou Y, Li D, *et al.* (2016) A long-acting FGF21 molecule, PF-05231023, decreases body weight and improves lipid profile in non-human primates and type 2 diabetic subjects. *Cell Metab* **23**:427–440.

215. Kim AM, Somayaji VR, Dong JQ, *et al.* (2017) Once-weekly administration of a long-acting fibroblast growth factor 21 analogue modulates lipids, bone turnover markers, blood pressure and body weight differently in obese people with hypertriglyceridaemia and in non-human primates. *Diabetes Obes Metab* **19**:1762–1772.

216. Davidsohn N, Pezone M, Vernet A, *et al.* (2019) A single combination gene therapy treats multiple age-related diseases. *Proc Natl Acad Sci U S A* **116**:23505–23511.

217. Shimomura I, Funahashi T, Takahashi M, *et al.* (1996) Enhanced expression of PAI-1 in visceral fat: Possible contributor to vascular disease in obesity. *Nat Med* **2**:800–803.

218. Juhan-Vague I, Alessi M-C, Mavri A, Morange PE. (2003) Plasminogen activator inhibitor-1, inflammation, obesity, insulin resistance and vascular risk. *J Thromb Haemost* **1**:1575–1579.

219. Tateya S, Tamori Y, Kawaguchi T, *et al.* (2010) An increase in the circulating concentration of monocyte chemoattractant protein-1 elicits systemic insulin resistance irrespective of adipose tissue inflammation in mice. *Endocrinology* **151**:971–979.

220. Lumeng CN, Bodzin JL, Saltiel AR. (2007) Obesity induces a phenotypic switch in adipose tissue macrophage polarization. *J Clin Invest* **117**:175–184.

221. Wentworth JM, Naselli G, Brown WA, *et al.* (2010) Pro-inflammatory CD11c+ CD206+ adipose tissue macrophages are associated with insulin resistance in human obesity. *Diabetes* **59**:1648–1656.

222. Degirolamo C, Sabba C, Moschetta A. (2016) Therapeutic potential of the endocrine fibroblast growth factors FGF19, FGF21 and FGF23. *Nat Rev Drug Discov* **15**:51–69.
223. Frasca D, Blomberg BB, Paganelli R. (2017) Aging, obesity, and inflammatory age-related diseases. *Front Immunol* **8**:1745.
224. Colella P, Ronzitti G, Mingozzi F. (2018) Emerging issues in AAV-mediated in vivo gene therapy. *Mol Ther Methods Clin Dev* **8**: 87–104.

Chapter 5

Hypothalamic-Sympathoneural-Adipocyte Axis Activation Targets Both Obesity and Cancer

Obesity Increases Cancer Risk and Mortality

The worldwide epidemic of obesity and global incidence of cancer are both rising.[1,2] Overweight and obesity are affecting one third of the world's population.[3] More alarmingly, 40 million children under the age of 5 were overweight or obese in 2019. Obesity is one of the most common etiological factors for chronic diseases.[4] In fact, overweight and obesity are leading risks for global deaths. Obesity increases the risk and morbidity of many types of cancer (postmenopausal breast, endometrial, renal, ovarian, esophagus, pancreas, prostate, hepatobiliary, and colorectal cancer).[5–9] Between 7% and 41% of certain cancer burdens are attributable to overweight and obesity. Obesity may account for 14% of all deaths from cancer, and 20% of those are in women.[9] It is estimated that obesity contributes to over 120,000 cancer-related deaths worldwide, increasing the risk of dying from cancer by 40% to 80%.[10–12]

Consequently, if people could maintain a normal body weight, many cancers could have been prevented. Unfortunately, sustained weight loss is not an easy task. Indeed, numerous studies have demonstrated that excessive weight gain can result in higher cancer rates, but the converse findings of weight loss causing lower cancer rates were much harder to find due to lack of successful weight loss modalities.[13,14] Lifestyle strategy and healthy diet can mitigate or slow the progression to obesity.[15] But both randomized and prospective

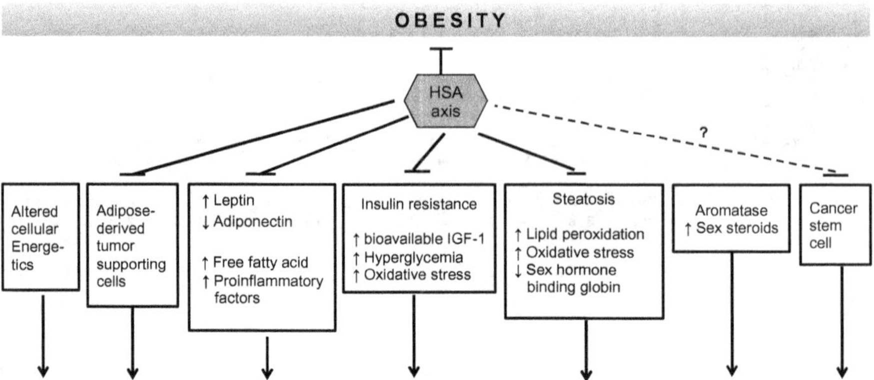

Fig. 5.1. Multiple mechanisms linking obesity to cancer can be inhibited by activating the hypothalamic-sympathoneural-adipocyte (HSA) axis.

studies demonstrate disappointing long-term outcome. Intensive lifestyle intervention achieves long-term weight loss in approximately 2% of obese diabetic patients with body mass index (BMI) of 30 at 10 years,[16] and is even less effective in patients with BMI above 35.[17] Metabolic or bariatric surgery can provide sustained weight loss,[18] and therefore help to establish a causal association between obesity and cancer. Longitudinal studies on bariatric surgery have demonstrated that successful weight loss lowers cancer rates and decreases cancer mortality.[17,19,20]

The mechanisms for the obesity–cancer association are multifactorial and include insulin resistance, increased growth factors and anabolic hormones, altered balance of adipokines, oxidative stress, inflammation, increased bioavailable sex hormones, deterioration in immune surveillance, and altered cellular energetic (**Fig. 5.1**).[21–23]

Hypothalamic-Sympathoneural-Adipocyte Axis Activation Targets Both Obesity and Cancer

As discussed in Chapters 2 and 3, we have used a mouse model of environmental enrichment (EE) to investigate how an active and engaging lifestyle influences metabolic health and cancer.[24–32] Our work has demonstrated that EE leads to anticancer and anti-obesity phenotypes via a specific neuroendocrine axis — hypothalamic-sympathoneural-adipocyte (HSA) axis.[24,25] EE stimulates brain-derived neurotrophic factor (BDNF) expression in the hypothalamus and thereby elevating the sympathetic tone preferentially to the white adipose tissue (WAT). The HSA axis activation leads to profound WAT remodeling, including reduced adipocyte size, induction of thermo-competent beige cells, and suppression of the production and release of leptin. These aspects of adipose remodeling are not interdependent but are all controlled by the β-adrenergic signaling.[24,25,28,33] The EE-induced anticancer and anti-obesity phenotypes are not attributable to physical exercise alone but can be largely reproduced by increasing BDNF expression in the hypothalamus.[24,25] Although not the sole component of the body's response to environmental stimuli, the HSA axis links physical and social environments to the regulation of adipose tissue function and energy balance, and thereby can influence the systemic internal environment through multi-organ crosstalk and ultimately alter cancer progression. Given the strong anticancer effects in animals of normal weight and the potent adipose remodeling in various models of obesity, we predict that the anticancer effect of HSA activation is likely to be even more robust in obese individuals.

In a B16 melanoma transplantation model, 3 weeks of EE results in approximate 70% decrease of melanoma mass in obese mice induced by high-fat diet feeding, a more pronounced effect compared to a 50% decrease in mice of normal weight in identical experimental setting except the diet.[24] The major adipokines, leptin and adiponectin, are recognized for their opposing influence on cancer risk and cancer biology.[34–36] Obesity is associated with higher leptin and lower adiponectin in circulation. Both animal and clinical data suggest that the altered balance of leptin to adiponectin — increased leptin/adiponectin ratio — may contribute to increased cancer risk associated with obesity.[37,38] Activation of the HSA axis leads to a reliable and sharp drop of leptin and sometimes a concomitant increase of adiponectin level, resulting in a favorable shift of leptin/adiponectin ratio. Our mechanistic studies have identified leptin as an important downstream component along with the HSA axis contributing to anticancer effect (see Chapter 2). In a follow-up study, we investigated the effects of EE on breast cancer development in obese models of varied leptin signaling.

Environmental Enrichment Inhibits Mammary Tumor Progression in Obesogenic Conditions

Breast cancer is the most common cancer for women worldwide,[39] and one of the leading causes of cancer-related deaths.[40,41] Obesity may be responsible for approximately one third of human mammary tumors.[42] Some clinical data suggest that weight loss reduces the risk of breast cancer for both pre- and postmenopausal women.[43] One study reports that a one unit reduction in BMI in the overweight and obese population can improve overall health and decrease the risk of colon and breast cancer.[44] Moreover, the cancer protective role of metabolic surgery is strongest for female obesity-related tumors.[22] We hypothesized that EE, a biobehavioral intervention highly effective in melanoma and colon cancer models, could influence breast cancer progression particularly in obesogenic conditions.

MMTV-PyMT Transgenic Mice

First, Grant Foglesong and colleagues used the mouse mammary tumor virus-the polyoma virus middle T antigen (MMTV-PyMT) transgenic mouse model to test the effects of EE on spontaneous breast cancer latency and growth.[45–47] PyMT is a potent oncogene. When driven by the MMTV long terminal repeat promoter/enhancer, its expression is restricted to the mammary tissue. The MMTV-PyMT transgenic mouse model has 100% of breast cancer penetrance in females positive for the transgene, and the mammary tumors become palpable at a predictable age. Although PyMT is not expressed in humans, the PyMT-induced tumors closely mimic the progression of human disease, therefore MMTV-PyMT transgenic mouse line is a widely used animal model to study breast cancer.

Hyperplasia of the mammary gland in MMTV-PyMT–positive mice becomes detectable as early as 3 weeks of age. Thus, EE and high fat diet (HFD) feeding (60% calorie from fat) were initiated immediately after weaning at an age of 3–4 weeks. Female MMTV-PyMT mice were randomized to live in either standard environment (SE) or EE for a total of 16 weeks. PyMT mice have been shown to somewhat resistant to diet-induced obesity (DIO). EE slightly slowed weight gain over the course of the study (**Fig. 5.2(a)**). Notably, 4 weeks of

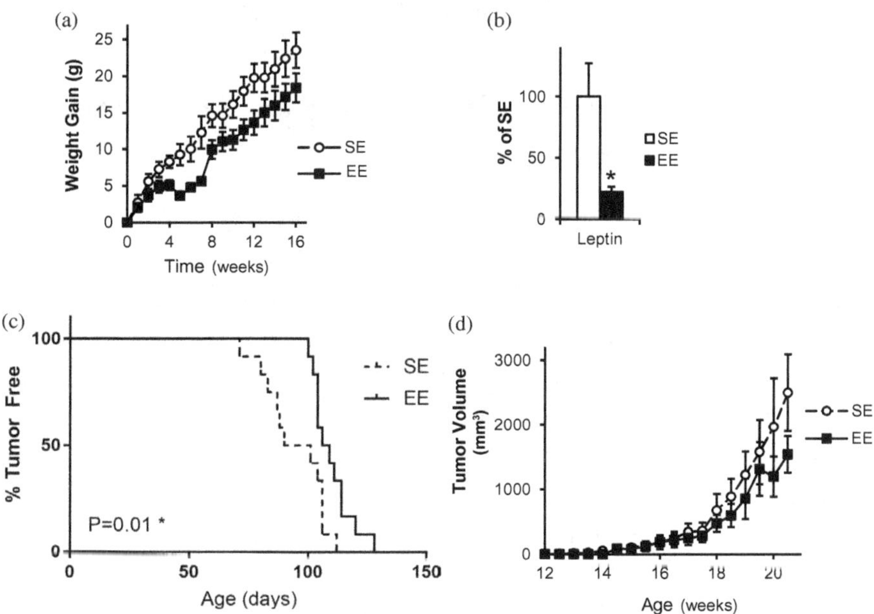

Fig. 5.2.　EE delays breast cancer onset in MMTV-PyMT transgenic mice fed a high-fat diet. (a) Weight gain. (b) Serum leptin levels 4 weeks post EE. (c) Kaplan-Meier analysis of latency of tum or occurrence. (d) Tumor volume. Data are mean ± SEM, *n* = 12 per group, *P* < 0.05. Reprinted from Foglesong *et al.* Enriched environment inhibits breast cancer progression in obese models with intact leptin signaling. Endocr Relat Cancer 2019, 5, 483–495, with permission of Bioscientifica Limited.

EE resulted in a significant decrease in circulating leptin level (**Fig. 5.2(b)**). The occurrence of mammary tumor was monitored daily by palpation. Mammary tumor latency was significantly lengthened in mice living in EE compared to their counterparts in SE, with a median difference of 12 days and the mean difference of 15 days (**Fig. 5.2(c)**). Tumor growth appeared to be slowed in EE but not reaching significance by the termination of the study (**Fig. 5.2(d)**).[48]

Tumor formation may occur in any or all of the 10 mammary glands in a MMTV-PyMT mouse. Once formed, the tumors progress very quickly, which may explain the large variability in the sum of tumor volume at study termination and the lack of significant difference. Nevertheless, EE resulted in significant inhibition on cancer onset in a highly aggressive form of breast cancer, suggesting implications in breast cancer prevention in obese individuals.

Wild Type Mice Engrafted with PyMT-Derived Primary Breast Cancer Cells

To investigate the effects of EE on mammary tumor growth, we shifted our focus to orthotopic transplantation models and also aimed to examine the role of leptin in tumorigenesis. Female C57BL/6 mice (6 weeks old) were randomly assigned to SE or EE housing, and fed with HFD. EE potently reduced HFD-induced weight gain and adiposity (**Fig. 5.3(a), (b)**). At 10-week EE, serum biomarkers showed a favorable pattern of change: an increase in adiponectin, decreases in leptin, triglyceride, and cholesterol, all indicating metabolic improvement (**Fig. 5.3(c)**). We harvested mammary tumors from a naïve female MMTV-PyMT mouse and isolated primary tumor cells. At 15-week EE, PyMT-derived mammary tumor cells were orthotopically implanted to the mammary gland. EE significantly inhibited the growth of engrafted mammary tumor (**Fig. 5.3(d)**).[48]

Gene expression profiling found EE upregulated the expression of *Bdnf*, its receptor *Ntrk2*, and other genes involved in regulation

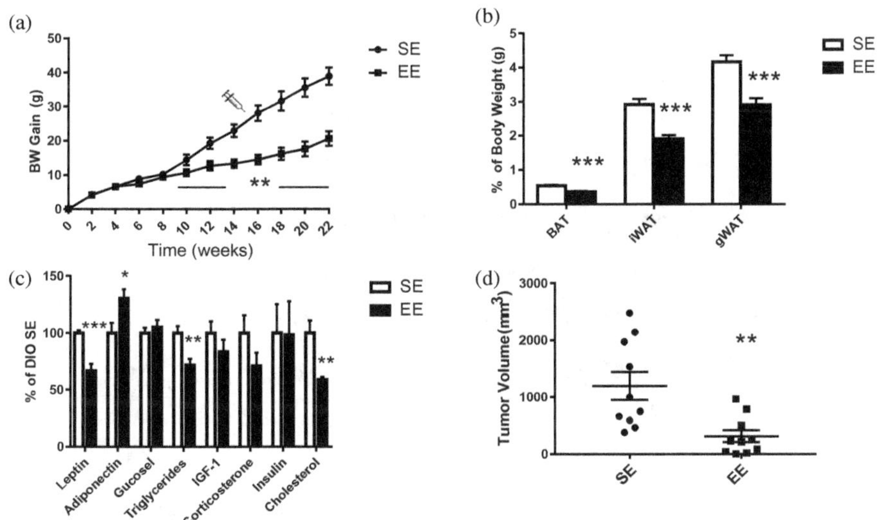

Fig. 5.3. EE attenuates DIO and mitigates breast cancer progression in wild type mice transplanted with PyMT-derived breast cancer cells. Mammary tumor cells were orthotopically implanted at 15-week EE. (a) Weight gain. Syringe indicates when tumor cells were inoculated. (b) Adiposity at euthanasia. (c) Serum biomarkers at euthanasia. (d) Tumor volume at euthanasia in DIO mice. Data are mean ± SEM, n = 10 per group, $*P < 0.05$, $**P < 0.01$, $***P < 0.001$. Reprinted from Foglesong *et al*. Enriched environment inhibits breast cancer progression in obese models with intact leptin signaling. Endocr Relat Cancer 2019, 5, 483–495, with permission of Bioscientifica Limited.

of energy homeostasis, meanwhile downregulated the expression of pro-inflammatory cytokines interleukin-1 and interleukin-6 in the hypothalamus. The messenger RNA (mRNA) levels of inflammatory markers such as plasminogen activator inhibitor-1 (*Pai-1*) and MCP-1 (encoded by *Ccl2*) were significantly suppressed in mammary fat.[48]

Leptin signaling has been implicated in breast cancer growth and progression.[49] Leptin binds to its receptor to activate multiple intracellular signaling including Janus kinase signal transducer and activator of transcription 3 (JAK2-STAT3), phosphatidylinositol 3-kinase-protein kinase B (PI3K-AKT), and mitogen-activated protein kinase (MAPK) pathways involved in various cellular activities.[50]

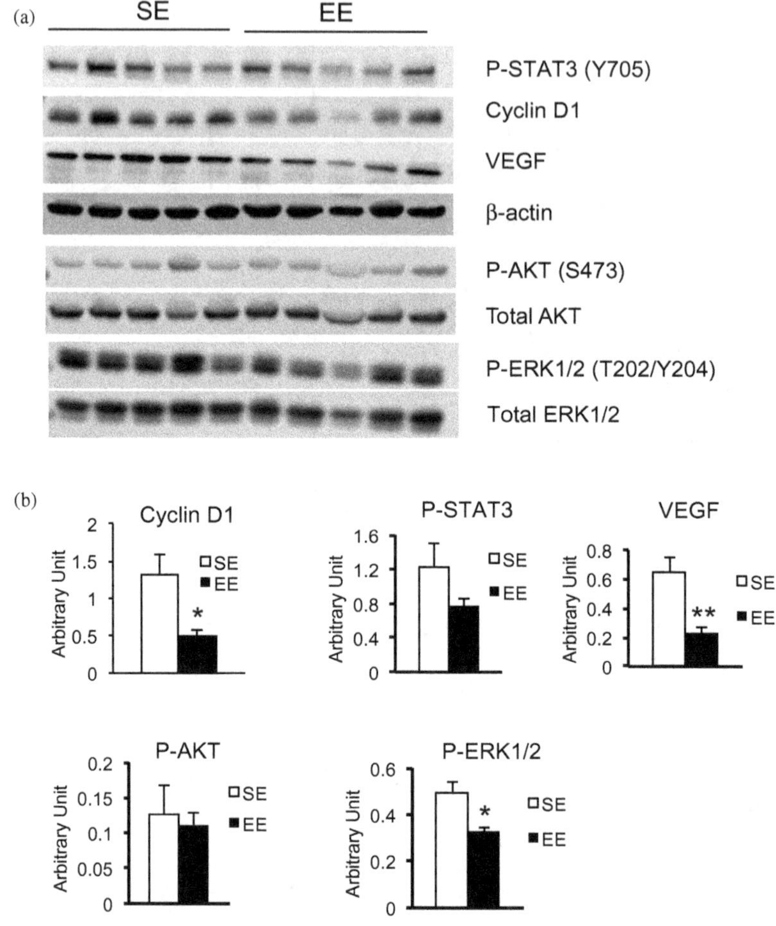

Fig. 5.4.   Western blotting of mammary tumors from DIO mice. (a) Western blotting. (b) Quantification of A. Data are mean ± SEM, $n = 5$ per group, *$P < 0.05$, ** $P < 0.01$. Reprinted from Foglesong *et al.* Enriched environment inhibits breast cancer progression in obese models with intact leptin signaling. En docr Relat Cancer 2019, 5, 483–495, with permission of Bioscientifica Limited.

We examined these signaling pathways in tumor samples from EE and SE mice by immunoblot (**Fig. 5.4**), and observed a trend of reduction of phospho-STAT3 together with a significant reduction of phospho-ERK1/2 signaling. Moreover, it is reported that leptin regulates Cyclin D1 in breast cancer cells *in vitro*[51] and in a transgenic mouse model of breast cancer.[52] The Cyclin D1 level in tumors from EE mice was significantly lower than those from SE mice consistent with slower tumor proliferation. Leptin has proangiogenic property, which is thought to contribute to tumor angiogenesis partially through induction of vascular endothelial growth factor (VEGF).[53,54] VEGF level was significantly reduced in EE tumors.[48]

Leptin-Deficient *ob/ob* Mice Engrafted with PyMT-Derived Primary Breast Cancer Cells

To test whether leptin is essential for EE effects on mammary tumorigenesis, leptin-deficient *ob/ob* mice were subjected to EE followed by orthotopic implantation of PyMT-derived primary breast cancer cells, mirroring the experiment conducted in wild type mice fed with HFD. EE exerted substantial metabolic benefits, including reduction of weight gain, improvement of glucose tolerance (**Fig. 5.5**), alleviation of hyperinsulinemia, and reduction of mammary fat mass. Of note, food consumption relative to body weight was higher in EE mice (**Fig. 5.5(b)**) suggesting reduced weight gain not due to suppression of food intake. Unexpectedly, *ob/ob* mice living in EE had significantly larger mammary tumors than their counterparts in SE (**Fig. 5.5(d)**), a finding opposite to that in wild type DIO mice (**Fig. 5.3(d)**).[48]

Gene expression analysis of the *ob/ob* mice showed a pattern distinct to DIO mice in the hypothalamus, mammary fat pads, and the tumors. For example, EE upregulated proangiogenic *Vegf* in the tumors, and pro-inflammatory *Il-1b* in the mammary fat, both opposing to the findings in DIO mice.[48]

Pathological examination found that tumors from EE *ob/ob* mice appeared to have larger areas of coagulative to liquefactive necrosis spanning multiple lobular structures and including the intervening stromal septa. Tumors from EE showed higher mitoses per field than that in SE group, but did not reach significance.[48]

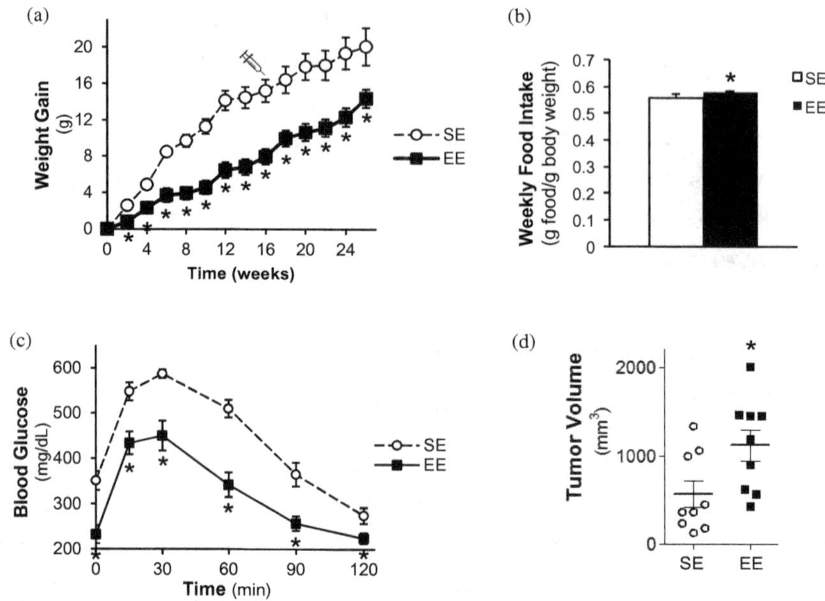

Fig. 5.5.   EE decreases weight gain and improves metabolism, but increases PyMT–derived breast cancer growth in the *ob/ob* mice fed a normal chow diet. (a) Weight gain; Syringe indicates when tumor cells were inoculated. (b) Food intake relative to body weight. (c) Glucose tolerance test. (d) Tumor volume at euthanasia. Data are mean ± SEM, $n = 9$ per group, $*P < 0.05$. Reprinted from Foglesong *et al.* Enriched environment inhibits breast cancer progression in obese models with intact leptin signaling. Endocr Relat Cancer 2019, 5, 483–495, with permission of Bioscientifica Limited.

Leptin, Breast Cancer, and EE

These results showed that both wild type DIO and *ob/ob* mice responded to EE displaying improved metabolism and attenuation of weight gain. However, the presence of functional leptin, specifically its drop following EE exposure, was necessary to impede PyMT-derived mammary tumor growth.[48] EE was effective at delaying the onset of spontaneous mammary tumor in the MMTV-PyMT mice, as well as suppressing engrafted PyMT-derived primary tumor growth in wild type DIO mice, both associated with a substantial drop in leptin levels. However, in the absence of functional leptin, EE accelerated

PyMT-derived mammary tumor progression in *ob/ob* mice, relative to SE. This result was unexpected and might seem paradoxical at first glance, but could be explained within the framework of the HSA axis activation.[24]

Our previous research reveals that activating the HSA axis preferentially increases sympathetic tone and norepinephrine release onto adipose tissue, a process essential to induce WAT remodeling, alleviation of obesity, and systemic metabolic improvements, as well as inhibitory effect on melanoma through the suppression of leptin production and release.[24,25] However, breast cancer is imbedded in mammary fat and therefore is directly exposed to the changes in leptin and norepinephrine within its microenvironment. Studies have demonstrated that stress hormones can modulate multiple components of the tumor microenvironment directly or indirectly to collectively support tumor initiation and progression.[55] Epinephrine and norepinephrine have been implicated in promoting the growth and metastatic potential of multiple types of cancer.[56]

We analyzed the amount of both stress hormones in the tumor, in the tumor-adjacent mammary fat, in the tumor-free mammary fat, and in the serum. Epinephrine is released predominantly from the adrenal medulla,[57] which has not been shown to be altered by EE or the HSA axis.[24] Consistent with previous findings, there was no change in epinephrine in response to EE exposure in either wild type DIO or *ob/ob* mice. Norepinephrine is released from sympathetic nerve terminal innervating various tissues including the adipose tissue.[58] EE increased norepinephrine levels in mammary fat and serum in the *ob/ob* mice but did not change in wild type DIO mice (**Fig. 5.6**), which might underscore the accelerated PyMT mammary tumor growth observed only in *ob/ob* mice. Notably, in our previous study when B16 melanoma cells were subcutaneously implanted to the flank of male *ob/ob* mice, EE had no effect on melanoma progression.[24] The inconsistency among different types of cancer might be caused by the location of tumor implantation: subcutaneous implantation of B16 melanoma cells distal to adipose

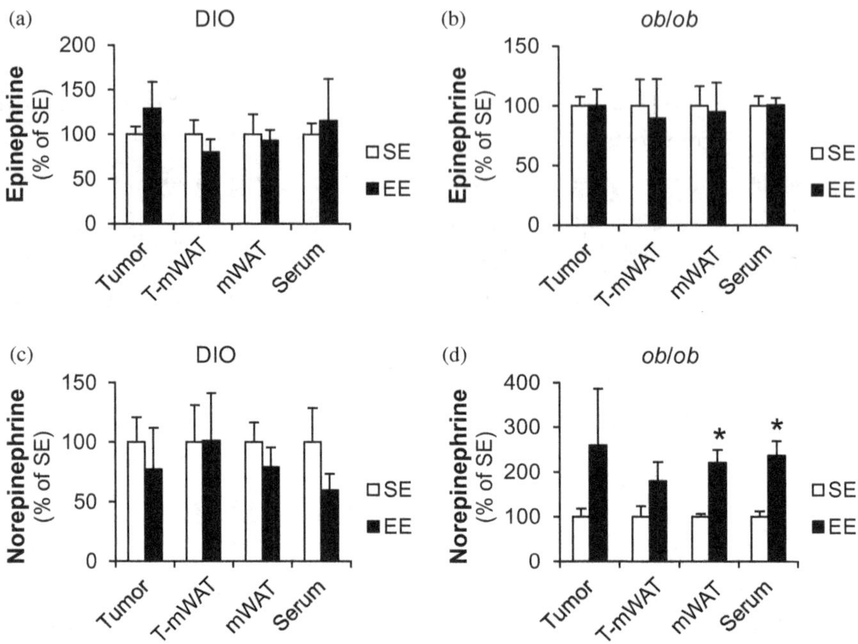

Fig. 5.6. Catecholamine analysis: (a) and (b), epinephrine; (c) and (d), norepinephrine, in tumor, tumor-associated mammary adipose tissue (T-mWAT), tumornaïve mammary adipose tissue (mWAT), and serum of wild type DIO mice and *ob/ob* mice on normal chow. Data are mean ± SEM, *n* = 9 per group, *P < 0.05. Reprinted from Foglesong *et al.* Enriched environment inhibits breast cancer progression in obese models with intact leptin signaling. Endocr Relat Cancer 2019, 5, 483–495, with permission of Bioscientifica Limited.

tissue versus direct mammary fat implantation of PyMT mammary tumor cells. But sex difference could not be ruled out.

Taken together, we propose that EE represents an active and sometimes challenging lifestyle,[26] serving as a unique and valuable model of eustress that is associated with adaptive responses and benign or beneficial effects on health.[59,60] In this framework, EE activates the HSA axis to stimulate norepinephrine release to adipose tissue, which in turn suppresses leptin production in adipose tissue leading to a substantial drop of circulating level of leptin.[24] We hypothesize that the overall impact on mammary tumor growth

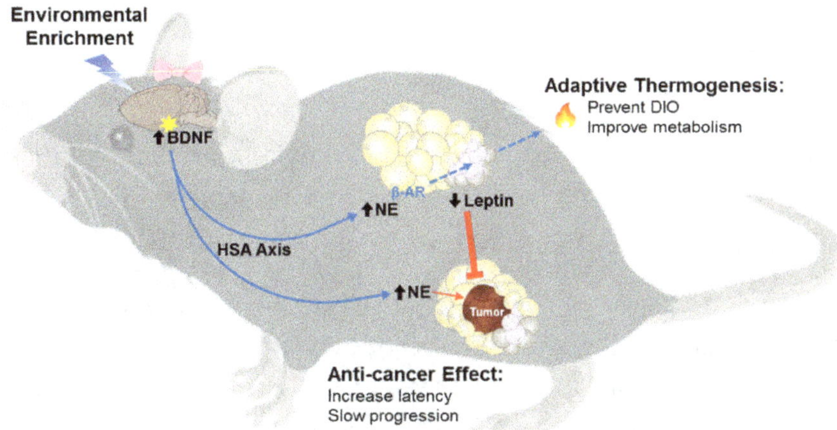

Fig. 5.7. The overall EE impact on mammary tumor depends on the balance between the elevation of norepinephrine and the drop of leptin driven by the HAS axis. At the presence of leptin signaling, the anticancer effect of leptin depletion outweighs the pro-cancer effect of norepinephrine, leading to inhibition of mammary tumor growth. At the absence of leptin such as *ob/ob* mice, the adverse effect of higher norepinephrine cannot be offset by the beneficial effect of a leptin reduction whereby resulting in increased mammary tumor growth. Figure credit to Grant Foglesong.

hinges on the balance between the elevation of norepinephrine and the drop of leptin. In animals with intact leptin signaling, the anticancer effect of leptin depletion may outweigh the pro-cancer effect of norepinephrine and the net impact is inhibition of mammary tumor growth. In the condition of leptin deficiency such as *ob/ob* mice, the pro-cancer effect of higher norepinephrine cannot be offset by the beneficial effect of a leptin drop, and therefore leading to acceleration of tumor growth associated with EE (**Fig. 5.7**). It is worth noting that the mammary tumor growth is slower in *ob/ob* mice compared to wild type mice on HFD regardless of housing conditions. Moreover, congenital leptin deficiency is extremely rare in humans.[61,62] Although homozygous *ob/ob* mice are useful to elucidate the roles of leptin and norepinephrine in mediating the EE effects on mammary tumor, the pro-cancer effect observed in *ob/ob* mice does not cause a substantial concern because the vast majority of obesity is associated with increased leptin levels in animals and humans.[48]

Hypothalamic Gene Transfer of BDNF Suppresses Breast Cancer Progression and Metastasis in Middle Age Obese Mice

In addition to environmentally activating the HSA axis via EE, we wanted to assess the effects of genetic activation of the HSA axis on obesity and breast cancer progression. Given the fact that postmenopausal obesity is associated with 50% higher risk of breast cancer,[63] we thought it would be more valuable to investigate this genetic approach in an age-relevant obesity model. In this gene therapy study,[64] we used a mammary gland medullary adenocarcinoma cell line EO771. The EO771 cells are estrogen receptor (ER)–positive and grow into solid tumors when implanted to the mammary fat pad of syngeneic immune-competent C57BL/6 female mice, and can eventually metastasize to other organs such as the intestinal mesentery, diaphragm, peritoneal wall, and the lung.[65,66]

We fed female C57BL/6 mice with HFD starting at age of 4 weeks to establish morbid obesity in older mice. It is thought that menopause occurs between 12 and 14 months of age in mouse.[67] Therefore, we conducted the gene therapy when mice reached 13 months of age and their body weights were roughly 60 g (**Fig. 5.8**). Obese middle age mice were randomly assigned to receive rAAV vector carrying HA-tagged human BDNF or green fluorescent protein (GFP) as a control. rAAV vectors were injected to the hypothalamus bilaterally via stereotaxic surgery. Immunohistochemical staining of the HA tag verified the transgene expression in the arcuate nucleus of hypothalamus (ARC), the ventromedial hypothalamus (VMH), and the dorsomedial hypothalamus (DMH) (**Fig. 5.8(c)**). These hypothalamic nuclei were targeted because BDNF expression was upregulated in these hypothalamic nuclei upon exposure to EE.[24,68]

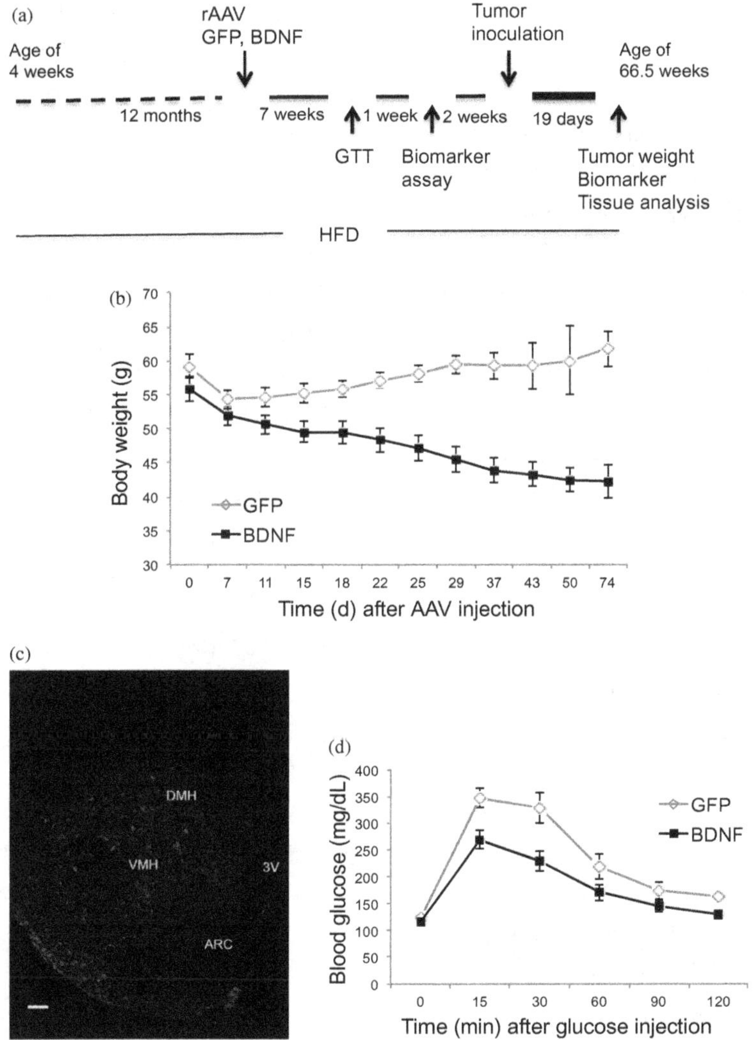

Fig. 5.8. Hypothalamic gene transfer of BDNF in middle age long-term DIO mice alleviates obesity and associated metabolic disturbance. (a) Timeline. (b) Body weight significantly lower in AAV-BDNF-treated mice compared to AAV-GFP-treated mice (repeated measures ANOVA [analysis of variance]). (c) Immunoreactivity to HA tag that is linked to BDNF transgene. Scale bar = 100 μm. (d) Glucose tolerance. Data are mean ± SEM, n = 13 for GFP, n = 12 for BDNF. Reprinted from Liu *et al.* Hypothalamic gene transfer of BDNF inhibits breast cancer progression and metastasis in middle age obese mice. Mol Ther 2014, 22, 1275–1284, with permission of American Society of Gene & Cell Therapy.

AAV-BDNF treatment led to ~2.5-fold increase of BDNF level in the hypothalamus without change of BDNF level in the circulation.

A battery of metabolic assessments was conducted (**Fig. 5.8(a)**). Mice receiving AAV-GFP initially lost weight due to surgery, quickly recovered, and then continued to gain weight (**Fig. 5.8(b)**). In contrast, BDNF-overexpressing mice lost ~30% of weight by 10-week post AAV injection (**Fig. 5.8(b)**). Our previous studies indicate that increased energy expenditure rather than food intake suppression causes weight loss and leanness associated with hypothalamic BDNF overexpression.[25,68] Similar to previous data of hypothalamic overexpression of BDNF in both lean and obese male mice, no decrease of food intake was observed in middle age female mice. A glucose tolerance test was performed 7 weeks after rAAV injection. BDNF-overexpressing mice showed markedly improved glucose tolerance (**Fig. 5.8(d)**), and 58% decrease in circulating leptin as well as 44% decrease in triglyceride in serum.[64]

At 10-week post AAV injection, the ER$^+$ EO771 breast cancer cells were injected to the right fourth mammary gland. Tumor progression did not affect body weight or food intake in both groups. The growth rate of tumor was slower in BDNF-overexpressing mice compared to GFP-expressing mice (**Fig. 5.9(a)**). The study was terminated 19 days after EO771 tumor cell implantation. BDNF treatment significantly decreased tumor weight by 44% compared to GFP mice (**Fig. 5.9(b)**). Importantly, 5 out of 12 GFP-expressing mice had visible metastasis while none of the 12 BDNF-overexpressing mice showed noticeable metastasis (**Fig. 5.9(b)**).

At sacrifice, the tumor-free body weight of BDNF-overexpressing mice was 31% less than GFP-expressing mice. Adiposity was reduced more pronouncedly by BDNF treatment, with subcutaneous, visceral, and mammary fat depots reduced by 47%, 58%, and 36%, respectively. Liver weight was decreased by 17%. Hepatic steatosis was substantially alleviated by BDNF treatment revealed by Oil Red O staining together with a hepatic gene expression signature including downregulation of lipogenic genes *Fasn* (encoding fatty acid

(a)

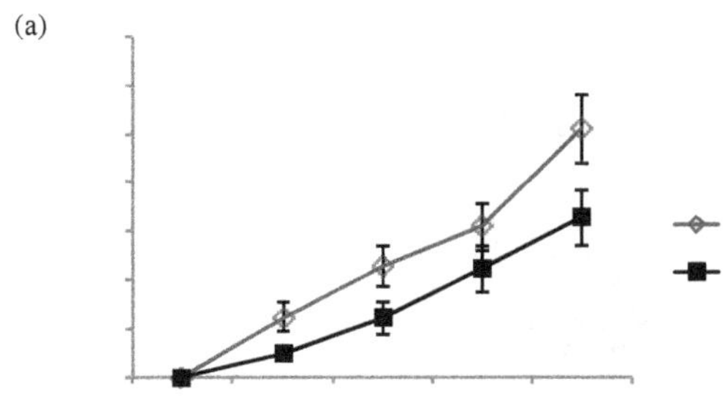

(b)

Group	Tumor weight	Metastasis
GFP	1.63±0.21 g	5/12
BDNF	0.91±0.15 g (P=0.01)	0/12

Fig. 5.9. Hypothalamic BDNF gene transfer suppresses EO771 mammary tumor progression. (a) Tumor volume significantly lower in AAV-BDNF-treated mice compared to AAV-GFP-treated mice (repeated measures ANOVA). (b) Tumor weight and metastasis incidence. Data are mean ± SEM, n = 12 per group. Reprinted from Liu *et al.* Hypothalamic gene transfer of BDNF inhibits breast cancer progression and metastasis in middle age obese mice. Mol Ther 2014, 22, 1275–1284, with permission of American Society of Gene & Cell Therapy.

synthase) and *Gpam* (encoding mitochondrial glycerol-3-phosphate acyltransferase) and upregulation of lipolytic gene *Cpt1a* (encoding carnitine palmitoyltransferase 1A).[64]

We measured various serum biomarkers prior to tumor implantation and at the sacrifice, and analyzed specific effects of the gene therapy, tumor presence, and the interaction between the two factors. Post-tumor levels of adiponectin, insulin-like growth factor 1 (IGF-1), and soluble leptin receptor were significantly lower than their pre-tumor levels regardless of gene therapy. Circulating leptin level was not influenced by tumor growth but markedly reduced in BDNF-overexpressing mice and maintained after tumor cell injection, once again highlighting leptin as a reliable readout of the HSA axis activation.[64]

We examined the mammary tumors using immunohistochemistry. The reduced tumor burden in BDNF-overexpressing mice was correlated to a decrease in cell proliferation marker PCNA

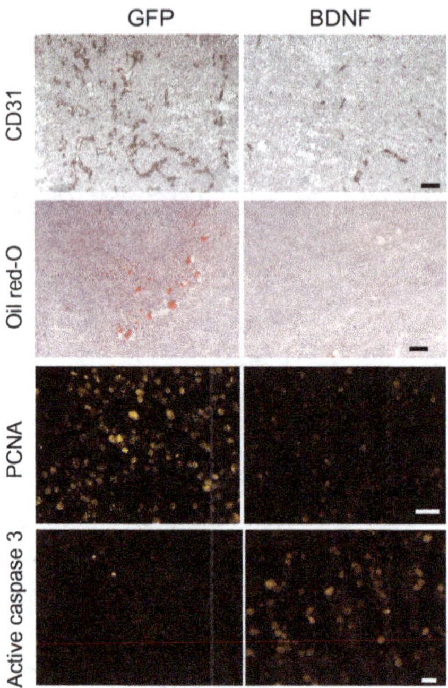

Fig. 5.10. Histology of EO771 mammary tumors. Scale bar = 50 μm. PCNA, proliferating cell nuclear antigen. Reprinted from Liu *et al.* Hypothalamic gene transfer of BDNF inhibits breast cancer progression and metastasis in middle age obese mice. Mol Ther 2014, 22, 1275–1284, with permission of American Society of Gene & Cell Therapy.

(proliferating cell nuclear antigen), a decrease in vascular marker CD31, whereas an increase in apoptosis marker active caspase 3. Moreover, immunostaining of the adipocyte marker perilipin and Oil Red O staining showed that BDNF treatment inhibited adipocyte infiltration of the mammary tumor and lipid accumulation within tumor (**Fig. 5.10**).[64]

Gene expression profile of the tumors showed downregulation of *Vegf* consistent with reduced tumor angiogenesis, and downregulation of several pro-inflammatory genes such as *Il1b*, *Pai1*, and *Socs3* (encoding suppressor cytokine signaling 3) in tumors collected from BDNF-overexpressing mice (**Fig. 5.11**). Leptin

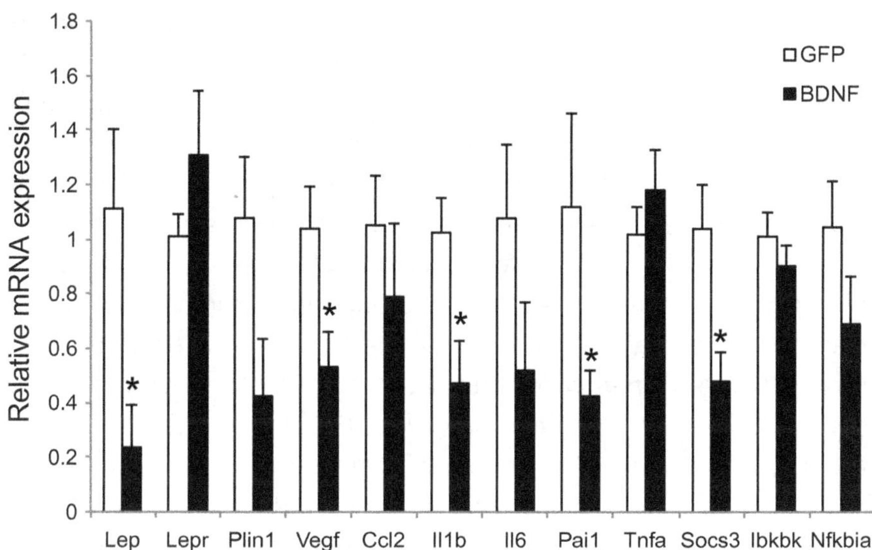

Fig. 5.11. Gene expression profile of EO771 mammary tumors. Data are mean ± SEM, *n* = 5 per group. *P < 0.05. Reprinted from Liu *et al.* Hypothalamic gene transfer of BDNF inhibits breast cancer progression and metastasis in middle age obese mice. Mol Ther 2014, 22, 1275–1284, with permission of American Society of Gene & Cell Therapy.

mRNA was downregulated by ~80% in the mammary tumors. But no leptin mRNA expression was detected in EO771 cells *in vitro*. Consequently, leptin mRNA detected in tumors is likely derived from tumor-infiltrating adipocytes. And the remarkable suppression of leptin expression in the tumors from BDNF-overexpressing mice reflects the elimination of adipocyte recruitment to the tumor, which is further supported by the reduction of adipocyte marker perilipin and lipid accumulation in the tumor. Zhang and colleagues report that tumors can recruit stromal progenitor cells from endogenous adipose tissue. The adipose-derived stromal cells can be incorporated into blood vessels or differentiate to adipocytes in an obesity-dependent manner.[69] Our data suggest that hypothalamic BDNF treatment could attenuate this process, thereby inhibiting the supportive properties of the tumor microenvironment (**Fig. 5.10**).[64]

Thaler and colleagues report that hypothalamic inflammation occurs within 1–3 days of HFD onset and prior to substantial weight gain, unlike the peripheral tissue inflammation that develops as a consequence of obesity. Although the signs of neuronal injury are temporarily subsided, prolonged HFD feeding can ultimately result in permanent inflammation and gliosis in the hypothalamus of mice.[70] Obesity-associated hypothalamic injury is also found in humans.[70] In this study, we profiled the hypothalamic gene expression of obese mice maintained on HFD for over 1 year, and compared to the lean mice fed with normal chow diet. Long-term HFD feeding induced inflammatory mediators including *Il1b*, *Il6*, and *Socs3* in the range of 2 to 4.5 folds. Hypothalamic gene transfer of BDNF significantly suppressed the expression of pro-inflammatory genes including *Il6*, *Socs3*, *Ccl2*, and *Nfkbia* (encoding nuclear factor of kappa light polypeptide gene enhancer in B cells inhibitor alpha) while did not alter *Il1b*, *Ikbkb* (encoding inhibitor of nuclear factor kappa B kinase subunit beta), and *Tnfa*. It is not known whether the anti-inflammatory effect is a consequence of BDNF-induced weight loss, or reversely, it contributes to the alleviation of obesity. BDNF has neuroprotective effects and its receptor TrkB is expressed in neurons, astrocytes, microglia, as well as immune cells.[71–73] We are interested in tackling this question as discussed more in Chapter 7.

In addition, multiple genes regulating energy balance were analyzed. Long-term HFD feeding altered expression of orexigenic *Agrp* (encoding agouti related peptide) and anorexigenic *Cartpt* expression (encoding cocaine-amphetamine–regulated transcript). The upregulation of *Agrp* may indicate the development of leptin resistance after long-term HFD feeding.[74] Insulin receptor expression was markedly downregulated in obese mice compared to lean mice indicating impaired insulin signaling in the hypothalamus. Notably, *Bdnf*, its receptor *Ntrk2*, and *Vgf*, a peptide regulating energy balance downstream of BDNF signaling,[25,68,75] were significantly downregulated in obese mice versus lean mice. This data suggests inhibition of BDNF signaling in the hypothalamus associated with

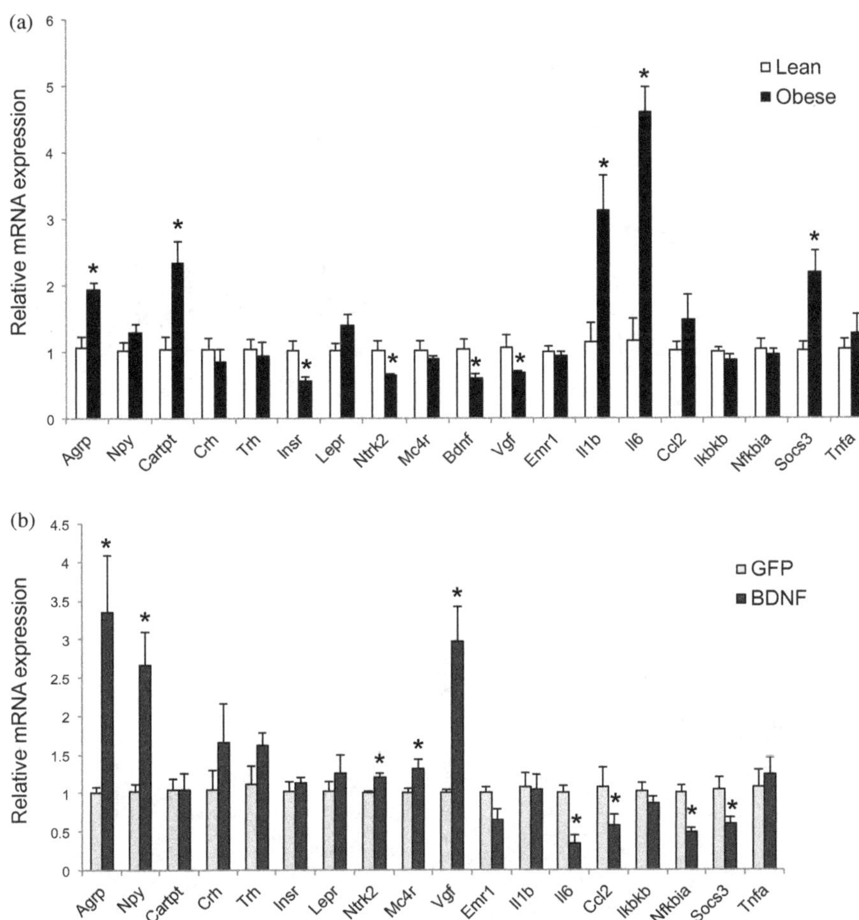

Fig. 5.12. Gene expression profile of the hypothalamus. (a) Gene expression profile of obese mice fed with HFD versus lean mice fed with normal chow diet. (b) Gene expression profile of AAV-BDNF-treated DIO mice compared to GFP-treated DIO mice. Data are mean ± SEM, $n = 5$ per group. *$P < 0.05$. Reprinted from Liu *et al* Hypothalamic gene transfer of BDNF inhibits breast cancer progression and metastasis in middle age obese mice. Mol Ther 2014, 22, 1275–1284, with permission of American Society of Gene & Cell Therapy.

DIO. Hypothalamic gene transfer of BDNF reversed the downregulation of *Bdnf*, *Ntrk2*, and *Vgf* associated with DIO (**Fig. 5.12**).[64]

To examine how hypothalamic overexpression of BDNF regulates mammary fat that is a microenvironment for mammary tumor,

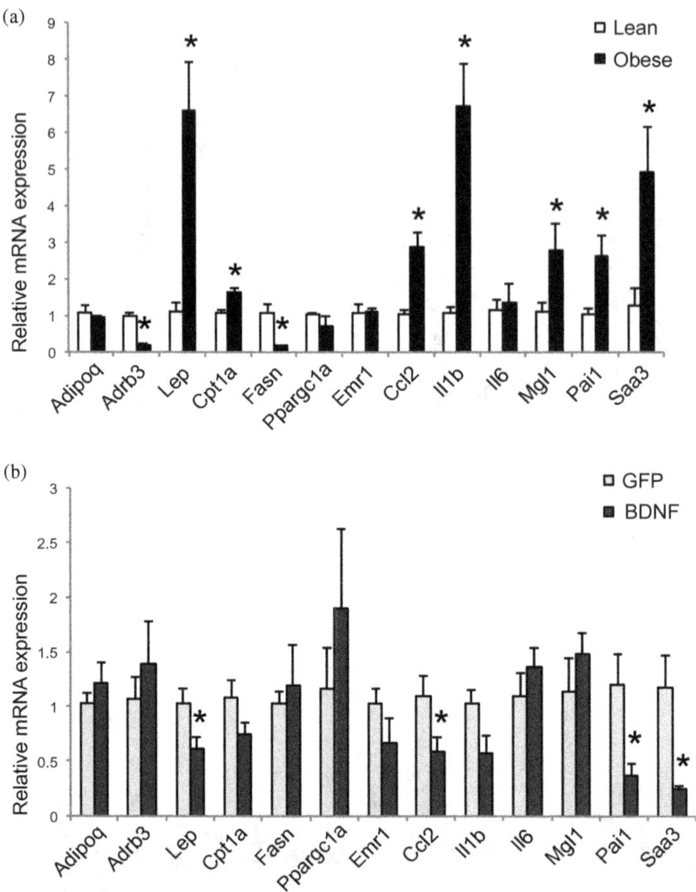

Fig. 5.13. Gene expression profile of the mammary fat. (a) Gene expression profile of obese mice fed with HFD versus lean mice fed with normal chow diet. (b) Gene expression profile of AAV-BDNF-treated DIO mice compared to GFP-treated DIO mice. Data are mean ± SEM, $n = 5$ per group. *$P < 0.05$. Reprinted from Liu *et al.* Hypothalamic gene transfer of BDNF inhibits breast cancer progression and metastasis in middle age obese mice. Mol Ther 2014, 22, 1275–1284, with permission of American Society of Gene & Cell Therapy.

we first analyzed the mammary fat gene expression after long-term HFD feeding compared to lean mice by quantitative reverse transcription polymerase chain reaction (qRT-PCR). DIO stimulated leptin expression more than 6 folds while had no effect on adiponectin expression (**Fig. 5.13(a)**). DIO downregulated β-adrenergic receptor 3 (encoded by *Adrb3*) expression by approximately 80%. Most notable changes in DIO mammary fat were the potent induction of a cluster of inflammatory mediators including *Ccl2, Il1b, Mgl1, Pai1,* and *Saa3* (encoding serum amyloid 3A) (**Fig. 5.13(a)**). Hypothalamic BDNF gene therapy significantly reduced the inflammation mediators such as *Ccl2, Pai1,* and *Saa3* (**Fig. 5.13(b)**). Consistent with the mRNA data, MCP-1 protein level in mammary fat was reduced in BDNF mice by 67%.[64]

Obesity is associated with chronic inflammation in the mammary gland and the pro-inflammatory molecules may play a key role in stimulating aromatase (encoded by *Cyp19* gene) expression leading to increased aromatase activity.[76] This obesity-inflammation-aromatase axis in the mammary gland and other fat depots has been proposed to explain the increased risk of hormone receptor–positive breast cancer in postmenopausal obesity and the impaired efficacy of aromatase inhibitors in treatment of breast cancer in obese individuals.[76,77] Our data demonstrate that hypothalamic BDNF gene transfer reduced several inflammatory mediators in mammary fat. The decrease of MCP-1 in the mammary fat was greater than that in the circulation. However, no increase of *Cyp19* transcription in the mammary fat was observed in the obese middle-aged ovary-intact mice compared to lean counterparts.[64] As a result, it is not surprising that BDNF treatment had no effect on *Cyp19* expression in mammary fat even at the presence of a strong anti-inflammatory effect in the current model. It appears DIO at middle age of 13 months unable to fully display the postmenopausal phenotypes observed in ovariectomized mice.[76] An ovariectomy obesity model may reveal the impact of BDNF treatment on aromatase.

In summary, our study demonstrates that hypothalamic gene transfer of BDNF to obese middle age female mice is effective at treating both obesity and breast cancer, evidenced by multiple outcomes including alleviation of obesity without decrease of food intake, improvement in glycemic control, amelioration of liver steatosis, inhibition of ER⁺ mammary tumor progression, blockade of adipocyte infiltration to tumor, and complete prevention of tumor metastasis. One of the key findings is that BDNF gene therapy markedly suppresses the inflammatory mediators in the circulation, the adipose tissue, the mammary tumor, and the hypothalamus.[64] These data suggest that genetic manipulation of a single molecule in the hypothalamus can influence multiple mechanisms implicated in the obesity–cancer association and potentially provides a target for the treatment of both diseases.

Hypothalamic Gene Transfer of BDNF Attenuates Preexisting Colon Cancer Growth in Obese Mice

To assess whether hypothalamic BDNF gene therapy could be effective in obese mice bearing tumors, we conducted a preliminary study using MC8 colon cancer implantation model. Male C57BL/6 mice were fed with HFD (45% calories from fat) starting at the age of 3 weeks until their body weight reached approximately 40 g. All mice received subcutaneous implantation of MC38 colon cancer cells on the flank (5×10^4 cells per mouse). Three days after colon cancer implantation, the mice were randomized to receive hypothalamic injection of AAV-autoBDNF (autoregulatory vector, see Chapter 4) or AAV-YFP as a control (bilateral injection, 5×10^9 viral genomic particle per injection). Mice were maintained on HFD throughout the experiment (**Fig. 5.14(a)**). Mice receiving AAV-YFP showed slight weight loss after stereotaxic surgery and then returned to the level prior to AAV injection. Mice receiving AAV-autoBDNF had larger weight loss than YFP mice as early as 7 days after AAV injection, and continued to lose weight until the termination of the experiment (**Fig. 5.14(b)**). Adiposity and liver weight were significantly reduced by BDNF treatment (**Fig. 5.14(e)**). The tumor growth rate was significantly decreased in mice receiving AAV-BDNF (**Fig. 5.14(c)**), and the final tumor weight at sacrifice (18-day post AAV injection, 21-day post MC38 implantation) was reduced by 21% compared to the YFP control (**Fig. 5.14(d)**).

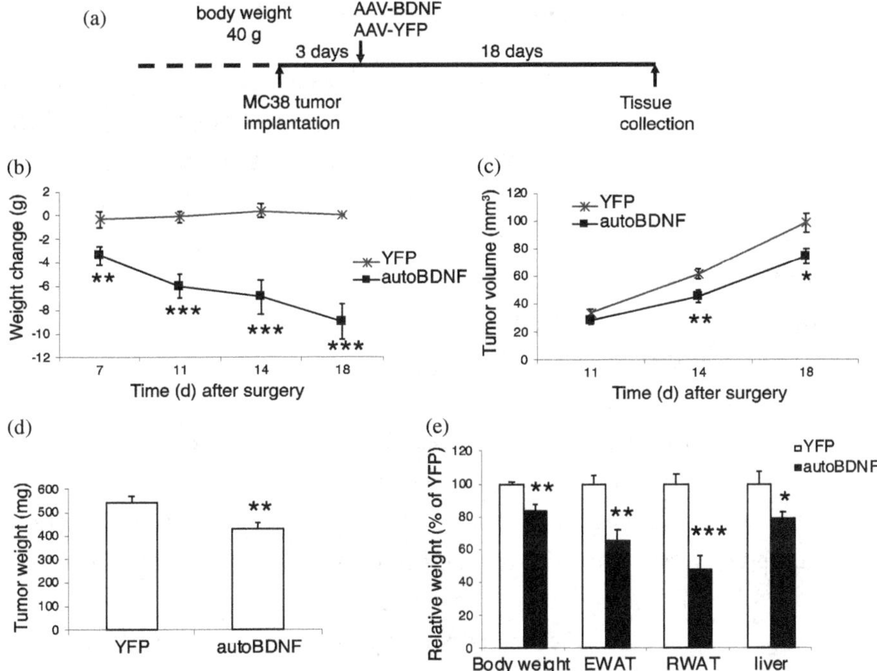

Fig. 5.14. Hypothalamic BDNF gene transfer inhibits preexisting colon cancer growth in obese mice. (a) Timeline. (b) Weight Change post AAV injection. (c) Tumor volume. (d) Tumor weight at sacrifice 18 days after tumor cell implantation. (e) Body weight and tissue weight at sacrifice. Data are mean ± SEM, $n = 5$ per group. $*P < 0.05$, $**P < 0.01$, $***P < 0.001$.

This preliminary study provides some data to evaluate the potential of activating the HSA axis in obese individuals with preexisting cancer as a treatment rather than preventive intervention. The anticancer effect, approximately 20% reduction of tumor mass, is not as remarkable as the findings from our published studies in which BDNF gene therapy is implemented several weeks prior to tumor implantation. It is worth noting that it takes at least several days for the transgene expression to take place after AAV1 vector injection, usually stabilizing at high level after 2 weeks. As such, the window of opportunity in this preliminary experiment might be too narrow to fully manifest the effects of gene therapy. Further testing in slow-growing cancer models is worthy of future investigation.

Summary and Future Directions

A wealth of evidence indicates that all aspects of obesity and associated metabolic syndrome negatively affect cancer progression, although it is unclear whether these effects are additive or synergistic.[15] Animal studies have demonstrated the remarkable systemic improvements in metabolism and overall health by environmental or genetic activation of the HSA axis. By resolving obesity and associated metabolic dysfunctions, activating this brain-fat axis should be particularly effective to obesity-associated cancer types, acting on multifactorial mechanisms (**Fig. 5.1**).

Altered balance of adipokines, specifically the leptin to adiponectin ratio, is one of the most reliable and prominent outcomes of the HSA axis action. Mechanistic studies have elucidated a critical role of leptin mediating the anticancer effect in both lean and obese states, via both local and systemic actions.

Adipokine-independent mechanisms may also exist and are likely to be revealed in obesity models. The chronically increased insulin levels have been associated with various cancers.[78–80] Activating HSA axis, environmentally by EE or genetically by hypothalamic BDNF gene transfer, can alleviate obesity-associated insulin resistance, hyperinsulinemia, dyslipidemia, and liver steatosis.[25,48,64,68] Both obesity and diabetes are risk factors for hepatocellular carcinoma.[81] Thus, liver cancer models are worthy of investigation.

An association between inflammation and cancer has been well established.[82] Obese adipose tissue is an effector of chronic low-grade inflammation and a source of local and circulating pro-inflammatory cytokines.[83,84] Both EE and hypothalamic BDNF gene transfer result in the suppression of select pro-inflammatory cytokines and chemokines in the circulation, the adipose tissue, and the hypothalamus. It is particularly interesting to investigate whether the central anti-inflammatory effect observed in the hypothalamus is the consequence of the alleviation of excessive adiposity in the periphery; or conversely, abolishing hypothalamic inflammation gives rise to reduction of adiposity and subsequently resolving peripheral inflammation. With regard to cancer, the overall anti-inflammatory effect of HSA axis action likely contributes to the inhibition of cancer progression. However, the precise role has not been delineated.

The notion that cancers arise from cells with stem cell–like properties continues to gain traction.[85] These cancer stem cells are thought to play critical roles not only in cancer initiation and maintenance, but also in tumor invasion, metastasis, drug resistance, and cancer recurrence.[85–88] Obesity is associated with increased levels of cytokines, many of which can facilitate self-renewal and survival of these particularly dangerous cancer stem cells.[84,89] Moreover, leptin and the leptin receptor have been implicated in the survival and growth of cancer stem cells.[10,90] Given the substantial suppression of both leptin and select cytokines, how the HSA axis may influence the cancer stem cells is an intriguing question that we intend to tackle.

Several cancers such as breast, ovarian, and endometrial are associated with altered sex steroids levels.[91] Insulin resistance and the compensatory hyperinsulinemia inhibit the hepatic production of sex hormone–binding globulin (SHBG) and thereby increasing the circulating levels of bioavailable sex hormones.[92] WAT is one of the major sources of extra glandular estrogen.[93] Other mechanisms implicated in obesity–cancer link include cellular energetics[94] and stromal contribution from cells originating within WAT.[95] The latter may be influenced by the HSA axis as EE is found to abrogate adipocyte infiltration of the mammary tumors in obesity model. Considering the potent remodeling of WAT upon EE exposure, how the HSA axis may affect cellular energetics and adipose stromal/vascular cell trafficking are fascinating topics worthy of further investigations. Moreover, our studies have demonstrated that hypothalamic BDNF orchestrates both innate and adaptive immune modulations associated with EE (see Chapter 6) in animals of normal body weight. We are currently investigating whether EE can lessen the deterioration in immune surveillance associated with obesity.

Upon updating the concept of cancer hallmarks, Hanahan and Weinberg have noted that the clinical responses to the hallmark-targeting cancer drugs are generally transitory followed by almost-inevitable relapses. One interpretation is that some cancer cells may survive a therapeutic agent targeting one key pathway by relying on other hallmark capabilities. Consequently, the combination of mechanism-guided therapies co-targeting multiple hallmarks is likely to be more effective and durable.[40] The HSA axis may have the capacity to influence multiple pathways implicated in obesity–cancer association (**Fig. 5.1**), and therefore represents an attractive target for combination therapy. Approaches targeting the upstream effector of this axis in the brain are likely more effective because of coordinated regulation of endocrine and immune systems, but are challenged by lack of noninvasive and specific CNS modulating modalities.

References

1. Pearson-Stuttard J, Zhou B, Kontis V, *et al.* (2018) Worldwide burden of cancer attributable to diabetes and high body-mass index: a comparative risk assessment. Lancet Diabetes Endocrinol 6:e6-e15.
2. I. U. A. Cancer_(UICC). (2008) World cancer declaration.
3. GBD Obesity Collaborators, Afshin A, Forouzanfar MH, *et al.* (2017) Health effects of overweight and obesity in 195 countries over 25 years. *N Engl J Med* **377**:13–27.
4. Fairs MAE, Attlee A. (2015) Obesity and cancer: What's the interconnection? *Adv Obes Weight Manag Control* **2**:2–7.
5. Reeves GK, Pirie K, Beral V, *et al.* (2007) Cancer incidence and mortality in relation to body mass index in the Million Women Study: Cohort study. *BMJ* **335**:1134.
6. Renehan AG, Tyson M, Egger M, *et al.* (2008) Body-mass index and incidence of cancer: A systematic review and meta-analysis of prospective observational studies. *Lancet* **371**:569–578.
7. Whitlock G, Lewington S, Sherliker P, *et al.* (2009) Body-mass index and cause-specific mortality in 900 000 adults: Collaborative analyses of 57 prospective studies. *Lancet* **373**:1083–1096.

8. Deng T, Lyon CJ, Bergin S, *et al.* (2016) Obesity, inflammation, and cancer. *Annu Rev Pathol* **11**:421–449.

9. Calle EE, Rodriguez C, Walker-Thurmond K, Thun MJ. (2003) Overweight, obesity, and mortality from cancer in a prospectively studied cohort of U.S. adults. *N Engl J Med* **348**:1625–1638.

10. Zheng Q, Dunlap SM, Zhu J, *et al.* (2011) Leptin deficiency suppresses MMTV-Wnt-1 mammary tumor growth in obese mice and abrogates tumor initiating cell survival. *Endocr Relat Cancer* **18**:491–503.

11. Ogden CL, Carroll MD, Kit BK, Flegal KM. (2014) Prevalence of childhood and adult obesity in the United States, 2011–2012. *JAMA* **311**:806.

12. Gallagher E, LeRoith D. (2015) Obesity and diabetes: The increased risk of cancer and cancer-related mortatlity. *Physiol Rev* **95**:727–48.

13. Ahn J, Schatzkin A, Lacey JV Jr, *et al.* (2007) Adiposity, adult weight change, and postmenopausal breast cancer risk. *Arch Intern Med* **167**:2091–2102.

14. Parker ED, Folsom AR. (2003) Intentional weight loss and incidence of obesity-related cancers: The Iowa Women's Health Study. *Int J Obes Relat Metab Disord* **27**:1447–1452.

15. Uzunlulu M, Telci Caklili O, Oguz A. (2016) Association between metabolic syndrome and cancer. *Ann Nutr Metab* **68**:173–179.

16. Knowler WC, Fowler SE, Hamman RF, *et al.* (2009) 10-year follow-up of diabetes incidence and weight loss in the Diabetes Prevention Program Outcomes Study. *Lancet* **374**:1677–1686.

17. Sjostrom L, Narbro K, Sjöström CD, *et al.* (2007) Effects of bariatric surgery on mortality in Swedish obese subjects. *N Engl J Med* **357**:741–752.

18. Buchwald H, Avidor Y, Braunwald E, *et al.* (2004) Bariatric surgery: A systematic review and meta-analysis. *JAMA* **292**:1724–1737.

19. Adams TD, Gress RE, Smith SC, *et al.* (2007) Long-term mortality after gastric bypass surgery. *N Engl J Med* **357**:753–761.

20. Renehan AG. (2009) Bariatric surgery, weight reduction, and cancer prevention. *Lancet Oncol* **10**:640–641.

21. Longo VD, Fontana L. (2010) Calorie restriction and cancer prevention: Metabolic and molecular mechanisms. *Trends Pharmacol Sci* **31**:89–98.

22. Ashrafian H, Ahmed K, Rowland SP, *et al.* (2011) Metabolic surgery and cancer: Protective effects of bariatric procedures. *Cancer* **117**:1788–1799.

23. Olson OC, Quail DF, Joyce JA. (2017) Obesity and the tumor microenvironment. *Science* **358**:1130–1131.

24. Cao L, Liu X, Lin E-JD, *et al.* (2010) Environmental and genetic activation of a brain-adipocyte BDNF/leptin axis causes cancer remission and inhibition. *Cell* **142**:52–64.

25. Cao L, Choi EY, Liu X, *et al.* (2011) White to brown fat phenotypic switch induced by genetic and environmental activation of a hypothalamic-adipocyte axis. *Cell Metab* **14**:324–338.

26. Cao L, During MJ. (2012) What is the brain-cancer connection? *Annu Rev Neurosci* **35**:331–345.

27. Cao L, Jiao X, Zuzga DS, *et al.* (2004) VEGF links hippocampal activity with neurogenesis, learning and memory. *Nat Genet* **36**:827–835.

28. During MJ, Liu X, Huang W, *et al.* (2015) Adipose VEGF links the white-to-brown fat switch with environmental, genetic, and pharmacological stimuli in male mice. *Endocrinology* **156**:2059–2073.

29. Foglesong GD, Huang W, Liu X, *et al.* (2016) Role of hypothalamic VGF in energy balance and metabolic adaption to environmental enrichment in mice. *Endocrinology* **157**:983–996.

30. Xiao R, Bergin SM, Huang W, *et al.* (2016) Environmental and genetic activation of hypothalamic BDNF modulates T-cell immunity to exert an anticancer phenotype. *Cancer Immunol Res* **4**:488–497.

31. McMurphy T, Huang W, Queen NJ, *et al.* (2018) Implementation of environmental enrichment after middle age promotes healthy aging. *Aging (Albany NY)* **10**:1698–1721.

32. Xiao R, Bergin SM, Huang W, *et al.* (2019) Enriched environment regulates thymocyte development and alleviates experimental autoimmune encephalomyelitis in mice. *Brain Behav Immun* **75**:137–148.

33. Queen NJ, Boardman AA, Patel RS, *et al.* (2020) Environmental enrichment improves metabolic and behavioral health in the BTBR mouse model of autism. *Psychoneuroendocrinology* **111**:104476.

34. Vona-Davis L, Rose DP. (2007) Adipokines as endocrine, paracrine, and autocrine factors in breast cancer risk and progression. *Endocr Relat Cancer* **14**:189–206.

35. Maccio A, Madeddu C, Gramignano G, *et al.* (2010) Correlation of body mass index and leptin with tumor size and stage of disease in hormone-dependent postmenopausal breast cancer: Preliminary results and therapeutic implications. *J Mol Med* **88**:677–686.
36. Paz-Filho G, Lim EL, Wong ML, Licinio J. (2011) Associations between adipokines and obesity-related cancer. *Front Biosci* **16**:1634–1650.
37. Nkhata KJ, Ray A, Dogan S, *et al.* (2009) Mammary tumor development from T47-D human breast cancer cells in obese ovariectomized mice with and without estradiol supplements. *Breast Cancer Res Treat* **114**:71–83.
38. Chen DC, Chung YF, Yeh YT, *et al.* (2006) Serum adiponectin and leptin levels in Taiwanese breast cancer patients. *Cancer Lett* **237**:109–114.
39. Kamangar F, Dores GM, Anderson WF. (2006) Patterns of cancer incidence, mortality, and prevalence across five continents: Defining priorities to reduce cancer disparities in different geographic regions of the world. *J Clin Oncol* **24**:2137–2150.
40. Hanahan D, Weinberg RA. (2011) Hallmarks of cancer: The next generation. *Cell* **144**:646–674.
41. Weigelt B, Peterse JL, van't Veer LJ. (2005) Breast cancer metastasis: Markers and models. *Nat Rev Cancer* **5**:591–602.
42. Vainio H, Kaaks R, Bianchini F. (2002) Weight control and physical activity in cancer prevention: International evaluation of the evidence. *Eur J Cancer Prev* **11 Suppl 2**:S94–100.
43. Moley KH, Colditz G. (2016) Effects of obesity on hormonally driven cancer in women. *Sci Transl Med* **8**:323ps3.
44. Verhaeghe N, De Greve O, Annemans L. (2016) The potential health and economic effect of a body mass index decrease in the overweight and obese population in Belgium. *Public Health* **134**:26–33.
45. Guy CT, Cardiff RD, Muller WJ. (1992) Induction of mammary tumors by expression of polyomavirus middle T oncogene: A transgenic mouse model for metastatic disease. *Mol Cell Biol* **12**:954–961.
46. Lin EY, Jones JG, Li P, *et al.* (2003) Progression to malignancy in the polyoma middle T oncoprotein mouse breast cancer model provides a reliable model for human diseases. *Am J Pathol* **163**:2113–2126.

47. Juncker-Jensen A, Rømer J, Pennington CJ, *et al*. (2009) Spontaneous metastasis in matrix metalloproteinase 3-deficient mice. *Mol Carcinog* **48**:618–625.

48. Foglesong GD, Queen NJ, Huang W, *et al*. (2019) Enriched environment inhibits breast cancer progression in obese models with intact leptin signaling. *Endocr Relat Cancer* **26**:483–495.

49. Ando S, Barone I, Giordano C, *et al*. (2014) The multifaceted mechanism of leptin signaling within tumor microenvironment in driving breast cancer growth and progression. *Front Oncol* **4**:340.

50. Ahima RS, Osei SY. (2004) Leptin signaling. *Physiol Behav* **81**:223–241.

51. Saxena NK, Vertino PM, Anania FA, Sharma D. (2007) Leptin-induced growth stimulation of breast cancer cells involves recruitment of histone acetyltransferases and mediator complex to CYCLIN D1 promoter via activation of Stat3. *J Biol Chem* **282**:13316–13325.

52. Zheng Q, Hursting SD, Reizes O. (2012) Leptin regulates cyclin D1 in luminal epithelial cells of mouse MMTV-Wnt-1 mammary tumors. *J Cancer Res Clin Oncol* **138**:1607–1612.

53. Newman G, Gonzalez-Perez RR. (2014) Leptin-cytokine crosstalk in breast cancer. *Mol Cell Endocrinol* **382**:570–582.

54. Rene Gonzalez R, Watters A, Xu Y, *et al*. (2009) Leptin-signaling inhibition results in efficient anti-tumor activity in estrogen receptor positive or negative breast cancer. *Breast Cancer Res* **11**:R36.

55. Antoni MH, Lutgendorf SK, Cole SW, *et al*. (2006) The influence of bio-behavioural factors on tumour biology: Pathways and mechanisms. *Nat Rev Cancer* **6**:240–248.

56. Szpunar MJ, Belcher EK, Dawes RP, Madden KS. (2016) Sympathetic innervation, norepinephrine content, and norepinephrine turnover in orthotopic and spontaneous models of breast cancer. *Brain Behav Immun* **53**:223–233.

57. Bartness TJ, Liu Y, Shrestha YB, Ryu V. (2014) Neural innervation of white adipose tissue and the control of lipolysis. *Front Neuroendocrinol* **35**:473–493.

58. Cannon B, Nedergaard J. (2004) Brown adipose tissue: Function and physiological significance. *Physiol Rev* **84**:277–359.

59. Milsum JH. (1985) A model of the eustress system for health/illness. *Behav Sci* **30**:179–186.

60. Selye H. (1974) *Stress without Distress.* McClelland and Stewart, Ltd., Toronto.

61. Farooqi IS, Matarese G, Lord GM, *et al.* (2002) Beneficial effects of leptin on obesity, T cell hyporesponsiveness, and neuroendocrine/metabolic dysfunction of human congenital leptin deficiency. *J Clin Invest* **110**:1093–1103.

62. Gibson WT, Farooqi IS, Moreau M, *et al.* (2004) Congenital leptin deficiency due to homozygosity for the Delta133G mutation: Report of another case and evaluation of response to four years of leptin therapy. *J Clin Endocrinol Metab* **89**:4821–4826.

63. Trentham-Dietz A, Newcomb PA, Egan KM, *et al.* (2000) Weight change and risk of postmenopausal breast cancer (United States). *Cancer Causes Control* **11**:533–542.

64. Liu X, McMurphy T, Xiao R, *et al.* (2014) Hypothalamic gene transfer of BDNF inhibits breast cancer progression and metastasis in middle age obese mice. *Mol Ther* **22**:1275–1284.

65. Gu JW, Young E, Patterson SG, *et al.* (2011) Postmenopausal obesity promotes tumor angiogenesis and breast cancer progression in mice. *Cancer Biol Ther* **11**:910–917.

66. Ewens A, Mihich E, Ehrke MJ. (2005) Distant metastasis from subcutaneously grown E0771 medullary breast adenocarcinoma. *Anticancer Res* **25**:3905–3915.

67. Siler LM. (1995) *Mouse Genetics: Concepts and Applications.* Oxford University Press, New York.

68. Cao L, Lin E-JD, Cahill MC, *et al.* (2009) Molecular therapy of obesity and diabetes by a physiological autoregulatory approach. *Nat Med* **15**:447–454.

69. Zhang Y, Daquinag AC, Amaya-Manzanares F, *et al.* (2012) Stromal progenitor cells from endogenous adipose tissue contribute to pericytes and adipocytes that populate the tumor microenvironment. *Cancer Res* **72**:5198–5208.

70. Thaler JP, Yi C-X, Schur EA, *et al.* (2012) Obesity is associated with hypothalamic injury in rodents and humans. *J Clin Investig* **122**:153–162.

71. Nagahara AH, Tuszynski MH. (2011) Potential therapeutic uses of BDNF in neurological and psychiatric disorders. *Nat Rev Drug Discov* **10**:209–219.

72. Givalois L, Arancibia S, Alonso G, Tapia-Arancibia L. (2004) Expression of brain-derived neurotrophic factor and its receptors in the median eminence cells with sensitivity to stress. *Endocrinology* **145**:4737–4747.

73. Schuhmann B, Dietrich A, Sel S, *et al.* (2005) A role for brain-derived neurotrophic factor in B cell development. *J Neuroimmunol* **163**:15–23.

74. Stofkova A, Skurlova M, Kiss A, *et al.* (2009) Activation of hypothalamic NPY, AgRP, MC4R, AND IL-6 mRNA levels in young Lewis rats with early-life diet-induced obesity. *Endocr Regul* **43**:99–106.

75. Bartolomucci A, La Corte G, Possenti R, *et al.* (2006) TLQP-21, a VGF-derived peptide, increases energy expenditure and prevents the early phase of diet-induced obesity. *Proc Natl Acad Sci USA* **103**:14584–14589.

76. Subbaramaiah K, Howe LR, Bhardwaj P, *et al.* (2011) Obesity is associated with inflammation and elevated aromatase expression in the mouse mammary gland. *Cancer Prev Res* **4**:329–346.

77. Bulun SE, Chen D, Moy I, *et al.* (2012) Aromatase, breast cancer and obesity: A complex interaction. *Trends Endocrinol Metab* **23**:83–89.

78. Gunter MJ, Hoover DR, Yu H, *et al.* (2009) Insulin, insulin-like growth factor-I, and risk of breast cancer in postmenopausal women. *J Natl Cancer Inst* **101**:48–60.

79. Trevisan M, Liu J, Muti P, *et al.* (2001) Markers of insulin resistance and colorectal cancer mortality. *Cancer Epidemiol Biomarkers Prev* **10**:937–941.

80. Jee SH, Ohrr H, Sull JW, *et al.* (2005) Fasting serum glucose level and cancer risk in Korean men and women. *JAMA* **293**:194–202.

81. Rossi M, Lipworth L, Dal Maso L, *et al.* (2009) Dietary glycemic load and hepatocellular carcinoma with or without chronic hepatitis infection. *Ann Oncol* **20**:1736–1740.

82. Coussens LM, Werb Z. (2002) Inflammation and cancer. *Nature* **420**:860–867.

83. Olefsky JM. (2009) IKKepsilon: A bridge between obesity and inflammation. *Cell* **138**:834–836.

84. Gilbert CA, Slingerland JM. (2013) Cytokines, obesity, and cancer: New insights on mechanisms linking obesity to cancer risk and progression. *Ann Rev Med* **64**:45–57.

85. Magee JA, Piskounova E, Morrison SJ. (2012) Cancer stem cells: Impact, heterogeneity, and uncertainty. *Cancer Cell* **21**:283–296.

86. Li X, Lewis MT, Huang J, *et al.* (2008) Intrinsic resistance of tumorigenic breast cancer cells to chemotherapy. *J Natl Cancer Inst* **100**:672–679.

87. Shafee N, Smith CR, Wei S, *et al.* (2008) Cancer stem cells contribute to cisplatin resistance in Brca1/p53-mediated mouse mammary tumors. *Cancer Res* **68**:3243–3250.

88. Balic M, Lin H, Young L, *et al.* (2006) Most early disseminated cancer cells detected in bone marrow of breast cancer patients have a putative breast cancer stem cell phenotype. *Clin Cancer Res* **12**:5615–5621.

89. Korkaya H, Liu S, Wicha MS. (2011) Breast cancer stem cells, cytokine networks, and the tumor microenvironment. *J Clin Invest* **121**:3804–3809.

90. Feldman DE, Chen C, Punj V, *et al.* (2012) Pluripotency factor-mediated expression of the leptin receptor (OB-R) links obesity to oncogenesis through tumor-initiating stem cells. *Proc Natl Acad Sci USA* **109**:829–834.

91. Eliassen AH, Hankinson SE. (2008) Endogenous hormone levels and risk of breast, endometrial and ovarian cancers: Prospective studies. *Adv Exp Med Biol* **630**:148–165.

92. Pugeat M, Crave JC, Elmidani M, *et al.* (1991) Pathophysiology of sex hormone binding globulin (SHBG): Relation to insulin. *J Steroid Biochem Mol Biol* **40**:841–849.

93. Flototto T, Djahansouzi S, Gläser M, *et al.* (2001) Hormones and hormone antagonists: Mechanisms of action in carcinogenesis of endometrial and breast cancer. *Horm Metab Res* **33**:451–457.

94. Ashrafian H. (2006) Cancer's sweet tooth: The Janus effect of glucose metabolism in tumorigenesis. *Lancet* **367**:618–621.

95. Zhang Y, Daquinag A, Traktuev DO, *et al.* (2009) White adipose tissue cells are recruited by experimental tumors and promote cancer progression in mouse models. *Cancer Res* **69**:5259–5266.

Environmental Enrichment Fine-Tunes Immunity in Cancer and Autoimmune Disease

Introduction

Accumulating evidence has revealed that environmental enrichment (EE) produces notable effects on both innate and adaptive immunity. This chapter summarizes our work in understanding how EE influences cancer immunity and autoimmunity and their respective mechanisms, and integrate into existing literature regarding the immune regulation by EE. These discoveries are fruits of collaborations with the lab of Dr. Michael Caligiuri. Run Xiao, a postdoc in our lab, and Stephen Bergin, then a MD/PhD student, and Anthony Mansour, a postdoc in Caligiuri lab, were instrumental to these projects focusing on EE regulation of immunity.

Environmental Enrichment Regulates Cancer T Cell Immunity via Hypothalamic BDNF

Our interest in how EE regulates T cell immunity stems from the observation of enhanced CD8 T cell cytotoxicity in the original discovery of the anticancer effect of EE.[1] Although the activation of a specific neuroendocrine axis, hypothalamic-sympathoneural-adipocyte (HSA) axis and the resulting sharp drop of circulating leptin had been identified as a key mechanism, we thought the modulation of an adaptive T cell immune response, particularly the cytotoxic T lymphocytes (CTLs), might also contribute critically to the anticancer effects of EE. Thus, we set out to test the hypothesis and investigate the mechanisms of CTL regulation responding to the complex stimuli provided by EE.[2]

CD8 T Cells Contribute to EE-Induced Tumor Inhibition

To test the hypothesis that increased CTL cytotoxicity and tumor infiltration play an important role in suppressing tumor growth in EE living, we conducted a CTLs depletion study (**Fig. 6.1**). Male C57BL/6 mice were randomized to live in SE or EE housing for a duration of 5 weeks when EE-associated metabolic changes are expected to occur. Indeed, serum leptin concentration in EE mice was ~70% lower than that in SE mice. Next, EE and SE mice were randomly assigned to receive intraperitoneal injection of either a CD8-depleting antibody or IgG control antibody. CD8-depleting antibody treatment completely eliminated CD8 T cells in blood. Twenty-four hours after the first dose of antibody, all mice received subcutaneous implantation of B16 melanoma on the flank (1 × 10⁵ melanoma cells per mouse). Antibodies were administered every 7 days till the termination of the study 18 days after melanoma implantation (**Fig. 6.1(a)**).[2]

EE mice receiving IgG control antibody displayed robust suppression of tumor growth, tumor mass ~80% less than that of SE mice receiving IgG, indicating administration of a control antibody not interfering with EE-induced tumor inhibition (**Fig. 6.1(b)**). In contrast, when CD8 T cells were eliminated by CD8-depleting antibody, the reduction of tumor mass associated with EE was weakened to ~50%, and importantly, this difference was not statistically significant between EE and SE mice receiving the same CD8-depleting antibody. Moreover, tumors in EE mice with CD8 depletion were approximately 150% larger than the tumors in EE mice without CD depletion (EE-anti-CD8 versus EE-IgG) (**Fig. 6.1(b)**). These data

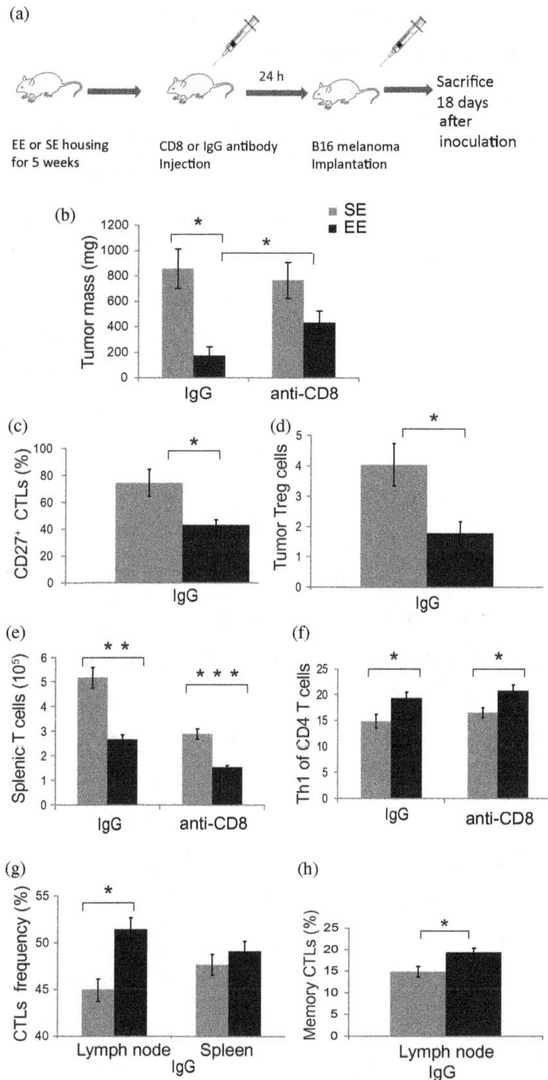

Fig. 6.1. CD8 T cells are required to exert EE's inhibition of tumor growth. (a) Study design of CD8 T-cell depletion experiment. (b) B16 melanoma mass. (c) Surface expression of CD27 proteins on tumor-infiltrating CTLs, cytotoxic lymphocytes. (d) Frequency of tumor-infiltrating Tregs. (e) T cell numbers in spleens. (f) Th1 helper T cells (CXCR3$^+$CCR4$^-$) in spleens. (g) Frequency of CTLs in lymph node and spleens. (h) Frequency of memory CTLs (CD44^{high}CD122$^+$). Data are mean ± SEM, n = 9–10 per group. *P < 0.05, **P < 0.01, ***P < 0.001. Reprinted from Xiao *et al.* Environmental and genetic activation of hypothalamic BDNF modulates T-cell immunity to exert an anticancer phenotype. *Cancer Immunol Res* 2016, 4(6), 488–497.

suggest an important role of CD8 T cells in EE-induced anticancer phenotype but not the sole effector.[2]

We examined the tumor immune microenvironment in EE versus SE, the two groups receiving IgG (EE-IgG versus SE-IgG). EE did not alter the frequency of tumor-infiltrating mononuclear cells or CD8 CTLs.[2] To assess whether EE can modulate CD8 cytotoxicity, we measured the surface expression of CD27 and PD-1 that are targets for clinical cancer immunotherapy.[3,4] CD27, a member of the tumor necrosis factor receptor superfamily, expresses on both naïve and long-lived CD8 T cells, but disappears on terminally differentiated effector CTLs with high expression of both granzyme B and perforin.[5–7] Tumor-infiltrating CTLs from EE mice showed a lower frequency of CD27 expression compared to the CTLs infiltrating SE tumors **(Fig. 6.1(c))**, indicating a higher proportion of differentiated effector CD8 T cells. However, EE did not alter the frequency of CTLs expressing PD-1 or the expression level of PD-1 on CTLs. T regulatory cells (Treg), a helper T cell that inhibits CTLs, was reduced in EE tumors **(Fig. 6.1(d))**.[2]

We also examined the immune changes in the secondary lymphoid tissues (SLT) such as spleen and lymph nodes. Total splenocyte and total splenic T cell numbers were reduced in EE mice **(Fig. 6.1(e))**, but the splenic CTLs showed greater tumor reactivity. Surface expression of chemokine receptors CXCR3 and CCR4 can be used to define the helper T cell type 1 (Th1) cells.[8,9] These Th1 cells (CXCR3$^+$CCR4$^-$CD4$^+$ T cells) enhance cellular immune response and induce CTL-mediated tumor eradication.[10] Polarization toward a Th1 phenotype was observed in the spleens from EE mice compared to their counterparts living in SE regardless of the status of CD8 T cell depletion **(Fig. 6.1(f))**. Moreover, EE increased the frequency of CTLs in the lymph nodes **(Fig. 6.1(g))**, associated with a greater proportion expressing a memory phenotype defined as CD44^{high}CD122$^+$ **(Fig. 6.1(h))**. These data collectively demonstrate that EE modulates T cell immunity as part of the overall cancer-inhibitory effects.[2]

EE Regulates Spleen/Lymph Node T Cell Phenotypes in the Absence of Cancer

In order to facilitate mechanistic studies, we sought to characterize the effects of EE on T cells in the SLTs without a challenge of tumor. Mice living in EE had fewer total splenocytes compared to mice living in SE. At 4-week EE exposure, the signature changes of EE such as upregulation of hypothalamic brain-derived neurotrophic factor (BDNF) expression and reduced weight gain were observed.[2] Next, we examined whether a short-term EE exposure was sufficient to affect T cells in the SLTs. Total T cell numbers showed a trend of reduction in the spleens of EE mice as early as 1-week EE, and this effect reached significance by 4-week EE (**Fig. 6.2(a)**). On the contrary, lymph nodes from EE mice were

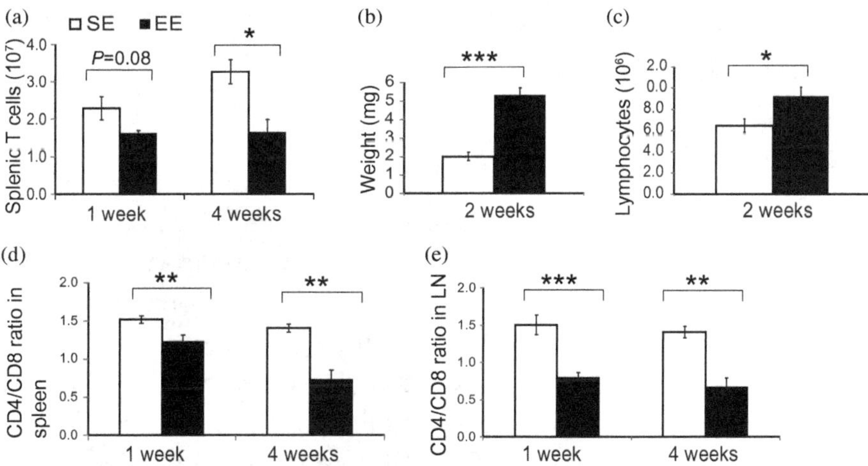

Fig. 6.2. Immune response to short- and long-term EE. (a) Total number of T cells in spleens. (b) Lymph node mass. (c) Total number of lymphocytes in lymph node. (d) CD4/CD8 ratio in spleen. (e) CD4/CD ration in lymph node following 1-week or 4-week EE exposure. Data are mean ± SEM, $n = 5$ per group. *$P < 0.05$, **$P < 0.01$, ***$P < 0.001$. Reprinted from Xiao *et al.* Environmental and genetic activation of hypothalamic BDNF modulates T-cell immunity to exert an anticancer phenotype. *Cancer Immunol Res* 2016, 4(6), 488–497.

measurably enlarged at 2-week EE, and contained significantly more lymphocytes (**Fig. 6.2(b), (c)**).

The frequency of single positive CD8 CTLs was higher in EE SLTs while the frequency of single positive CD4 T cells was lower, leading to a depressed CD4/CD8 ratio that persisted to 4-week EE. The reduced CD4/CD8 ratio was also found in lymph nodes at both time points (**Fig. 6.2(d), (e)**). These changes were largely similar to the findings in the aforementioned melanoma experiment. A noted difference was that EE increased the frequency of memory CTLs in tumor-bearing mice but not in tumor-free mice.[2] This data suggests that T cells might respond differently in the context of health and disease. In other words, EE may condition mice to launch a more potent immune response when encountering a tumor challenge.

Mechanisms of EE Regulation of T Cell Immunity in the Secondary Lymphoid Tissues

Hypothalamic BDNF

Because hypothalamic BDNF drives the HSA axis critical for the anti-obesity and anticancer effects of EE, we investigated whether hypothalamic BDNF also mediated the T cell changes associated with EE using similar tools characterized in previous studies.[1,11] Adeno-associated viral (AAV)-mediated overexpressing BDNF in the hypothalamus reproduced the T cell phenotypic changes associated with EE, namely lower total splenocyte number, higher CTL frequency, and reduced CD4/CD8 ratio in the SLT (**Fig. 6.3**). Of note, the immune modulation was independent of the effect on body weight because these immune changes were observed at 3-week after AAV-BDNF injection when significant change in body weight had not occur.[2]

Conversely, mice received hypothalamic injection of either an AAV vector carrying a microRNA against *Bdnf* or a microRNA

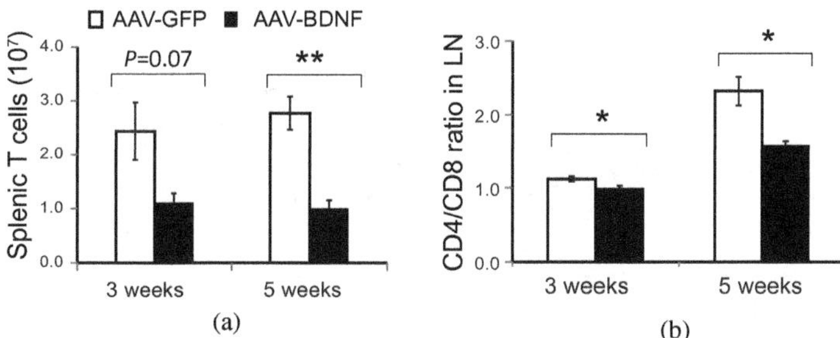

Fig. 6.3. Hypothalamic overexpressing BDNF reproduces the T-cell phenotypes induced by EE. (a) TCRβ⁺ T cells in spleens 3 or 5 weeks post AAV-BDNF injection and living in SE. (b) The T-cell CD4/CD8 ration in lymph node 3 weeks post AAV injection. Data are mean ± SEM, n = 5 per group. *P < 0.05, **P < 0.01. Reprinted from Xiao *et al.* Environmental and genetic activation of hypothalamic BDNF modulates T-cell immunity to exert an anticancer phenotype. *Cancer Immunol Res* 2016, 4(6), 488–497.

targeting a scrambled sequence as control. After recovery from stereotaxic surgery, mice receiving each AAV vector were split to live in either SE or EE for 5 weeks. Knockdown of *Bdnf* specifically in the hypothalamus led to increase in total splenocytes and T cell numbers in mice living in SE. Importantly, preventing the EE-induced upregulation of hypothalamic *Bdnf* abolished the EE-induced CTL changes such as the shift to CTLs within SLT (**Fig. 6.4**). The gain-of- and loss-of-function studies collectively demonstrate hypothalamic BDNF as a key brain mediator of the T cell regulatory effects associated with EE.[2]

Sympathetic nervous system (SNS)

All primary and secondary immune organs are sympathetically innervated from sympathetic postganglionic neurons.[12,13] The main sympathetic neurotransmitter norepinephrine binds to either α- or β-adrenergic receptors expressed on the surface of immune or lymphoid stromal cells, which results in changes in gene expression of various immune cell–derived factors.[14,15] We have previously

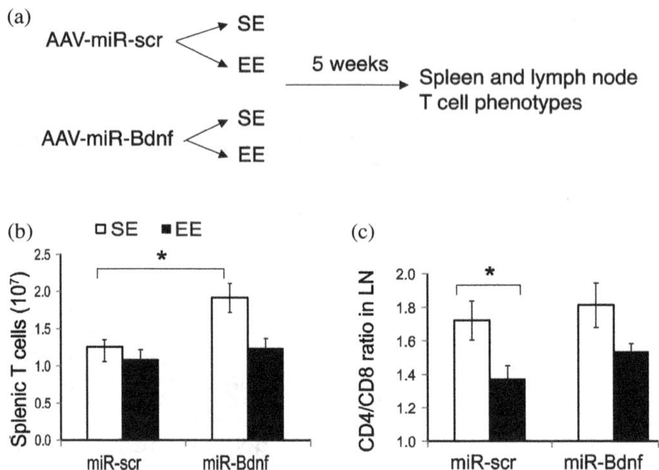

Fig. 6.4. Hypothalamic *Bdnf* knockdown inhibits EE-induced T cell modulation. (a) Experimental design. (b) Total splenic T cells. (c) The T-cell CD4/CD8 ratio in lymph node. Data are mean ± SEM, *n* = 5–8 per group. *P < 0.05. Adapted from Xiao *et al.* Environmental and genetic activation of hypothalamic BDNF modulates T-cell immunity to exert an anticancer phenotype. *Cancer Immunol Res* 2016, 4(6), 488–497.

demonstrated that administration of a nonspecific β-blocker propranolol abrogates the metabolic effects as well as the anticancer effect induced by EE. We employed the similar approach and found that propranolol supplied in drinking water completely blocked the key feature of CTL change associated with EE — depressed CD4/CD8 ratio.[2] This data suggests intact SNS signaling is required for EE's T cell regulation.

Hypothalamus-pituitary-adrenal (HPA) axis

Glucocorticoids play an important role in regulating the inflammatory and immune response and have been widely used in medicine to treat diseases caused by various inflammatory and autoimmune disorders.[16] All immune cells express glucocorticoid receptors (GR), and thereby responsive to glucocorticoids released upon activation of

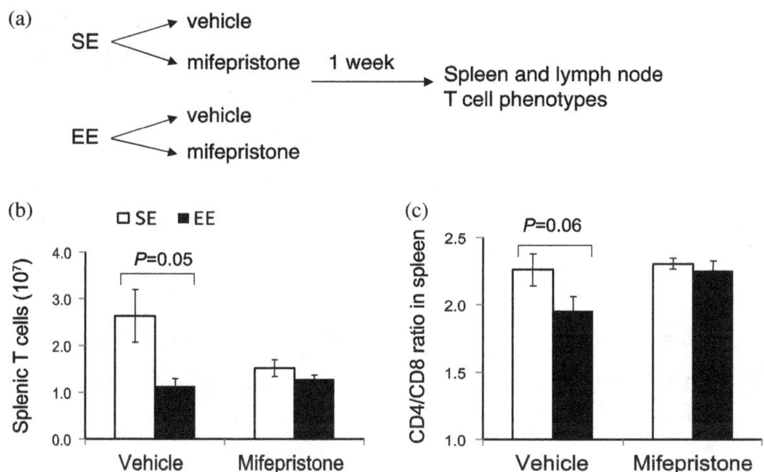

Fig. 6.5.   Cortisol receptor antagonist mifepristone blocks the EE effect on CD4/CD8 ratio. (a) Experimental design. (b) Total splenic T cells. (c) The XT-cell CD4/CD8 ration in spleen. Data are mean ± SEM, n = 5 per group. Adapted from Xiao *et al.* Environmental and genetic activation of hypothalamic BDNF modulates T-cell immunity to exert an anticancer phenotype. *Cancer Immunol Res* 2016, 4(6), 488–497.

the HPA axis.[17] In light of a mild but significant increase in circulating concentration of corticosterone associated with EE, we investigated whether the HPA axis activation is involved in the T cell modulation. Mice were randomized to SE or EE housing, and administered either a GR antagonist mifepristone[18] or solvent as vehicle control by daily oral gavage for 1 week. Mifepristone antagonized some EE-induced immune changes such as the reduction of splenic T cell numbers and the reduced CD4/CD8 ratio (**Fig. 6.5**), suggesting a role of the HPA axis.[2]

In summary, these data demonstrate that CTLs contribute substantially to the anticancer phenotype of an EE in an orthotropic melanoma model because depletion of CD8 T cells partially but significantly attenuated the reduction of tumor mass in EE. The tumor microenvironment contained more activated CTLs while fewer Tregs in animals living in EE. In tumor-bearing animals, EE significantly enlarged lymph node and increased the proportion of CD8 CTLs, consistent with previous finding of enhanced CD8 tumor-killing activity *in vitro*. Overall, EE leads to a favorable immune microenvironment of tumor, consistent with reports that increased proportions of CD8 T cells and decreased Tregs correlate with a better prognosis of cancer.[19,20] In the absence of tumor, EE induced early changes in T cell homeostasis in SLT characterized as a reduction of the total number of splenic T cells and a skew to CTLs (decreased CD4/CD8 ratio). One regulatory mechanism is the upregulation of BDNF expression in the hypothalamus, which activates both the SNS and the HPA axis.[2]

EE Boosts Natural Killer Cell Immunity Against Cancer

Natural killer (NK) cells are innate immune cells that constitute the first line of defense against microbial pathogens and a variety of cancers[21,22] as they are able to recognize and lyse malignant cells without prior antigen specificity.[23] NK cells are highly responsive to internal or external stimuli.[24,25] Several animal studies have shown that EE enhances NK cell cytotoxicity in tumor-free mice based on an *in vitro* splenocyte cytotoxicity assay.[1,26] A recent study has shown that minimal cage enrichment by providing an igloo can enhance the activation of NK cells and thereby contributing to tumor suppressing effect in a murine ovarian cancer model.[27] This surprising finding has yet been validated by other labs or in additional mouse strains and cancer models.

Song and colleagues have characterized EE effects on NK cells in more details and demonstrated that NK cell–mediated immunity plays a critical role in EE-induced tumor inhibition in murine models of pancreatic cancer and lung cancer.[28] Tumor-infiltrating NK cells from EE mice has a distinct pattern of surface markers in comparison to those in SE mice. Significantly higher expression of activating cell surface markers CD107a[29] and NKG2D receptor[30] on tumor-infiltrating NK cells is consistent with enhanced capability to lyse tumor cells. Furthermore, a greater number of CCR5+ NK cells is observed in pancreatic tumors of EE mice, suggesting an enhanced regulation of tumor infiltration.[28]

NK cells are heterogeneous with regard to their phenotype, function, and anatomic distribution. NK cells are thought to develop primarily in the bone marrow, but can also develop and mature in SLTs such as spleen, lymph nodes, and tonsils.[31,32] NK cell precursors circulate in the blood and reside in the spleen, lymph nodes, and other peripheral nonlymphoid organs where they continue to develop and mature.[33] The maturation of NK cells is critical for the acquisition of robust effector functions and for the immune response to tumors. Mouse NK cells undergo a maturation process that can be defined by the expression of the surface markers CD27 and CD11b: stage I, precursor (CD11b^{low}, CD27^{low}); stage II, immature (CD11b^{low}, CD27^{high}); stage III, proinflammatory (CD11b^{high}, CD27^{high}); and stage IV, cytotoxic (CD11b^{high}, CD27^{low}).[34]

The NK cell development is regulated by both genetic and environmental factors.[32,35] Meng and colleagues report that EE promotes the terminal maturation of NK cells both within the bone marrow and peripherally in the spleen and blood.[36] Additionally, EE increases CD27+ stage II immature and stage III proinflammatory NK cell proliferation in the bone marrow and blood.[36] The authors report that removal of spleen attenuates the tumor suppressing effect of EE supporting a role of NK cell immunity in EE's anticancer effect. Blockade of sympathetic signaling either by nonselective β blocker propranolol[1,36] or by chemical sympathectomy[37] eliminates these NK modifications and antitumor effects of EE, indicating the involvement of SNS.

In line with inhibitory effects of EE on peripheral tumors, EE exposure has been shown to slow the growth rate and reduce tumor size, as well as to extend survival of mice receiving orthotopic glioma implantations.[38] The authors propose both immune and nonimmune mechanisms underlying the suppression of glioma. The former is EE stimulation of BDNF, which directly acts on the glioma (see Chapter 2). And the latter is EE-induced NK cell accumulation and activation via an increase of the cytokine interleukin (IL)-15. IL-15 supports NK cell development and triggers their proliferation, motility, activation, and cytotoxic effector molecule expression.[39,40] Garofalo and colleagues report higher cerebral level of IL-15 in EE mice correlated with smaller glioma mass. Brain infusion of IL-15 protein increases the frequency of NK cell infiltrating the glioma. NK cell depletion attenuates the tumor-inhibitory effect and survival benefits induced by EE or exogenous IL-15.[38] These encouraging results may facilitate clinical trials testing the effect of IL-15 in patients suffering from malignant glioma.

EE Promotes NK Cell Maturation via Hypothalamic BDNF

In agreement with literature, we also observed that EE promoted NK cell maturation in the spleen. We were interested in teasing out a central mechanism of this EE-induced NK effect and zoomed in to the hypothalamic BDNF because of its essential roles in driving the metabolic outcome and T cell modulation associated with EE. We wanted to explore whether EE is effective in other indications involving NK cells.

Congenital or iatrogenic deficiency of NK cell numbers has been associated with an increased incidence of life-threatening infections.[41,42] Studies have shown that rapid and robust NK cell recovery early after hematopoietic cell transplant is associated with less relapse, non-relapse mortality, and improved survival.[43,44] Conversely, abrogation of NK cell maturation has been observed in progression of acute myeloid leukemia (AML).[45,46] These reports suggest clinical implications of NK cell recovery and NK cell maturation.[47] Hence, identifying factors that control NK cell development and reconstitution is relevant to improving clinical outcomes following hematopoietic stem cell transplantation and treatment of AML. We conducted a study to examine whether EE influenced NK cell reconstitution and maturation following their *in vivo* depletion and whether hypothalamic BDNF mediates EE-induced NK phenotypes.[48]

Anti-asialo GM1 antibody is commonly used to deplete NK cells in animal studies of NK cell functions. We first verified the depletion efficacy and found a single dose of anti-asialo GM1 eliminated both splenic and bone marrow NK cells by over 95% compared to a control group injected with IgG isotype. Time course monitoring revealed it took approximately 23 days to recover the blood NK cell level to ~50%, comparable to the recovery rate reported in literature.[49] At 23-day post anti-asialo GM1 injection, the frequency of NK cells remained >50% lower in bone marrow and spleen compared to isotype IgG control group.[48]

To examine how EE influences NK cell recovery and maturation, male C57BL/6 mice, 4 weeks old, were injected with anti-asialo GM1 antibody, and then randomly assigned to live in SE or EE housing for 23 days. At 23 days of EE or SE housing, the frequency of splenic NK cells was 2-fold higher in EE mice compared to their counterparts in SE (**Fig. 6.6(a)**) together with a significant increase in absolute number of splenic NK cells (**Fig. 6.6(b)**). In addition, EE significantly increased the NK cell proportion in the bone marrow and the blood by 1.5-fold and 2.5-fold, respectively. Hypothalamic BDNF expression was upregulated in EE groups.[48]

In terms of NK maturation, the EE mice displayed a shift toward more mature NK subsets in the spleen characterized as significantly lower percentage of Stage I and Stage II immature splenic NK cells, higher percentage of Stage IV mature subset (**Fig. 6.6(c)**). Of note, unlike the spleen, EE did not have similar effect on NK maturation in either bone marrow or the blood, suggesting distinct mechanisms

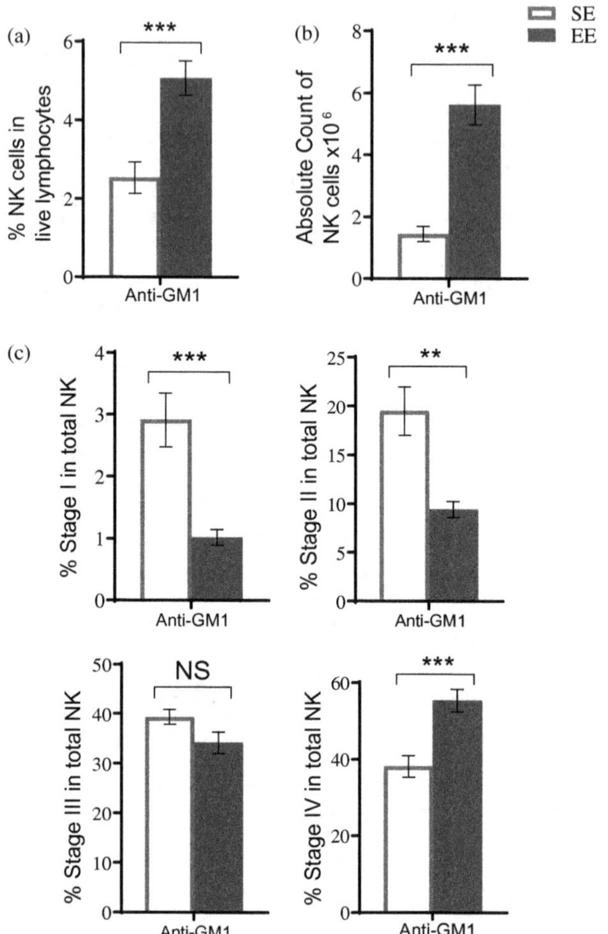

Fig. 6.6. EE enhances splenic NK cell maturation following NK cell depletion by anti-asialo GM1 treatment. (a) Frequency and (b) absolute number of splenic NK cells (Lin NK1.1$^+$CD49b$^+$) assessed in mice housed in SE or EE 23 days after anti-asialo GM1 treatment on day 0. (c) Percentage of splenic NK cells from each of four stages of NK cell maturation. Data are mean ± SEM, n = 5 for SE, n = 7 for EE. $**P < 0.01$, $***P < 0.001$, NS, nonsignificant. Reprinted from Mansour *et al.* Enriched environment enhances NK cell maturation through hypothalamic BDNF in male mice. *Eur J Immunol* 2021, 51(3), 557–556, with permission of John Wiley and Sons.

govern different tissues in modulating the maturation or migration of NK cells.[48]

Because changes of NK maturation were found neither in the bone marrow nor in the blood at 3-week EE exposure, we thought these changes likely take place in the SLTs. Hence, we investigated whether hypothalamic BDNF controls EE modulation of NK maturation in the SLTs. Overexpressing BDNF in the hypothalamus resulted in a significant decrease in the Stage II while a significant increase in Stage IV NK cells in both the spleen and lymph nodes. On the other hand, preventing the upregulation of hypothalamic BDNF expression was sufficient to block the shift of NK cell stages induced by EE.[48] This study not only identifies one key brain molecule mediating the EE's regulation of peripheral NK cell maturation but also add evidence to the notion that hypothalamic BDNF serves as a center hub linking environmental stimuli and peripheral metabolic and immune phenotypes. It will be intriguing to investigate whether EE or overexpressing BDNF can mitigate the impaired NK cell maturation in patients and mice with AML[45,46,50] or other clinically relevant conditions.

The downstream effectors in the hypothalamic BDNF-SNS pathway mediating EE modulation of NK cells remain unknown. Given the enhanced NK maturation and cytotoxicity associated with EE, we speculate that IL-15 might be a downstream effector in the periphery as the case in the brain.[38] Although a published study finds no change of circulating IL-15 in EE mice,[36] we think it is worthy of examining whether EE influences different forms of IL-15 in the circulation and in various tissues and organs. Moreover, cytokine profile analysis of serum samples should be further explored in order to discover potential effectors downstream of the neuro-immune regulatory pathway.

Exercise influences NK functions dependent on multiple factors such as the exercise regime, duration, and intensity.[51–53] Our research has repeatedly demonstrated physical activity alone unable to account for the beneficial effects on systemic metabolism, aging, and cancer associated with EE. However, the contribution of exercise to the EE-induced immune phenotypes has not been interrogated, which certainly requires future investigations.

EE Regulates Adipose Resident NK Cell via Hypothalamic BDNF-Adipocyte IL-15 Axis

Given the profound adipose remodeling and regulation of T cells and NK cells in SLT by EE, we naturally turned eyes to the immune populations residing in the adipose tissue. There is rising interest in the adipose immune microenvironment because of its significant consequences for both normal adipose tissue physiology and for the tumor immune microenvironment as well as cancer progression.[54] Many different immune cell populations reside in adipose tissue including myeloid and lymphoid cells. Both adaptive and innate lymphocytes play important roles in adipocyte physiology and response to stress such as cold exposure and high-fat diet (HFD) feeding.[55–60] However, little is known about how one's physical and social environment may influence the adipose tissue immune microenvironment, and no data published about EE effects. Hence, we explored how EE affects the composition of white adipose tissue (WAT) immune microenvironment and discovered an expansion of WAT NK cells in mice living in the EE.[61]

We first examined the immune cell composition of the inguinal WAT (iWAT, a surrogate for subcutaneous fat) and the epididymal WAT (eWAT, a surrogate for visceral fat) after 2-week exposure to EE at that time body weight was not different but both fat pad masses were reduced in EE mice. We isolated the stromal vascular fraction (SVF) of adipose tissue that contains both nonimmune cells (endothelial cells, fibroblasts, and preadipocytes) and immune cells,[62] and performed flow cytometry to screen cellular changes in the immune populations residing in WAT (**Table 6.1**). EE had no effect on the percentage of CD45[+] immune cells within the SVF of either

Table 6.1   Flow Cytometry Panels

Cell	Flow Layout	Panel
LIN-	CD45+Lineage-	Innate lymphocyte
NK	CD45+Lineage-NK1.1+CD127-/dim	Innate lymphocyte
Macrophage (Macro)	CD45+F480+SiglecF-	Macrophage
M1	CD45+F480+SiglecF-CD11C+CD206-	Macrophage
M2	CD45+F480+SiglecF-CD11C-/dimCD206+	Macrophage
DN (M0)	CD45+F480+SiglecF-CD11C-CD206-	Macrophage
Eosinophil (Eos)	CD45+F480-SigletF+	Macrophage
T cell (T)	CD45+CD3+	Adaptive lymphocyte
CD4 T cell	CD45+CD3+CD4+CD8-	Adaptive lymphocyte
Treg	CD45+CD3+CD4+CD25+	Adaptive lymphocyte
CD8 T cell	CD45+CD3+CD4-CD8+	Adaptive lymphocyte
B cell (B)	CD45+CD3-CD19+	Adaptive lymphocyte

eWAT or iWAT. EE was associated with an increase in the abundance of NK cells (defined as CD45$^+$ LIN (CD3 CD19)$^-$ NK1.1$^+$) in both fat depots (**Fig. 6.7(a), (b)**). The NK cell numbers calibrated to fat depot mass were significantly higher in EE mice compared to SE mice (**Fig. 6.7(c)**). Mild effects on myeloid populations were observed but in a fat depot–dependent fashion. CD8 T cell abundance was decreased in both iWAT and eWAT of EE mice (**Fig. 6.7(a), (b)**).[61]

As the increase in the frequency of NK cells was significant in both subcutaneous and visceral fat depots, we decided to investigate NK cell as our first attempt to understanding how EE regulates adipose immune microenvironment. To search for regulatory factors, we profiled gene expression of isolated mature adipocytes after a 2-week exposure of EE including cytokines known to be involved in NK regulation. NK cell development and homeostasis are dependent on the presence of the cytokine IL-15.[63–65] IL-15 and IL-2 share

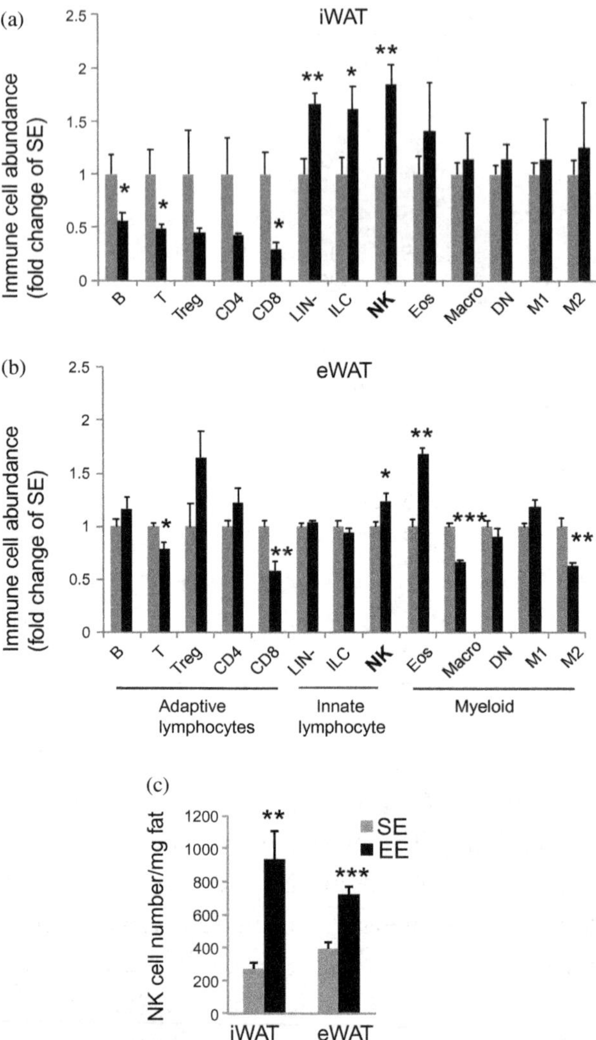

Fig. 6.7. EE alters adipose immune microenvironment. (a) Fold change of immune cell composition in subcutaneous iWAT. (b) Fold change of immune cell composition in visceral eWAT. (c) Total NK cell numbers in iWAT and eWAT after 2-week EE exposure. Data are mean ± SEM, $n = 5$ per group. *$P < 0.05$, **$P < 0.01$ ***$P < 0.001$. Reprinted from Environmental activation of a hypothalamic BDNF-adipocyte IL-15 axis regulates adipose-natural killer cells, Bergin *et al. Brain Behav Immun* 2021, 95, 477–488, with permission from Elsevier.

many structural features including the use of the two shared receptor (R) subunits (IL-2/IL-15Rβ and IL-2/IL-15Rγ) and similar intracellular signaling. The cytokine-specific receptor α subunit, IL-15Rα, is the high-affinity form of the IL-15 receptor.[66] The main action mode of IL-15 is through *trans-* presentation, meaning IL-15 is *trans* presented as IL-15/IL-15Rα complex expressed on the antigen-presenting cells (activated monocytes and dendritic cells) to the IL-2R/IL-15Rβ, and γ heterodimer expressed on effector NK, T, and B cells.[67–69] Adipocytes can be another source of IL-15.[70] We found that EE upregulated expression of *Il15* and *Il15ra* in mature adipocytes isolated from both iWAT and eWAT, but not in the SVF, while the IL-2/15R (*Il2rg*) was not changed (**Fig. 6.8(a)**). Immunoblot confirmed the increase of IL-15 protein levels in adipocytes (**Fig. 6.8(b)**).[61]

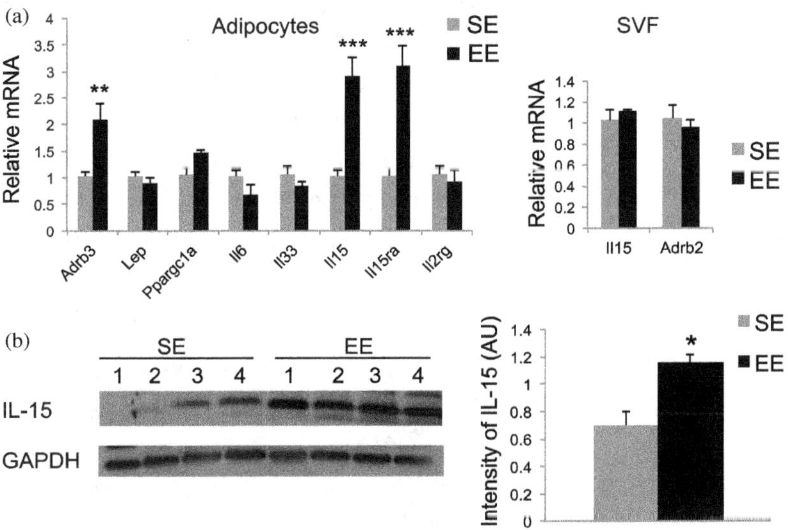

Fig. 6.8.   EE induces gene expression changes in adipose tissue. (a) EE upregulates *Il15* and its receptor expression in adipocytes but not the stromal vascular fraction (SVF). (B) Western blot of iWAT and quantification. Each number represents an individual mouse. Data are mean ± SEM, *n* = 5 per group in (a), *n* = 4 per group in (b). *P < 0.05, **P < 0.01 ***P < 0.001. Reprinted from Environmental activation of a hypothalamic BDNF-adipocyte IL-15 axis regulates adipose-natural killer cells, Bergin *et al. Brain Behav Immun* 2021, 95, 477–488, with permission from Elsevier.

We hypothesized that adipocyte-derived IL-15 directly mediates the expansion of adipose NK cells seen in EE. To test this hypothesis, we generated a microRNA to knockdown murine *Il15* (named miR-Il15), and a control microRNA targeting a scrambled sequence against no known gene (named miR-scr). We then used our newly characterized adipose-tropic AAV serotype Rec2 vector (see Chapter 4) to knockdown *Il15* expression in the mature adipocytes.[71,72] We injected mice with either Rec2-miR-Il15 or Rec2-miR-scr, and then randomly placed half of each vector group to live in EE or SE (**Fig. 6.9(a)**). After 4-week EE housing, eWAT mass was lower in EE mice than their counterparts in the SE housing regardless of injection with miR-Il15 or miR-scr (**Fig. 6.9(b)**). The drop of the serum leptin level is a reliable metric for EE-induced metabolic phenotypes.[1,11,73] Both miR-Il15 and miR-scr mice living in EE showed a significant reduction in circulating leptin level (**Fig. 6.9(c)**). Moreover, miR-Il15 did not interfere with the EE-induced upregulation of *Bdnf* in the hypothalamus, the upstream effector of the HSA axis (**Fig. 6.9(d)**). However, gene delivery of miR-Il15 to adipocytes prevented the EE-induced upregulation of adipocyte *Il15* mRNA (**Fig. 6.9(e)**) and attenuated the upregulation of adipocyte *Il15ra* mRNA (**Fig. 6.9(f)**). Importantly, adipocyte *Il15* knockdown reduced the adipose NK cell frequency in the SE-housed mice (miR-Il15/SE versus miR-scr/SE) and abolished the expansion of adipose NK cells in the EE-housed mice (miR-Il15/EE versus miR-Il15/SE) (**Fig. 6.9(g)**).[61]

To test whether increasing the expression of *Il15* can mimic EE effect on adipose NK cells, we generated a Rec2 vector to preferentially overexpress *Il15* in the visceral fat (named AS/Rec2-IL15). A vector containing the same expression cassette but lacking a transgene was used as control (named AS/Rec2-empty). Mice, intraperitoneally injected with either AS/Rec2-IL15 or AS/Rec2-empty, were housed in SE for 3 weeks. The two groups did not differ in body weight or tissue mass of thymus, spleen, iWAT, or eWAT. No significant changes of eWAT SVF cell number, serum levels of IL-15

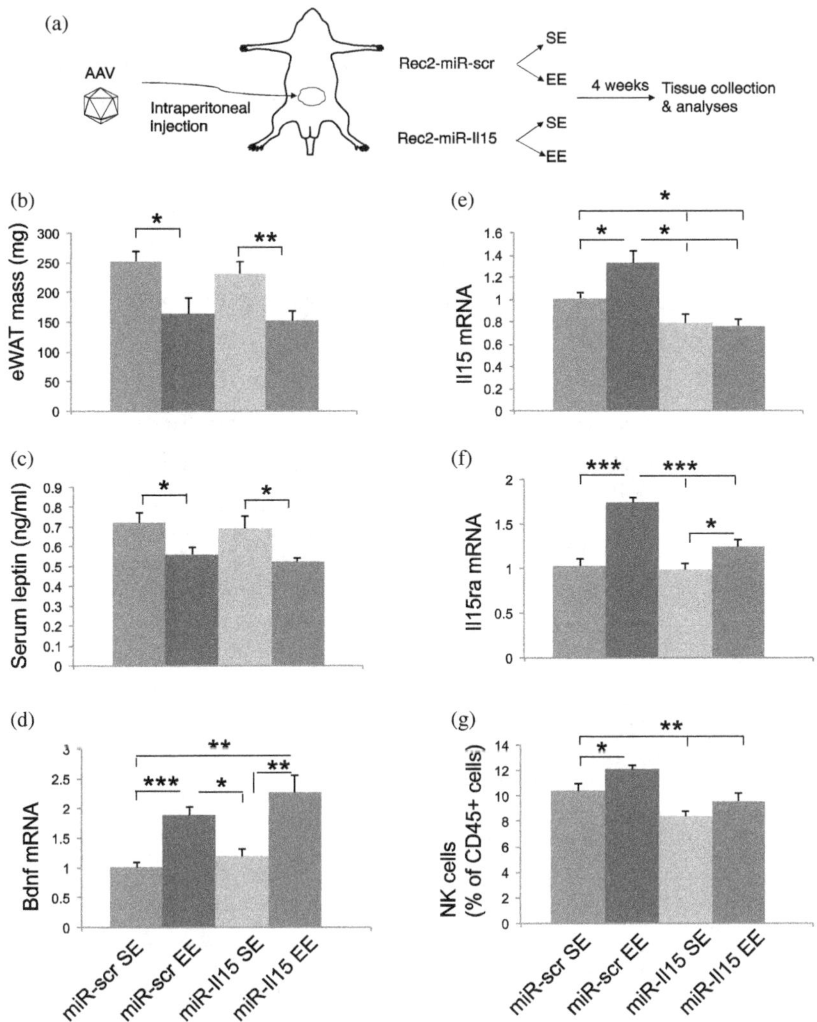

Fig. 6.9. AAV-mediated IL-15 knockdown in adipocytes selectively inhibits EE regulation of adipose NK cells. (a) Experimental design (b) eWAT mass after Intraperitoneal injection of AAV vector and EE housing. (c) Serum leptin levels. (d) Hypothalamic *Bdnf* expression. (e) eWAT adipocyte Il15 expression. (f) eWAT adipocyte *Il15ra* expression. (g) eWAT NK cells abundance. Data are mean ± SEM, *n* = 7–8 per group. *P < 0.05, **P < 0.01 ***P < 0.001. Reprinted from Environmental activation of a hypothalamic BDNF-adipocyte IL-15 axis regulates adipose-natural killer cells, Bergin *et al. Brain Behav Immun* 2021, 95, 477–488, with permission from Elsevier.

or leptin were observed. However, mice injected with AS/Rec2-IL15 showed a robust overexpression of *Il15* mRNA and protein in eWAT adipocytes, and a 2-fold increase in adipose NK cells. Of note, no changes in spleen or blood NK cells were observed.[61] These data suggest that AAV-mediated overexpression of *Il15* in visceral fat adipocytes results in a primarily local increase in NK cells restricted within the transduced fat depot.

Additional mechanistic studies demonstrated that the adipocyte IL-15 change induced by EE was downstream of the HSA axis.[61] We propose a hypothalamic BDNF-sympathoneural-adipocyte IL-15 axis as a regulatory mechanism through which EE increases NK cell abundance in both subcutaneous and visceral fat depots in lean animals (**Fig. 6.10**). This notion of hypothalamic BDNF-adipocyte IL-15 axis is supported by several lines of evidence:

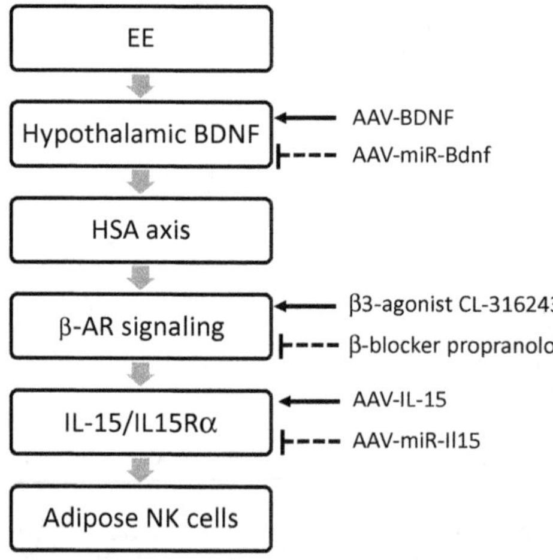

Fig. 6.10. Mechanisms of EE-induced adipose NK cell modulation. EE upregulates BDNF expression in the hypothalamus and subsequently elevates sympathetic tone to the adipose tissue. The resulting activation of β-adrenergic receptor signaling induces IL-15 and its receptor expression in adipocytes, whereby stimulating adipose resident NK cells. Gain- and loss-of-function studies identify each major component of the brain BDNF-adipose IL-15 axis.

1. Hypothalamic overexpression of BDNF replicated the EE-induced expansion of adipose NK cells whereas inhibition of BDNF signaling from the hypothalamus via TrkB.T1 reversed this effect.

2. Signaling through the SNS serves as the link between hypothalamic BDNF and WAT. The administration of a β blocker propranolol prevented the expansion of adipose NK cells in the EE. Conversely, the use of a β3-specific agonist CL-316243 induced a robust increase of adipocyte *Il15* and Il15ra expression and concordant higher abundance of adipose NK cells, thereby reproducing the EE effect on adipose NK cell.

3. Adipocyte-derived IL-15 is the final effector of this axis. EE upregulated *Il15* and *Il15ra* expression only in the mature adipocytes but not in the SVF. Knockdown of adipocyte *Il15* sufficiently blocked the EE effect on adipose NK cells whereas adipocyte overexpression of IL-15 expanded the adipose NK cell population in SE without affecting blood-circulating or spleen NK cells.

Taken together, these findings suggest EE shapes the innate immune microenvironment within WAT driven by a defined brain-fat axis.

We always have this question in mind when a mechanistic pathway is discovered from EE research: can this molecular pathway be exploited to improve health or treat disease? With regard to adipose NK cells, we asked whether adipocyte IL-15 could be targeted to mobilize adipose NK cells against a tumor at distal location. In a proof-of-concept study, we injected mice with either AS/Rec2-Il15 or AS/Rec2-empty (2×10^{10} vg per mouse). Six weeks after intraperitoneal injection of AAV vectors, B16 melanoma cells were implanted subcutaneously on the flank (10^5 cells per mouse) (**Fig. 6.11(a)**). At 18-day post tumor inoculation, tumor mass in AS/Rec2-Il15-treated mice was 64% smaller compared to AS/Rec2-empty-treated mice (**Fig. 6.11(b, c)**). The reduction of tumor mass was not associated

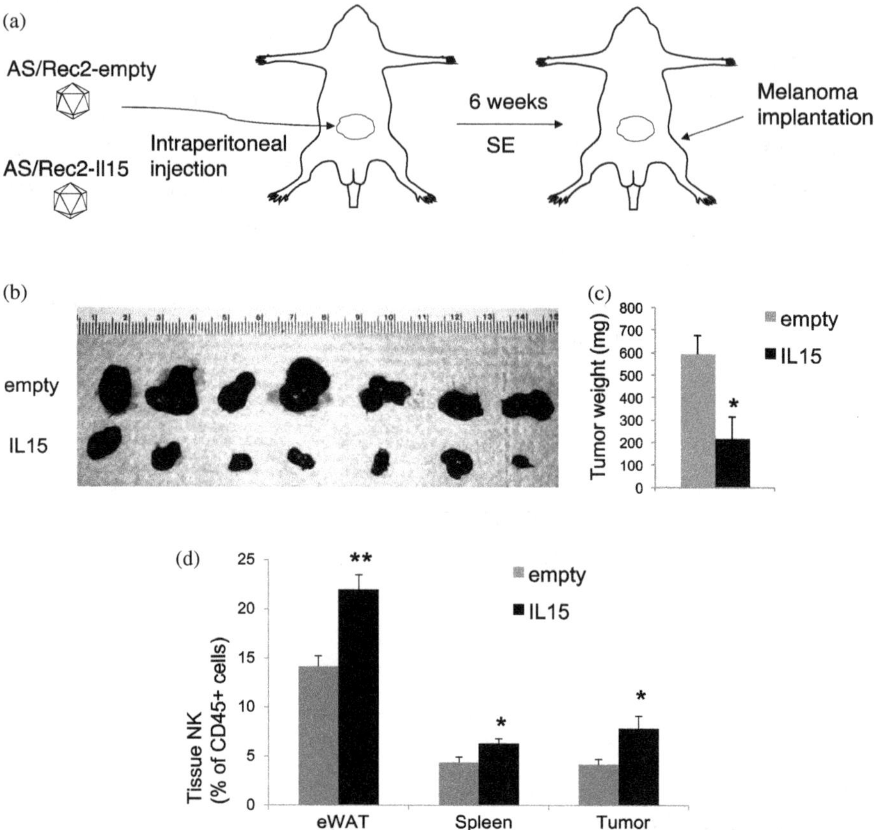

Fig. 6.11. Adipose tissue gene transfer of IL-15 stimulates adipose NK cells and inhibits tumor growth. (a) Experimental design. (b) V16 melanomas dissected 18 days after tumor cell implantation. (c) Tumor weight. (d) NK cell abundance in eWAT, spleen, and tumor. Data are mean ± SEM, $n = 7$ per group. *$P < 0.05$, **$P < 0.01$. Reprinted from Environmental activation of a hypothalamic BDNF-adipocyte IL-15 axis regulates adipose-natural killer cells, Bergin *et al. Brain Behav Immun* 2021, 95, 477–488, with permission from Elsevier.

with a change of serum IL-15 level, but was associated with an increase of NK cells within eWAT, in the spleen, and in the tumor (**Fig. 6.11(d)**). It is worth noting that adipocyte-specific overexpression of IL-15 did not alter splenic NK cells in the absence of a tumor but did significantly increase splenic NK cells when challenged with a distal tumor.[61] These data suggest that targeting the adipocyte to enhance cellular immunity, either with direct gene transfer of IL-15 or through activation of hypothalamic BDNF, may be a possible strategy for enhancing NK cell antitumor activity for cancer treatment.

Adipose Tissue–Oriented Cancer Gene Therapy

In a separate gene therapy project, we investigated the therapeutic efficacy of an adipose-targeting AAV vector expressing an IL-15/IL-15Rα complex. This idea is based on the *trans*-presentation type of action mode of IL-15. IL-15 binds its receptor α chain IL-15Rα on the surface of antigen presenting cells (APCs). The resulting IL-15/IL-15Rα complex binds to the IL2/IL-15Rβ/γc receptor across the immunologic synapse, and thereby stimulating neighboring effector cells such as NK cells and CD8 T cells. *Trans*-presentation requires close cell–cell contact and enables context-dependent activation of effector cells.[74]

Recombinant IL-15 protein has been shown to stimulate NK cells, leading to enhanced antitumor activity in animal studies as a single agent or in combination with vaccines and drug treatments.[75] However, administration of IL-15 protein has shown several limitations including a short half-life, poor tolerability, and low biological activity *in vivo*,[76,77] possibly contributing to modest antitumor responses in the first clinical trial.[78] To overcome these limitations, IL-15/IL-15Rα complex or derivatives of IL-15/IL-15Rα complex (claimed as super-agonist), such as ALT-803, have been developed.[79,80] Recent studies have shown that ALT-803 superior to IL-15 alone largely due to its extended half-life and longer persistence in tissues, leading to enhanced antitumor effects in preclinical studies including multiple myeloma,[81] bladder cancer,[79] glioblastoma,[82] and breast cancer.[83] Moreover, recent clinical trials have shown that ALT-803 induces several clinical responses in patients with ovarian cancer,[84] non–small cell lung cancer,[85] advanced melanoma, renal cell, head and neck cancer,[86] or hematological malignancies who relapse after allogeneic hematopoietic cell transplantation.[87] Despite an extended half-life, ALT-803 requires repeated administration every 5–7 days, and skin rashes at the subcutaneous administration site occur in many patients.[87] Hence, alternative approaches aiming to sustained delivery of IL-15/IL-15Rα complex may improve therapeutic efficacy and eliminate adverse effects.

We were encouraged by the promising results that IL-15 gene delivery to visceral fat induced adipose NK cell expansion and suppressed the growth of subcutaneously implanted melanoma, and therefore expanded the adipose-oriented gene therapy to IL-15/IL-15Rα complex.[88] We synthesized an IL-15/IL-15Rα complex transgene by linking IL-15 and IL-15Rα with a 2A sequence,[89–91] and used the dual-cassette adipose-targeting rAAV vector for gene delivery to the visceral fat via intraperitoneal administration. This gene therapy was evaluated in two cancer models: a subcutaneous implantation of Lewis lung cancer (LLC) and a metastatic model with intraperitoneal injection of B16-F10 melanoma[92] (**Fig. 6.12**).

A single intraperitoneal injection of the therapeutic vector (AS/Rec2-IL-15/IL-15Rα complex, 2×10^{10} vg per mouse) led to 65% higher IL-15/IL-15Rα complex protein level in the serum compared to mice receiving a vector with the identical backbone without a transgene (AS/Rec2-empty, 2×10^{10} vg per mouse). In visceral fat, IL-15/IL-15Rα complex gene delivery doubled the frequency of NK cells and tripled the absolute number of NK cells, with no effects on the frequency of T cells or the CD4/CD8 ratio. Moreover, IL-15/IL-15Rα complex treatment resulted in a >2-fold increase in the frequency and absolute number of NK cells in the spleen, and a shift toward mature NK subsets by decreasing the Stage II immature subset meanwhile increasing Stage IV cytotoxic subset. CD69 expression on NK cells was not changed. Gene therapy had no effects on IFN-γ secretion from NK, CD4, or CD8 cells *in vitro*, suggesting the NK cells not activated in tumor-free animals.[92]

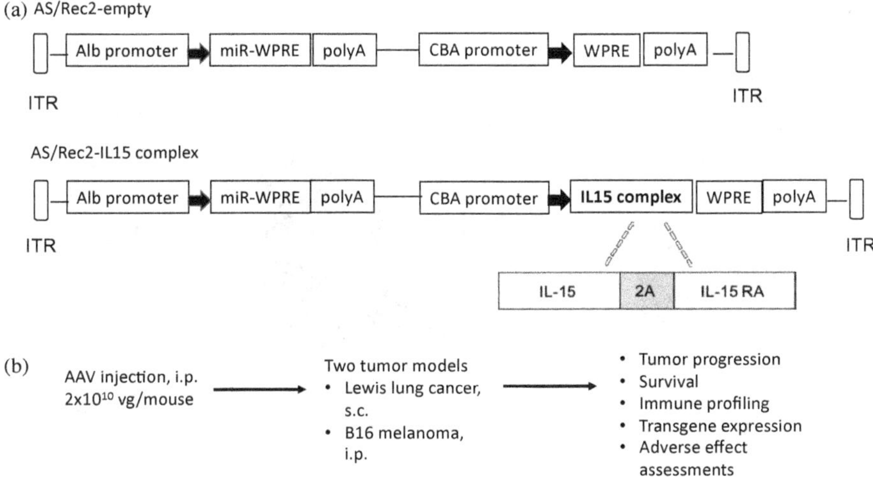

Fig. 6.12. Targeting fat for cancer immune therapy. (a) Schematic of AAV vector. (b) Study designs.

Adverse effects have been reported with administration of IL-15 protein or IL-15 superagonist such as weight loss, hypothermia, and liver injury.[93–95] In this preclinical study, we monitored the mice for 5 weeks after AAV injection to assess adverse effects, and found no changes in behavior, body weight, food intake, body temperature, liver function panel, spleen weight and total splenocyte counts, or complete blood count with differentials. These data suggest an excellent safety profile of adipose-oriented IL-15 gene therapy, which is associated with approximately 2-fold increase of NK cells in spleen and visceral fat.[88] It is reported that four repeated intraperitoneal infusions of IL-15/IL-15Rα complex protein result in a 16-fold increase in NK cells associated with toxicity and organomegaly.[95] Hepatic IL-15/IL-15Rα complex gene therapy via intravenous injection leads to ~50-fold increase in NK cells associated with organomegaly.[80,96] These data from literature and our study suggest a milder but sustained increase of IL-15/IL-15Rα complex level without the spike by protein injection may avoid measurable toxicity.

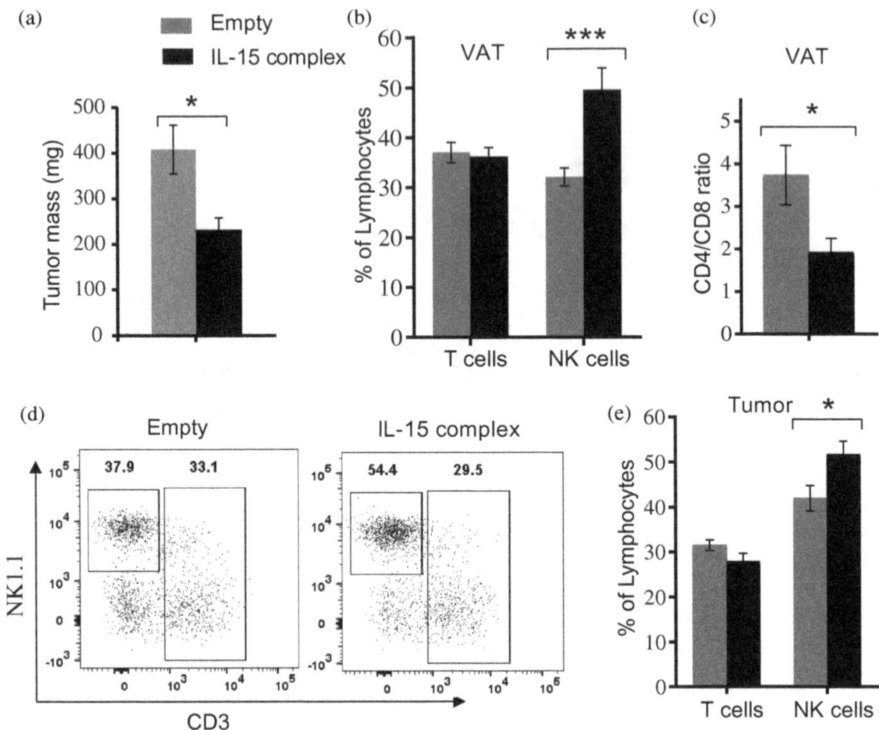

Fig. 6.13. Adipocyte IL-15 complex gene therapy suppresses LLC growth. (a) LLC tumor mass. (b) Percentage of NK cells and T cells in visceral WAT (VAT). (c) CD4/CD8 ratio in VAT. (d) Representative flow cytometry of NK and T cells in tumor. (e) Percentage of NK and T cells in tumor. Data are mean ± SEM, n = 10 per group. *P < 0.05, ***P < 0.001. Reprinted from Xiao *et al.* Adipocytes: a novel target for IL-15/IL-15R α cancer gene therapy. *Mol Ther* 2019, 27(5), 922–932, with permission of American Society of Gene & Cell Therapy.

To test the effect of visceral fat gene therapy on the growth of a distant tumor, we implanted LLC cells subcutaneously to mice 5 weeks after AAV injection. IL-15/IL-15Rα complex gene therapy led to 50% reduction in tumor mass (**Fig. 6.13**), associated with immune changes including ~25% increase in NK frequency in tumor infiltrating lymphocytes (TILs), 2-fold increase in NK frequency in the spleen, shifting to Stage IV cytotoxic NK subset, and reduced CD4/CD8 ratio. Similar stimulation of NK cells was found in the visceral fat as well.[88]

Next, we determined the effect on survival in a metastasis model in which B16-F10 melanoma cells were intraperitoneally implanted 5 weeks after AAV injection. The gene therapy significantly prolonged the median survival by ~40% (**Fig. 6.14(a)**).

In a separate experiment, IL-15/IL-15Rα complex treatment resulted in reduced tumor burden as evidenced by 60% lower luciferase signal intensity that tagged the tumor cells by 10 days after melanoma implantation (**Fig. 6.14(b, c)**). The suppression of tumor progression was associated with an increase of NK cells in the spleen, visceral fat, tumor site, and peripheral blood, and a shift to mature NK subset (**Fig. 6.15(a, c)**). In this metastatic model, IL-15/IL-15Rα complex gene therapy significantly increased the expression of CD44 on CD4 and CD8 T cells, a marker indicative of effector memory T cells[97,98] (**Fig. 6.15(b)**). The NK, CD4, and CD8 T cells harvested from IL-15/IL-15Rα complex-treated mice showed a significant increase of IFN-γ secretion upon *in vitro* stimulation suggesting an activated state (**Fig. 6.15(e)**). Among TILs, IL-15/IL-15Rα complex-treated mice showed ~4-fold increase in NK frequency and ~50% increase in CD8 T cell frequency (**Fig. 6.15(a), (d)**). These immune alterations collectively suggest an enhanced antitumor immunity of NK cells and CD8 T cells in animals receiving IL-15/IL-15Rα complex gene therapy.[88]

This is the first proof-of-concept study on a molecular therapy targeting the adipose tissue for cancer immune therapy. We are encouraged by the promising results, and intend to expand the adipose IL-15/IL-15Rα complex gene therapy to additional cancer models, and to assess the therapeutic efficacy in established cancer models as well as oncogene-induced cancer models.

We are aware of many questions to be addressed in order to assess the translation potential. For example, obesity is associated with an increased risk of numerous types of cancers and with a poorer prognosis.[99–101] Adipose dysfunction including disturbance of adipose resident immune cells is observed in obese individuals, which is thought to be a mechanism of the obesity–cancer link. Thus, it is important to investigate the immune, metabolic, and anticancer

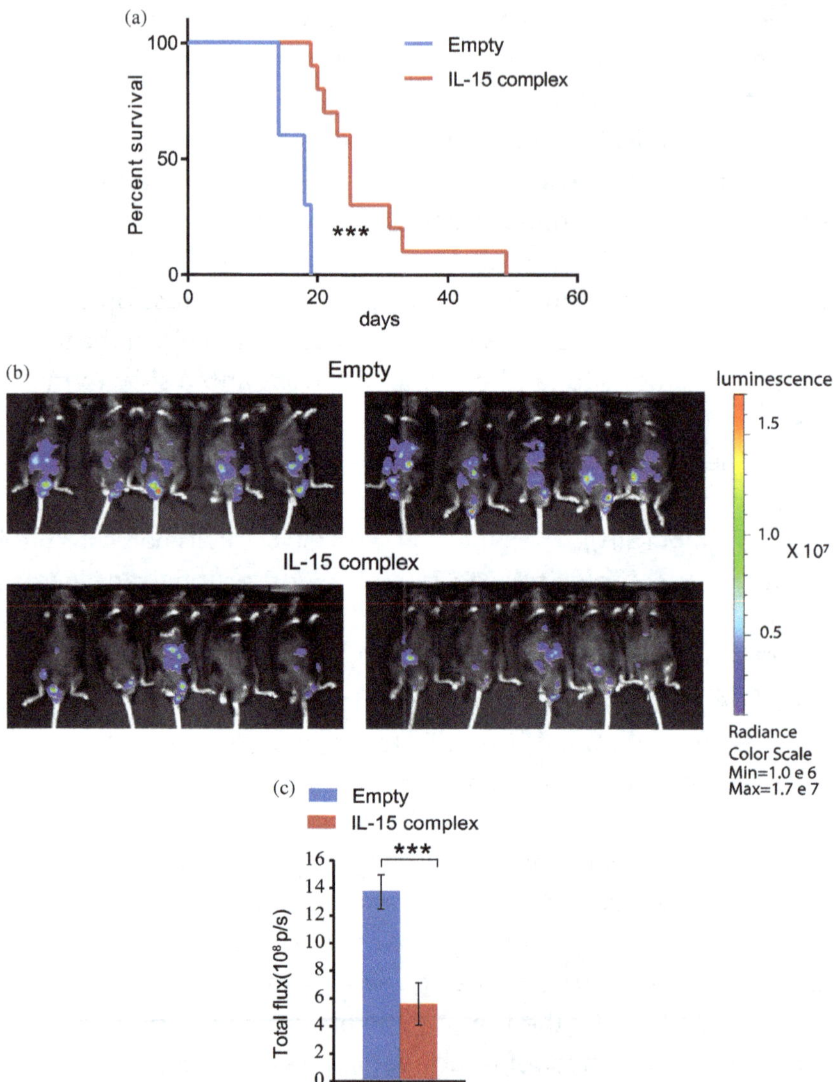

Fig. 6.14. Adipocyte IL-15 complex gene therapy extends survival in a pre-clinical mouse model of metastatic melanoma. (a) Keplan–Meier survival curve analysis of mice treated with AAV vectors, followed by Intraperitoneal injection of B16-F10 melanoma cells. (b) *In vivo* bioluminescence imaging of luciferase-expressing B16-F10 at day-10 post tumor implantation in a separate experiment. (c) Total bioluminescence activity (photons per second). Data are mean ± SEM, *n* = 10 per group. **P < 0.01. Reprinted from Xiao *et al.* Adipocytes: a novel target for IL-15/IL-15Rα cancer gene therapy. *Mol Ther* 2019, 27(5), 922–932, with permission of American Society of Gene & Cell Therapy.

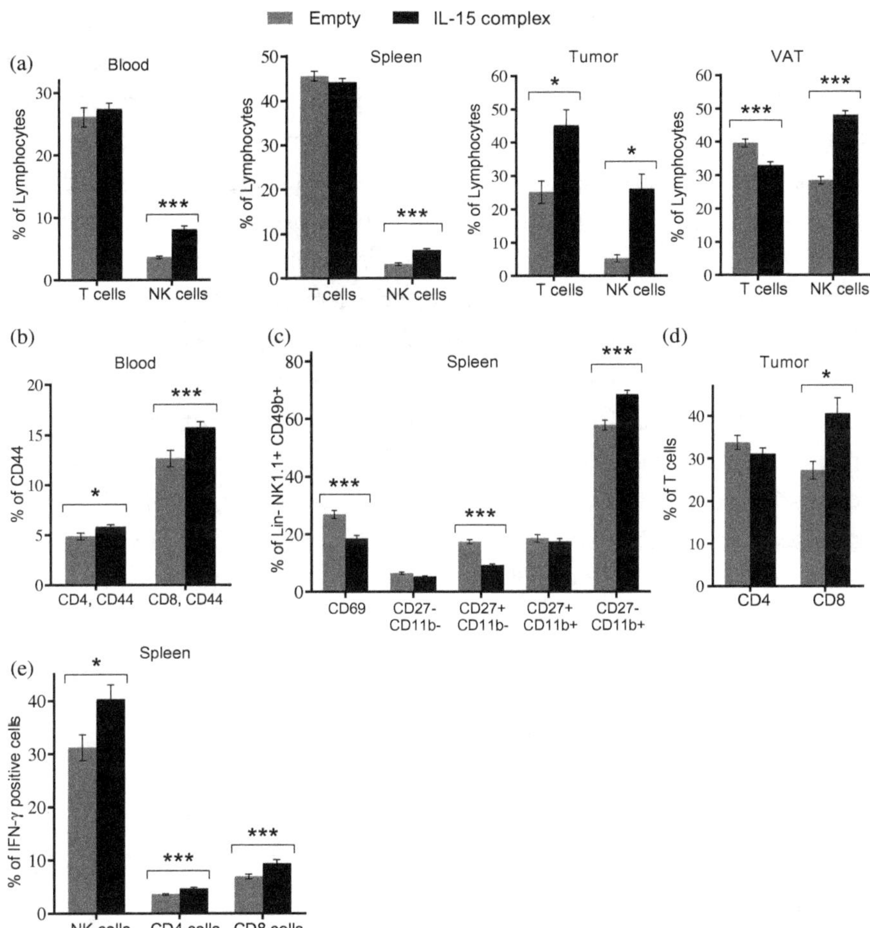

Fig. 6.15. Adipocyte IL-15 complex gene therapy enhances antitumor immunity in mice bearing B16-F10 melanoma. (a) Percentage of NK and T cells in blood, spleen, tumor, and VAT. (b) CD44 expression on CD4 or CD8 T cells in blood. (c) Percentage of CD69 and NK cell maturation stages of splenic NK cells. (d) Percentage of CD4 and CD8 T cells in tumor. (e) IFN-γ expression in splenic NK and T cells after 6-hr *in vitro* stimulation. Data are mean ± SEM, *n* = 10 per group. *P < 0.05, ***P < 0.001. Reprinted from Xiao *et al.* Adipocytes: a novel target for IL-15/ IL-15Rα cancer gene therapy. *Mol Ther* 2019, 27(5), 922–932, with permission of American Society of Gene & Cell Therapy.

effects of adipose IL-15/IL-15Rα complex gene therapy in the context of obesity. On the other hand, patients with advanced cancer may have low fat reserves, which may limit the success of adipose gene therapy. Moreover, a recent study reports that continuous treatment with IL-15 can cause NK cell exhaustion and functional impairment.[102] It remains to be seen whether the current gene therapy approach would result in NK cell exhaustion. Additionally, there are some concerns about tumor formation in the context of prolonged exposure to high-level endogenous IL-15 such as a genetic-modified mouse line overexpressing IL-15.[103] Long-term monitoring of adipose gene transfer will address this concern. A regulatory strategy or rescue approach may improve the safety of gene therapy. In this sense, adipose tissue as the target of gene transfer might be of advantage compared to liver because fat could be removed in the worst scenario when transgene expression causes serious concerns.

Immune and Nonimmune Mechanisms of Anticancer Effects of EE

A decade of research has demonstrated that EE, representing an active social, mental, and physical life, confers on mice a tumor-resistant phenotype, through multifactorial mechanisms. We are able to tease out both metabolic and immune mechanisms important for controlling tumor progression. As summarized in **Fig. 6.16**, EE induces BDNF expression in the hypothalamus and thereby elevating sympathetic tone preferentially to the WAT. The subsequent WAT remodeling includes (1) the suppression of leptin expression and release contributing to the suppression of cancer progression, (2) upregulation of phosphatase and tensin homolog (PTEN) contributing to decrease of adipocyte size, and (3) the stimulation of VEGF contributing to the induction of beige cells, elevated energy balance, and resistance to obesity.[1,11,73,104–106] The alleviation of obesity and related metabolic syndromes may in turn inhibit cancer progression

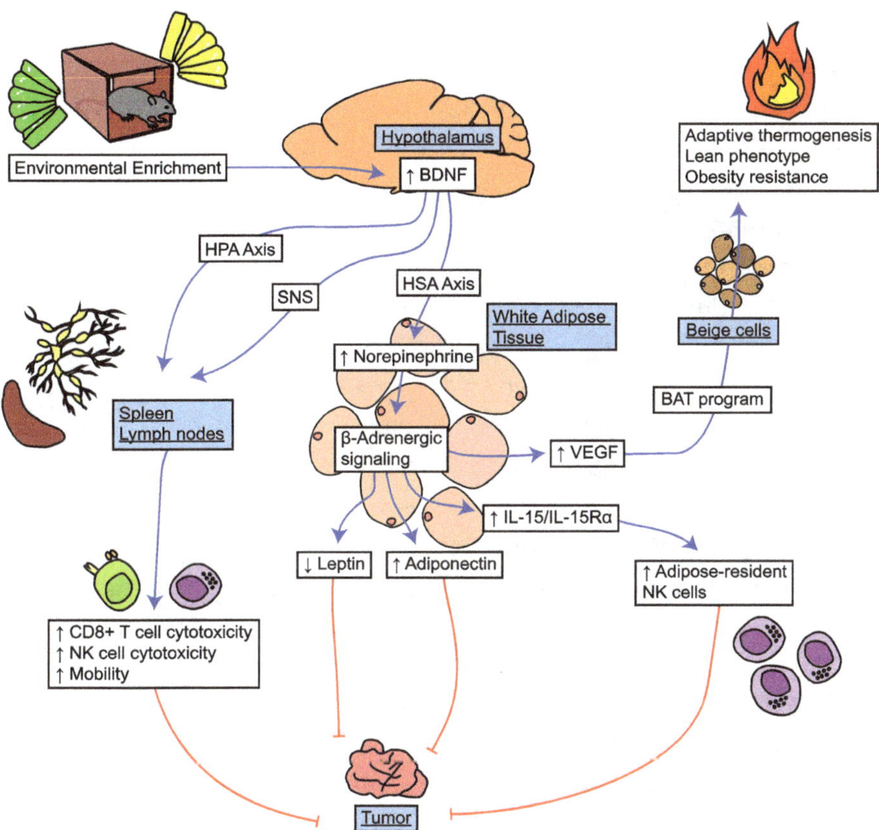

Fig. 6.16. Immune and nonimmune mechanisms of EE's anticancer effects driven by hypothalamic BDNF. Adapted from Hassan *et al*. Regulation of aging and cancer by environmental activation of a hypothalamic-sympathoneural-adipocyte axis. *Transl Cancer Res* 2020, 9(9), 5687–5699.

via multiple mechanisms (see Chapter 5). In addition to metabolic benefits, hypothalamic BDNF plays a critical role in regulating immune effector cells important for antitumor immunity associated with EE.[107–109] Specifically, EE modulates T cell homeostasis in the SLT and enhances CTL activity in the tumor microenvironment.[108] Additionally, EE promotes NK cell maturation, modifies NK activating surface receptors, increases NK cell infiltration of tumors, and enhances NK cell cytotoxicity against cancer cells.[1,36,37,48,110] Blocking one of these metabolic or immune effects of EE can significantly attenuate but not fully abolish the EE-induced tumor inhibition, which underscores the strength of EE to interfere with multiple cancer-promoting capabilities. Hence, targeting hypothalamic BDNF, the driver of many of EE's peripheral benefits, is likely more effective and durable with respect to cancer prevention and treatment (**Fig. 6.16**).

Some data suggest that the immune responses and the metabolic responses might be parallel but the precise relationship between the two phenotypes and whether EE could influence immune cell metabolism require further investigations. It is also plausible that the metabolic and immune phenotypes are intertwined particularly in the context of excessive accumulation of fat and metabolic stress. EE alters the composition of immune microenvironment in the WAT in lean mice while its effects in obesogenic conditions remain unexplored. Obesity is associated with accumulation of large number of macrophages in the WAT and their polarization toward proinflammatory state, which has been implicated as a link between obesity and local and systemic insulin resistance. Therefore, it is interesting to investigate how EE may influence adipose macrophages and the subsequent contributions to local and systemic insulin sensitivity, inflammation, and tumor microenvironment. In addition, augmentation of adipokine balance is one of the main features of EE, including decreased leptin levels and increased adiponectin levels. These adipokines play important roles in the communication between the neuroendocrine and immune systems.[111–114] The role of leptin is worthy of further investigation in the EE-induced immune modulations.

Besides the BDNF-centric pathways discussed here, additional immune and nonimmune mechanisms of EE's anticancer phenotypes have been elucidated in various models of cancer (see Chapter 2). More is certainly to come following the awareness of the profound impact of social and physical environment among cancer research community.

EE Regulates Thymocyte Development and Protects Against Autoimmunity

Apart from T cells in the SLT, we have expanded research on EE's immune modulations to the primary lymphoid organ thymus. Thymocyte selection is responsible for the development of a self-tolerant T cell repertoire capable of responding to foreign antigens. The selective processes require occupancy of the T cell receptor (TCR) by peptide-loaded MHC-encoded molecules (self pMHC). The bone marrow–derived primitive thymocyte precursors lacking expression of TCR, CD4 or CD8 molecules — double negative (DN) cells — pass beta-selection to differentiate into CD4 CD8 double positive (DP) cells. DP thymocytes undergo lineage commitment, maturing into single positive (SP) cells through positive and negative selection. Briefly, the majority of DP thymocytes fail to express TCR with sufficient avidity to rescue them from a default death pathway (positive selection).[115,116] Thymocytes expressing TCRs with high avidity for self over a certain threshold (autoreactive thymocytes) are then eliminated by apoptosis (negative selection).[115,116] As a result, only thymocytes bearing TCRs with intermediate avidity for self are rescued and differentiate into CD4 SP cells or CD8 SP cells. Mature SP T cells exit the thymus, enter circulation, and reside in SLT and other tissues.[115] Studies including ours have found that EE can influence T cell development at each step of the way from thymus to spleen.

EE Regulates Thymocyte Development and Egression

We found that 1-week exposure to EE led to a significant reduction in thymic mass in juvenile mice independent of sex.[117] This thymic involution persisted at least for 3 months associated with lower total number of thymocytes in EE. Nevertheless, pathological examination noted no overt histologic differences in thymuses between EE and SE mice beyond the smaller size found in EE. We examined whether

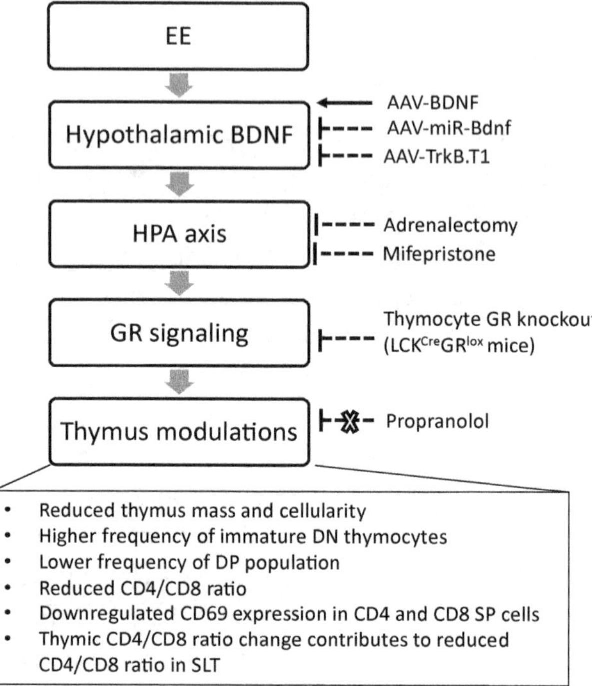

Fig. 6.17. Mechanisms of EE-induced thymic modulation. EE upregulates BDNF expression in the hypothalamus and subsequently elevates the HPA axis. Adrenal gland-derived glucocorticoid receptor to exert effects on thymus mass, thymus cellularity, thymocyte maturation and selection, and egression. Gain- and loss-of-function studies identify each major component of the brain BDNF-HPA-thymocyte GR pathway.

EE affected the distribution of thymocytes at different differential stages. EE increased the frequency of immature DN thymocytes, but decreased the DP population. Among SP populations, EE elevated the frequency of CD8 SP T cells, leading to a reduced CD4/CD8 ratio. EE decreased the absolute numbers of DP and CD4 SP T cells (**Fig. 6.17**).

Expression of the surface protein CD69 retains SP T cells within the thymus, and SP cells downregulate CD69 expression prior to emigration to the SLT.[118] EE downregulated the expression of CD69 on CD4 SP cells as early as 1 week of EE, whereas a reduction of CD69 expression on CD8 SP cells occurred after 4 weeks of EE,[117] suggesting EE might influence the egression of mature SP T cells. To assess whether the thymic changes contribute to the depressed CD4/CD8 ratio in SLT,[108] we subjected RAG2-GFP mice to EE or SE for 2 weeks. In RAG2-GFP mice, GFP is expressed in T cells that have recently undergone TCR rearrangement and therefore tracks recent thymic emigrants in SLT.[119] In the SLT, we observed a significantly reduced CD4/CD8 ratio only among GFP-positive T cells in EE but not among GFP-negative T cells. These data indicate that some of the SLT T cell alterations arise from the thymic modulation by EE (**Fig. 6.17**).

Hypothalamic BDNF Mediates the EE-Induced Thymic Phenotypes

The hypothalamus is composed of a number of discrete nuclei including the arcuate (ARC), paraventricular (PVH), ventromedial (VMH), dorsomedial (DMH), and lateral hypothalamic area (LHA). The ARC nucleus integrates signals from the brainstem and the periphery to play a critical role in regulation of food intake. The PVH nucleus regulates the HPA axis through the release of corticotropin-releasing hormone (CRH).[120] EE upregulates *Bdnf* expression in the ARC and VMH/DMH, and subsequently activates the HSA axis leading to leanness.[1,11].

To investigate whether BDNF and the HPA axis are involved in the EE's thymic modulation, we isolated the PVH, ARC, and VMH/DMH by microdissection after 2-week EE exposure and found significant upregulation of *Bdnf* expression in the VMH and ARC nuclei. Hypothalamic overexpression of BDNF reproduced, whereas hypothalamic knockdown of BDNF reversed EE-induced thymic phenotypes, supporting the notion that EE's thymic effects are also mediated by the hypothalamic BDNF (**Fig. 6.17**). It is worth noting, differing from the SLT immune phenotypes, sympathetic signaling was not critical for EE-induced thymic phenotypes as β blocker failed to antagonize these EE effects.[117]

HPA Signaling Is Essential for EE's Modulation of Thymus

Activation of the HPA axis is an adaptive response to acute and chronic stress, and our data suggest that EE mildly activates the HPA axis.[1] Along the HPA axis, hypothalamic CRH stimulates secretion of adrenocorticotrophin hormone (ACTH) in the anterior pituitary, which stimulates glucocorticosteroid (GC) production in the adrenal glands. In this study, significant upregulation of *Crh* was found in the PVH nucleus and increased serum corticosterone level was observed after 1 week of EE exposure, indicative of activation of the HPA axis. We then used two paradigms to evaluate the role of the HPA axis in EE-induced thymic phenotypes.

First, in order to investigate whether adrenal gland-derived GC is essential, we used mice undergone an adrenalectomy (ADX) with sham surgery as a control. Both ADX and sham surgery mice were randomized to live in SE or EE for 5 weeks. Most of the thymic modulations associated with EE were observed in sham surgery mice. In contrast, ADX completely eliminated the EE-induced effects on thymus, including thymus mass, thymus cellularity, thymocyte maturation and selection, and CD69 expression on SP cells (**Fig. 6.17**).[117]

Second, to investigate whether thymocytes are directly regulated by HPA activation induced by EE, we used a conditional knockout mouse strain *LCK^{Cre}GR^{lox}* (*GR^{lck-Cre}*), in which the GR gene is specifically deleted in the thymocytes prior to selection and therefore their DP and SP cells are unable to respond to GC.[121] After 5-week EE exposure, the *GR^{lck-Cre}* mice did not display any of the EE-induced thymic changes found in wild type (WT) mice (**Fig. 6.17**), indicating the EE's thymic modulation via thymocyte GR signaling.[117]

EE's Thymic Modulation Contributes to Protection Against Experimental Autoimmune Encephalomyelitis (EAE)

EAE is a murine model of multiple sclerosis (MS), an inflammatory demyelinating disease of the central nervous system (CNS). It is characterized by mononuclear cell infiltration into the CNS and degeneration of the myelin sheath surrounding neuronal axons. CD4 T cells are critically involved in the immune pathogenesis of EAE.[122] EAE protocol typically uses myelin oligodendrocyte glycoprotein (MOG35-55)/CFA emulsion and pertussis toxin to induce EAE symptoms which are scored based on 0–10 scale for motor dysfunction: 0, no clinical signs; 1, partially limp tail; 2, paralyzed tail; 3, hind limb paresis, uncoordinated movement; 4, one hind limb paralyzed; 5, both hind limbs paralyzed; 6, hind limbs paralyzed, weakness in forelimbs; 7, hind limbs paralyzed, one forelimb paralyzed; 8, hind limbs paralyzed, both forelimbs paralyzed; 9, Moribund; 10, death.

In our studies, EE mice showed significantly lower clinic score compared to SE mice (**Fig. 6.18(a)**). The attenuation of EAE development was supported by diminishing inflammatory foci or CD4 T cell infiltration and less demyelination in lumbar spinal cord sections from EE mice (**Fig. 6.18(b)**).[117] We examined the thymic changes on day 34 after MOG immunization at which time the recovery of symptom was plateaued. Interestingly, EE increased total thymocyte numbers (**Fig. 6.18(c)**), elevated CD4/CD8 ratio (**Fig. 6.18(d)**), and increased frequency of CD69-expressing SP cells (**Fig. 6.18(e)**) in the EAE disease model, opposing to the signature changes associated with EE in naïve mice. We thought these opposite changes might reflect the attenuation of EAE-induced thymic changes (in other words, indicators of autoimmunity). For instance, EAE mice living in SE had lower frequency of CD69-expressing CD4 cells (40%) compared to normal mice in SE (60%–70%), whereas EAE mice living in EE showed milder drop of CD69 expression (50%).[117]

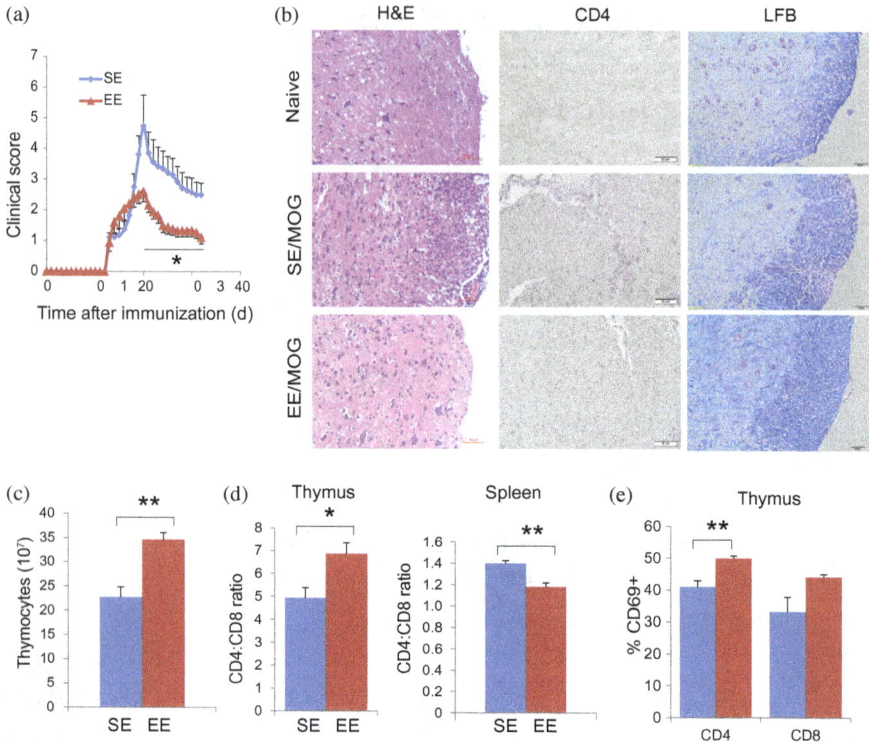

Fig. 6.18. EE alleviates EAE symptoms associated with immune modulations. (a) The EAE clinical score of SE and EE mice. (b) Histology and immunohistochemistry of spinal cords. LFB indicates demyelination. (c) Thymocytes counts. (d) The CD4/CD8 ration in thymus and spleen. (e) CD69 expression on CD4 or CD8 SP cells in thymus. Data are mean ± SEM, n = 8–10 per group. *P < 0.05, **P < 0.01. Reprinted from Xiao *et al.* Enriched environmental regulates thymocyte development and alleviates experimental autoimmune encephalomyelitis. *Brain Behav Immun* 2019, 75, 137–148, with permission from Elsevier.

To clarify whether EE can counter EAE-induced thymic disturbance, we repeated the EAE experiment to examine thymic changes at 10 days after MOG immunization prior to the occurrence of clinical symptoms (**Fig. 6.19**). At this earlier stage of EAE course, MOG immunization resulted in reduction of thymus mass and cellularity and depressed CD4/CD8 ratio (SE-EAE compared to SE-Sham).

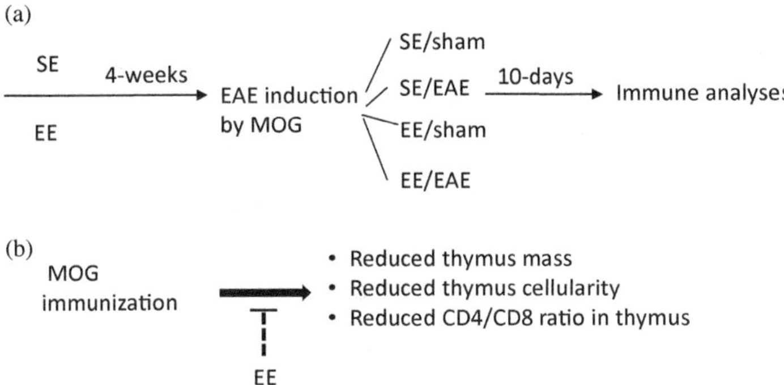

Fig. 6.19. EE affects immune response in the early stage of EAE prior to clinical symptoms. (a) Experimental design. (b) Immune outcomes. EE attenuates EAE-induced thymic changes.

EE attenuated these EAE-induced changes (EE-EAE compared to EE-Sham). We profiled CD4 cell subpopulations (Treg, Th1, Th2, and Th17 cells) because they are thought to be the main pathogenic T cells in EAE.[123–126] In the absence of MOG immunization, EE had no significant effects on CD4 subsets in the thymus. In contrast, EE increased Treg frequency and reduced Th1 frequency in the thymus of EAE mice. In spleen, EE reduced both Treg and Th1 cell percentages in EAE mice.[117]

To address the question whether EE's thymic modulation accounts for the protection against EAE, we employed two approaches. First, we repeated the EAE experiment using $GR^{lck-Cre}$ mice that failed to respond to EE-induced thymic regulation. WT mice and $GR^{lck-Cre}$ mice were housed in SE or EE for 4 weeks followed by MOG immunization, and remained in their corresponding housing till sacrifice 27 days after MOG immunization around the peak of EAE progression. EE significantly improved clinical outcome in WT mice (**Fig. 6.20(a)**) while this protection was completely lost in $GR^{lck-Cre}$ mice. In fact, $GR^{lck-Cre}$ mice regardless of living in SE or EE, showed worse clinic scores compared to WT-EE mice (**Fig. 6.20(a)**).

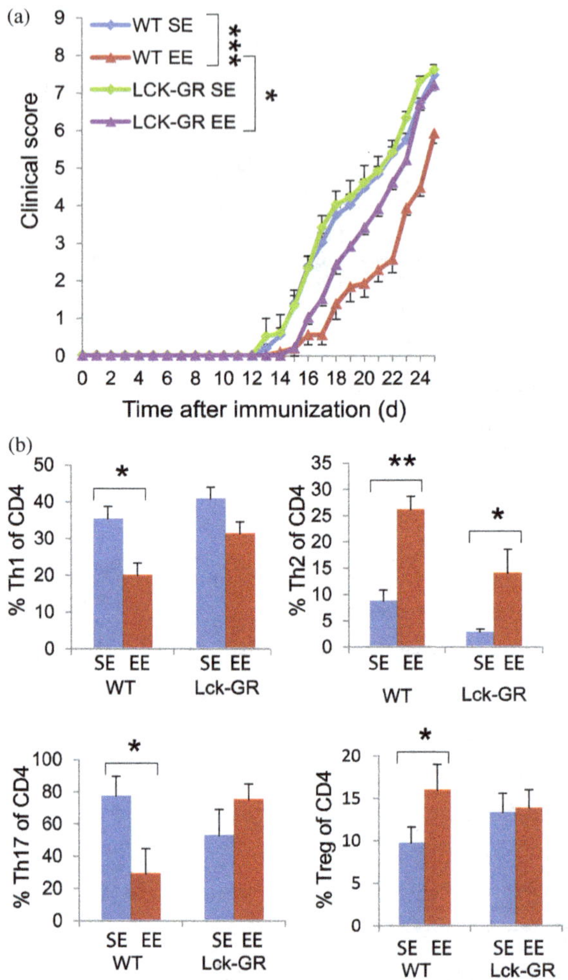

Fig. 6.20. Thymocyte-specific GR knockout prevents EE-induced immune modulations and attenuates EAE protection associated with EE. (a) The EAE clinical score of WT and GR knockout mice in SE or EE housing. (b) Frequency of CD4 subsets in brain and spinal cord. Data are mean ± SEM, *n* = 10–11 per group. *P < 0.05, **P < 0.01, P < 0.001. Reprinted from Xiao *et al.* Enriched environmental regulates thymocyte development and alleviates experimental autoimmune encephalomyelitis. *Brain Behav Immun* 2019, 75, 137–148, with permission from Elsevier.

Coincidently, the EE-associated thymic changes (thymus mass and cellularity, CD4 subsets) observed in WT mice were abrogated in $GR^{lck\text{-}Cre}$ mice. The *in vitro* stimulation of splenocytes harvested from EAE mice showed reduced levels of IFN-γ, IL4, and IL17 as well as Treg frequency only in WT-EE mice but not in $GR^{lck\text{-}Cre}$ mice.[117] In the brain and spinal cord, EE led to a reduction of pathogenic Th1 and Th17 cell populations and an increase in Th2 and Treg cell populations in WT mice (WT-EE versus WT-SE) (**Fig. 6.20(b)**). The majority of these changes diminished in $GR^{lck\text{-}Cre}$ mice (**Fig. 6.20(b)**).[117]

Next, we performed an adoptive transfer experiment to evaluate the contribution of thymic modulation to EE-induced alleviation of EAE. WT mice were immunized with MOG and maintained in SE housing. Ten days later, the MOG-immunized mice were randomized to receive infusion of thymocytes harvested from mice (without MOG immunization) that had been exposed to either 2-week EE or 2-week SE housing. Adoptive transfer of thymocytes from EE mice significantly improved clinical score and inhibited spinal cord inflammation in the MOG-immunized mice living in SE housing.[117]

Mechanisms of EE-Induced Thymic Modulation

Unlike other major organs, the primary lymphoid organ thymus is highly dynamic, capable of undergoing multiple rounds of dramatic involution followed by rapid restoration.[127] Chronic thymic involution is primarily related with age, whereas acute thymic involution can be caused by physiological and psychological stressors, infection, pregnancy, cancer, and cancer treatment.[127] We have described an EE-induced thymic involution without immunosenescence in early adult life of mice. EE can regulate thymocyte maturation and selection at several stages. The main features include reducing thymocyte numbers, lowering the DP cells and CD4/CD8 SP ratio, and facilitating emigration of CD4 T cells. These EE-induced thymic phenotypes are sex-independent in young mice. One mechanism has been identified that originates from the hypothalamic BDNF, whose stimulation by EE upregulates *Crh* expression and thereby activating the HPA axis and the ensuring mild but significant increase of circulating GC. The adrenal gland-derived GC directly acts on GR expressed in thymocytes resulting in the aforementioned thymic phenotypic changes associated with EE (**Fig. 6.17**). This is in line with the literature that enhanced GR signaling in T cells affects thymocyte development characterized by lower DP cells and higher CD8 frequency.[128] Unlike many of peripheral effects such as anticancer, anti-obesity phenotypes as well as T cell modulation of SLT,[1,11,108] EE exerts thymic modulation without the requirement of the SNS but dependent on the HPA axis. This finding is consistent with literature suggesting immature thymocytes more susceptible to GC-induced apoptosis than mature thymocytes or peripheral T cells.[117]

It might appear paradoxical that EE, exerting diverse health benefits, is associated with thymic involution. Age-related thymic involution — progressive regression in thymus size and diminishment of thymic structure — is evolutionarily and conservatively maintained in vertebrates.[129] Thymic involution can be associated with immunosenescence concomitant with greater susceptibility to infections and increased propensity for autoimmune diseases and cancers in aged population.[130] Studies have shown that early life programming of the thymus is crucial for T cell development and the impact is long-lasting.[131] However, most of these studies are nutritional.[132] Our work reveals an EE-induced thymic involution without immunosenescence in juvenile and young adults when the thymic development is very sensitive to early events.[132] The long-term impact warrants future investigation.

How to interpret the HPA axis activation induced by EE in absence of an immunocompromised state? Endogenous GC is required for a robust adaptive immune response because of its promotion of selection for T cells that have sufficient avidity for self. In fact, the absence of thymocyte GC signaling results in an immunocompromised state.[121] We will discuss the notion that EE is a unique model of eustress/hormesis[133] in Chapter 8. Briefly, classical stress literature notes that departures from homeostasis can be "eustressful" or "distressful" and that health impacts vary accordingly. Eustress is referred to milder and/or briefer challenges that induce a positive or healthy adaptation. Indeed, EE recapitulating a socially, mentally, and physically active lifestyle, leads to a mild (within the physiological range) but significant increase in circulating GC. The activation of the HPA axis is required for the EE-induced immune regulations, and the higher GC level in EE is not associated with an immunosuppressive state but instead an enhanced anticancer immunity.[1,108] Study has shown that GCs inhibit naïve CD8 T cells but have little impact on activated CD8 T cells and do not inhibit the antitumor activity.[134] Of note, EE manifests dual-modal immune benefits: on the one hand enhancing antitumor activity of NK cells and CTLs[1,107,108] in tumor-bearing animals, and on the other hand inhibiting autoimmune responses in EAE.[117] It is interesting to study the EE's effects on other T-cell-mediated events such as graft-versus-host disease and cancer immunotherapy with adoptive cell transfer.[135]

Implications of EE's Thymic Modulation in Animal Models of Multiple Sclerosis

MS is an inflammatory and degenerative disease of the CNS. Its pathogenesis is thought to involve autoimmunity, and stressful life events may potentially trigger disease exacerbation.[136] Animal studies using an EAE model implicate a decreased HPA function in increased susceptibility and severity of the disease. Experimental and clinical evidence has shown that both hyper- and hypo-activity of the HPA axis are associated with more severe courses of MS.[136] Our studies have demonstrated that EE can lessen the maximal disability, reduce the cumulative clinical scores, and accelerate recovery. EE's thymic modulation contributes critically to the improvement of functional outcome in EAE. Notably, some immune alterations depend on whether or not there is an immune challenge, lending support to the notion that EE can train or fine-tune the immune system to be more adaptive when facing a challenge.

Multiple Mechanisms Underlie the EE's Protection Against EAE

Studies have elucidated protective mechanisms beyond the thymus effects, majority of which focusing on the CNS. It is reported that EE mobilizes neural progenitor cells from the subventricular zone to migrate to demyelinating lesions, and thereby favoring functional recovery.[137] A recent report shows that EE inhibits neuroinflammation during EAE by reducing proinflammatory cytokine (IL-1β, TNF-α, and IL-6) expression and by increasing the expression of anti-inflammatory molecules (TGF-β, arginase-1) at CNS lesions.[138] The latter may link to a shift of microglia/macrophages toward an anti-inflammatory M2 phenotype.[139] Another interesting finding is that EE stimulates the secretion of exosomes from immune cells, resulting in promotion of CNS myelination.[140] Moreover, CNS-specific autoimmune T cells have been identified as important players of brain plasticity,[141] which may trigger interest in their potential involvement in EE's protection against EAE. It is plausible that various mechanisms are connected or interdependent, and work together to protect against EAE. Whether an overarching mechanism exists remains to be seen.

Impact of EE on Other Immune Cell Populations

B Cells

Relative to T cells and NK cells, how EE impacts B cell has been poorly characterized. B cells originate from hematopoietic stem cells in the bone marrow and emigrate to SLT where complete development takes place.[142] B cells are the center of the humoral immunity arm of the adaptive immune system, and are responsible for the production and secretion of antigen-specific antibodies.[143] Gurfein and colleagues report that EE increases splenic B cell frequencies and decreases T cell frequencies, resulting in an increased B/T lymphocyte ratio.[144] However, when EE mice are subjected to unpredictable chronic mild stress, an opposite effect occurs — a decreased splenic B/T lymphocyte ratio due to reduced B cell frequency and increased T cell frequency. EE mice exhibit a lower frequency of immature B cells (defined as B220+, CD93+) and germinal B cells (defined as B220+, IgD−, CD95+) than SE mice. This study demonstrates that EE can modulate splenic B cell composition and may elicit different, sometimes even opposing, immunomodulatory impact contingent on whether or not there is a challenge. Similarly, we have noted that EE's thymic modulation is also context-dependent, that is, with or without MOG immunization to induce EAE.

Myeloid Cells

Myeloid cells including granulocytes and monocytes are differentiated descendants from common myeloid progenitors derived from hematopoietic stem cells in the bone marrow. Myeloid cells are constantly provided to all tissues through circulation and can be rapidly recruited into local tissues upon pathogen invasion. At infection site, myeloid cells are activated for phagocytosis and for secreting inflammatory cytokines to play major roles in innate immunity.[145] Fewer data are available with regard to EE-induced peripheral myeloid changes in the absence of infection.

Brod and colleagues report that 2-week EE exposure does not alter total numbers of blood leukocytes or individual leukocyte populations.[146] However, EE results in significant alteration in the relative frequencies of leukocyte populations — higher proportion of neutrophils and a correspondingly lower proportion of lymphocytes — suggesting myeloid cells are responsive to EE. The authors have evaluated the effects of EE on inflammatory immune responses in two models of acute inflammation: zymosan-induced peritonitis (ZIP) allowing the characterization of leukocyte egress into the peritoneal cavity, and the cecal ligation and puncture (CLP) to produce sepsis.[146] In both models, EE mice exhibit enhanced neutrophil and macrophage influx into peritoneal cavity. Peritoneal macrophages isolated from EE mice have shown enhanced phagocytic capacity. In CLP model, EE mice display improved capability of clearing systemic bacterial infection. In parallel, transcriptome analysis of whole blood of EE animals demonstrates a significantly altered gene expression profile indicative of enhanced immunity and immunoprotection.

Unlike the peripheral myeloid cells, more is known about EE impact on microglial. Microglial cells are myeloid cells residing in the CNS and contribute to immune defense and neuronal homeostasis.[147] Our research has shown that EE influences microglial morphology and gene expression in middle age or older mice,[148,149] which will be discussed in Chapter 7.

Impacts of EE on Viral Infection

There are handful studies reporting the effect of EE on viral infection and the majority focuses on neuroprotection and behavioral outcome.[150–155] One study shows that EE mice recover faster from encephalitis (intranasal infection of Piry virus), display milder behavioral disturbance, and have a lesser degree of microgliosis whereas more infiltrating T cells in the infected areas compared to SE mice.[152]

Another study reports that EE attenuates hippocampal neuroinflammation and improves cognitive function during peripheral infection with H1N1 influenza.[156] One concern of the robustness of this study is that single housing was used as the control group, which might be inappropriate because social isolation is known to impair immune function.[157] Gurfein and colleagues report that EE alters splenic immune cell composition (T cells, B cells) and enhances secondary influenza vaccine responses in mice.[158] Of note, the EE paradigm used in this study only provided larger space and nesting materials but without toys and running wheels with a purpose to reduce stress. In fact, they observed increased weight gain and decreased corticosterone level in the atypical EE, which are opposite to our findings in an EE providing social, physical, and cognitive stimuli.[1,11,108,117]

Summary and Future Direction

EE can affect cytokines, various immune components and glial cells suggesting EE as an immunomodulatory intervention and a model to study neuroimmune mechanisms.[159–161] However, the immunomodulatory role of EE has received less attention than its neurobiological and behavioral effects. More recently, we have expanded research from investigating the metabolic effects of EE to characterizing EE-induced immune phenotypes. EE reduces the CD4/CD8 ratio in the spleen and lymph node and enhances tumor-infiltrating CD8 T cells contributing to EE-induced anticancer effect via both the SNS and the HPA axis.[108] On the other hand, EE regulates thymocyte maturation and selection, CD4/CD8-lineage choice, and T cell export mediated by the HPA axis and dependent on GR expressed on thymocyte. In an EAE model of MS, EE alleviates symptoms, inhibits spinal cord inflammation through regulation of type 1 T-helper cells, and prevents EAE-induced thymic disturbance.[117] In addition, EE enhances NK cell maturation in the spleen and promotes NK cell reconstitution after NK cell depletion in mice.[48] EE also modulates NK cells residing in the adipose tissue via adipocyte-derived IL-15.[61] Gene delivery of IL-15/IL-15Rα complex to the adipose tissue activates adipose resident NK cells resulting in suppression of tumor growth and significant survival benefits.[88] Interestingly, our mechanistic studies have shown that these diverse immunomodulatory effects of EE are mediated by hypothalamic BDNF via the SNS, the HPA axis, or the HSA axis in a tissue- and cell-type-specific manner.

We will continue to investigate the roles of hypothalamic BDNF in orchestrating multiple processes through which EE alters the body's major adaptive systems — nerve, endocrine, and immune systems. We are particularly interested in understanding how EE influences the adipose immune microenvironment in health and disease, and the underlying regulatory mechanisms. Current projects are focused on adipose resident T cells and adipose resident macrophages.

Covid-19 pandemic has drawn our attention to research on EE and viral infection. Overall, few studies have examined EE effects on viral infection or vaccine response, and none published in the context of aging despite a clear link between aging and impaired response to vaccination. And the mechanisms remain largely unknown. Based on a decade of successful research with regard to the metabolic, immune, and behavioral benefits of EE across life span, we are well-equipped to investigate whether a bio-behavioral intervention may mitigate various age-related functional declines and thereby enhancing vaccination efficacy. Our first step is to determine whether and how EE modulates response to influenza vaccination in older mice and to identify underlying mechanisms. We will approach this research with a unique perspective focusing on hypothalamic BDNF-driven neuroendocrine and immune pathways. This project might shed lights on how the complex neuroendocrine-immune pathways interact with lifestyle factors, and provide urgently needed lessons for Covid-19 pandemic that is caused by an influenza-like RNA virus (SARS-CoV-2), and the major risk factors such as old age, obesity, diabetes, and impaired immune responses[162] can be addressed with an EE mediated by neuroimmune and neurometabolic pathways in animal models (also see Chapter 7).

References

1. Cao L, Liu X, Lin E-JD, *et al.* (2010) Environmental and genetic activation of a brain-adipocyte BDNF/leptin axis causes cancer remission and inhibition. *Cell* **142**:52–64.

2. Xiao R, Bergin SM, Huang W, *et al.* (2016) Environmental and genetic activation of hypothalamic BDNF modulates T-cell immunity to exert an anticancer phenotype. *Cancer Immunol Res* **4**:488–497.

3. van de Ven K, Borst J. (2015) Targeting the T-cell co-stimulatory CD27/CD70 pathway in cancer immunotherapy: Rationale and potential. *Immunotherapy* **7**:655–667.

4. Nomi T, Sho M, Akahori T, *et al.* (2007) Clinical significance and therapeutic potential of the programmed death-1 ligand/programmed death-1 pathway in human pancreatic cancer. *Clin Cancer Res* **13**:2151–2157.

5. Laidlaw BJ, Cui W, Amezquita RA, *et al.* (2015) Production of IL-10 by CD4(+) regulatory T cells during the resolution of infection promotes the maturation of memory CD8(+) T cells. *Nat Immunol* **16**:871–879.

6. Cui W, Liu Y, Weinstein JS, *et al.* (2011) An interleukin-21-interleukin-10-STAT3 pathway is critical for functional maturation of memory CD8+ T cells. *Immunity* **35**:792–805.

7. Baars PA, Sierro S, Arens R, *et al.* (2005) Properties of murine (CD8+) CD27-T cells. *Eur J Immunol* **35**:3131–3141.

8. Kim CH, Rott L, Kunkel EJ, *et al.* (2001) Rules of chemokine receptor association with T cell polarization *in vivo*. *J Clin Invest* **108**:1331–1339.

9. Zhang S, Lukacs NW, Lawless VA, *et al.* (2000) Cutting edge: Differential expression of chemokines in Th1 and Th2 cells is dependent on Stat6 but not Stat4. *J Immunol* **165**:10–14.

10. Janssen EM, Droin NM, Lemmens EE, *et al.* (2005) CD4+ T-cell help controls CD8+ T-cell memory via TRAIL-mediated activation-induced cell death. *Nature* **434**:88–93.

11. Cao L, Choi EY, Liu X, *et al.* (2011) White to brown fat phenotypic switch induced by genetic and environmental activation of a hypothalamic-adipocyte axis. *Cell Metab* **14**:324–338.

12. Nance DM, Sanders VM. (2007) Autonomic innervation and regulation of the immune system (1987-2007). *Brain Behav Immun* **21**:736–745.

13. Klein RL, Wilson SP, Dzielak DJ, *et al.* (1982) Opioid peptides and noradrenaline co-exist in large dense-cored vesicles from sympathetic nerve. *Neuroscience* **7**:2255–2261.

14. Kin NW, Sanders VM. (2006) It takes nerve to tell T and B cells what to do. *J Leukoc Biol* **79**:1093–1104.

15. Kenney MJ, Ganta CK. (2014) Autonomic nervous system and immune system interactions. *Compr Physiol* **4**:1177–1200.

16. Liberman AC, Budziñski ML, Sokn C, *et al.* (2018) Regulatory and mechanistic actions of glucocorticoids on T and inflammatory cells. *Front Endocrinol* **9**:235.

17. Miller AH, Spencer RL, Pearce BD, *et al.* (1998) Glucocorticoid receptors are differentially expressed in the cells and tissues of the immune system. *Cell Immunol* **186**:45–54.

18. Bourgeois S, Pfahl M, Baulieu EE. (1984) DNA binding properties of glucocorticosteroid receptors bound to the steroid antagonist RU-486. *EMBO J* **3**:751–755.

19. Facciabene A, Motz GT, Coukos G. (2012) T-regulatory cells: Key players in tumor immune escape and angiogenesis. *Cancer Res* **72**:2162–2171.

20. Preston CC, Maurer MJ, Oberg AL, *et al.* (2013) The ratios of CD8+ T cells to CD4+CD25+ FOXP3+ and FOXP3- T cells correlate with poor clinical outcome in human serous ovarian cancer. *PLoS One* **8**:e80063.

21. Zitvogel L, Tesniere A, Kroemer G. (2006) Cancer despite immunosurveillance: Immunoselection and immunosubversion. *Nat Rev Immunol* **6**:715–727.

22. Bozzano F, Marras F, De Maria A. (2017) Natural killer cell development and maturation revisited: Possible implications of a novel distinct Lin(-)CD34(+)DNAM-1(bright)CXCR4(+) cell progenitor. *Front Immunol* **8**:268.

23. Morvan MG, Lanier LL. (2016) NK cells and cancer: You can teach innate cells new tricks. *Nat Rev Cancer* **16**:7–19.

24. Schedlowski M, Jacobs R, Stratmann G, *et al.* (1993) Changes of natural killer cells during acute psychological stress. *J Clin Immunol* **13**:119–126.

25. Long EO, Rajagopalan S. (2002) Stress signals activate natural killer cells. *J Exp Med* **196**:1399–1402.

26. Benaroya-Milshtein N, Hollander N, Apter A, *et al.* (2004) Environmental enrichment in mice decreases anxiety, attenuates stress

responses and enhances natural killer cell activity. *Eur J Neurosci* **20**:1341–1347.

27. Takai D, Abe A, Miura H, *et al.* (2019) Minimum environmental enrichment is effective in activating antitumor immunity to transplanted tumor cells in mice. *Exp Anim* **68**:569–576.

28. Song Y, Gan Y, Wang Q, *et al.* (2017) Enriching the housing environment for mice enhances their NK cell antitumor immunity via sympathetic nerve–dependent regulation of NKG2D and CCR5. *Cancer Res* **77**:1611–1622.

29. Alter G, Malenfant JM, Altfeld M. (2004) CD107a as a functional marker for the identification of natural killer cell activity. *J Immunol Methods* **294**:15–22.

30. Wensveen FM, Jelencic V, Polic B. (2018) NKG2D: A master regulator of immune cell responsiveness. *Front Immunol* **9**:441.

31. Abel AM, Yang C, Thakar MS, Malarkannan S. (2018) Natural killer cells: Development, maturation, and clinical utilization. *Front Immunol* **9**:1869.

32. Yu J, Freud AG, Caligiuri MA. (2013) Location and cellular stages of natural killer cell development. *Trends Immunol* **34**:573–582.

33. Gregoire C, Chasson L, Luci C, *et al.* (2007) The trafficking of natural killer cells. *Immunol Rev* **220**:169–182.

34. Chiossone L, Chaix J, Fuseri N, *et al.* (2009) Maturation of mouse NK cells is a 4-stage developmental program. *Blood* **113**:5488–5496.

35. Vosshenrich CA, Di Santo JP. (2013) Developmental programming of natural killer and innate lymphoid cells. *Curr Opin Immunol* **25**:130–138.

36. Meng Z, Liu T, Song Y, *et al.* (2019) Exposure to an enriched environment promotes the terminal maturation and proliferation of natural killer cells in mice. *Brain Behav Immun* **77**:150–160.

37. Song Y, Gan Y, Wang Q, *et al.* (2017) Enriching the housing environment for mice enhances their NK cell antitumor immunity via sympathetic nerve-dependent regulation of NKG2D and CCR5. *Cancer Res* **77**:1611–1622.

38. Garofalo S, D'Alessandro G, Chece G, *et al.* (2015) Enriched environment reduces glioma growth through immune and non-immune mechanisms in mice. *Nat Commun* **6**:1–13.

39. Fehniger TA, Caligiuri MA. (2001) Interleukin 15:Biology and relevance to human disease. *Blood* **97**:14–32.
40. Carson WE, Giri JG, Lindemann MJ, *et al.* (1994) Interleukin (IL) 15 is a novel cytokine that activates human natural killer cells via components of the IL-2 receptor. *J Exp Med* **180**:1395–1403.
41. Mace EM, Orange JS. (2019) Emerging insights into human health and NK cell biology from the study of NK cell deficiencies. *Immunol Rev* **287**:202–225.
42. Ullah MA, Hill GR, Tey S-K. (2016) Functional reconstitution of natural killer cells in allogeneic hematopoietic stem cell transplantation. *Front Immunol* **7**:144.
43. Savani BN, Mielke S, Adams S, *et al.* (2007) Rapid natural killer cell recovery determines outcome after T-cell-depleted HLA-identical stem cell transplantation in patients with myeloid leukemias but not with acute lymphoblastic leukemia. *Leukemia* **21**:2145–2152.
44. Bergerson RJ, Williams R, Wang H, *et al.* (2016) Fewer circulating natural killer cells 28 days after double cord blood transplantation predicts inferior survival and IL-15 response. *Blood Adv* **1**:208–218.
45. Mundy-Bosse BL, Scoville SD, Chen L, *et al.* (2016) MicroRNA-29b mediates altered innate immune development in acute leukemia. *J Clin Invest* **126**:4404–4416.
46. Scoville SD, Nalin AP, Chen L, *et al.* (2018) Human AML activates the aryl hydrocarbon receptor pathway to impair NK cell development and function. *Blood* **132**:1792–1804.
47. Chang YJ, Zhao XY, Huang XJ. (2008) Effects of the NK cell recovery on outcomes of unmanipulated haploidentical blood and marrow transplantation for patients with hematologic malignancies. *Biol Blood Marrow Transplant* **14**:323–334.
48. Mansour AG, Xiao R, Bergin SM, *et al.* (2020) Enriched environment enhances NK cell maturation through hypothalamic BDNF in male mice. *Eur J Immunol* **51**:557–566.
49. Nishikado H, Mukai K, Kawano Y, *et al.* (2011) NK cell-depleting anti-asialo GM1 antibody exhibits a lethal off-target effect on basophils *in vivo*. *J Immunol* **186**:5766–5771.
50. Hughes T, Briercheck EL, Freud AG, *et al.* (2014) The transcription factor AHR prevents the differentiation of a stage 3 innate lymphoid cell subset to natural killer cells. *Cell Rep* **8**:150–162.

51. Idorn M, Hojman P. (2016) Exercise-dependent regulation of NK cells in cancer protection. *Trends Mol Med* **22**:565–577.
52. Pedersen L, Idorn M, Olofsson GH, *et al.* (2016) Voluntary running suppresses tumor growth through epinephrine- and IL-6-dependent NK cell mobilization and redistribution. *Cell Metab* **23**:554–562.
53. Zimmer P, Schenk A, Kieven M, *et al.* (2017) Exercise induced alterations in NK-cell cytotoxicity - methodological issues and future perspectives. *Exerc Immunol Rev* **23**:66–81.
54. Deng T, Liu J, Deng Y, *et al.* (2017) Adipocyte adaptive immunity mediates diet-induced adipose inflammation and insulin resistance by decreasing adipose Treg cells. *Nat Commun* **8**:15725.
55. Nussbaum JC, Van Dyken SJ, von Moltke J, *et al.* (2013) Type 2 innate lymphoid cells control eosinophil homeostasis. *Nature* **502**:245–248.
56. Molofsky AB, Nussbaum JC, Liang H-E, *et al.* (2013) Innate lymphoid type 2 cells sustain visceral adipose tissue eosinophils and alternatively activated macrophages. *J Exp Med* **210**:535–549.
57. O'Sullivan TE, Rapp M, Fan X, *et al.* (2016) Adipose-resident group 1 innate lymphoid cells promote obesity-associated insulin resistance. *Immunity* **45**:428–441.
58. Wensveen FM, Jelenčić V, Valentić S, *et al.* (2015) NK cells link obesity-induced adipose stress to inflammation and insulin resistance. *Nat Immunol* **16**:376–385.
59. Brestoff JR, Kim BS, Saenz SA, *et al.* (2015) Group 2 innate lymphoid cells promote beiging of white adipose tissue and limit obesity. *Nature* **519**:242–246.
60. Lee MW, Odegaard JI, Mukundan L, *et al.* (2015) Activated type 2 innate lymphoid cells regulate beige fat biogenesis. *Cell* **160**:74–87.
61. Bergin SM, Xiao R, Huang W, *et al.* (2021) Environmental activation of a hypothalamic BDNF-adipocyte IL-15 axis regulates adipose-natural killer cells. *Brain Behav Immun* **95**:477–488.
62. Riordan NH, Ichim TE, Min W-P, *et al.* (2009) Non-expanded adipose stromal vascular fraction cell therapy for multiple sclerosis. *J Transl Med* **7**:29.
63. Giri JG, Kumaki S, Ahdieh M, *et al.* (1995) Identification and cloning of a novel IL-15 binding protein that is structurally related to the alpha chain of the IL-2 receptor. *EMBO J* **14**:3654–3663.

64. Kennedy MK, Glaccum M, Brown SN, *et al.* (2000) Reversible defects in natural killer and memory Cd8 T cell lineages in interleukin 15–deficient mice. *J Exp Med* **191**:771–780.

65. Cooper MA, Bush JE, Fehniger TA, *et al.* (2002) In vivo evidence for a dependence on interleukin 15 for survival of natural killer cells. *Blood* **100**:3633–3638.

66. Waldmann TA. (2015) The shared and contrasting roles of IL2 and IL15 in the life and death of normal and neoplastic lymphocytes: Implications for cancer therapy. *Cancer Immunol Res* **3**:219–227.

67. Dubois S, Mariner J, Waldmann TA, Tagaya Y. (2002) IL-15Rα recycles and presents IL-15 in trans to neighboring cells. *Immunity* **17**:537–547.

68. Mortier E, Woo T, Advincula R, *et al.* (2008) IL-15Rα chaperones IL-15 to stable dendritic cell membrane complexes that activate NK cells via trans presentation. *J Exp Med* **205**:1213–1225.

69. Guimond M, Freud AG, Mao HC, *et al.* (2010) In vivo role of Flt3 ligand and dendritic cells in NK cell homeostasis. *J Immunol* **184**:2769–2775.

70. Liou YH, Wang S-W, Chang C-L, *et al.* (2014) Adipocyte IL-15 regulates local and systemic NK cell development. *J Immunol* **193**:1747–1758.

71. Huang W, Liu X, Queen NJ, Cao L. (2017) Targeting visceral fat by intraperitoneal delivery of novel AAV serotype vector restricting off-target transduction in liver. *Mol Ther Methods Clin Dev* **6**:68–78.

72. Huang W, Queen NJ, McMurphy TB, *et al.* (2019) Adipose PTEN regulates adult adipose tissue homeostasis and redistribution via a PTEN-leptin-sympathetic loop. *Mol Metab* **30**:48–60.

73. During MJ, Liu X, Huang W, *et al.* (2015) Adipose VEGF links the white-to-brown fat switch with environmental, genetic, and pharmacological stimuli in male mice. *Endocrinology* **156**:2059–2073.

74. Stonier SW, Ma LJ, Castillo EF, Schluns KS. (2008) Dendritic cells drive memory CD8 T-cell homeostasis via IL-15 transpresentation. *Blood* **112**:4546–4554.

75. Waldmann TA. (2006) The biology of interleukin-2 and interleukin-15: Implications for cancer therapy and vaccine design. *Nat Rev Immunol* **6**:595.

76. Kobayashi H, Carrasquillo JA, Paik CH, *et al.* (2000) Differences of biodistribution, pharmacokinetics, and tumor targeting between interleukins 2 and 15. *Cancer Res* **60**:3577–3583.
77. Zamai L, Ponti C, Mirandola P, *et al.* (2007) NK cells and cancer. *J Immunol* **178**:4011–4016.
78. Conlon KC, Lugli E, Welles HC, *et al.* (2015) Redistribution, hyper-proliferation, activation of natural killer cells and CD8 T cells, and cytokine production during first-in-human clinical trial of recombinant human interleukin-15 in patients with cancer. *J Clin Oncol* **33**:74.
79. Gomes-Giacoia E, Miyake M, Goodison S, *et al.* (2014) Intravesical ALT-803 and BCG treatment reduces tumor burden in a carcinogen induced bladder cancer rat model; a role for cytokine production and NK cell expansion. *PLoS One* **9**:e96705.
80. Rubinstein MP, Kovar M, Purton JF, *et al.* (2006) Converting IL-15 to a superagonist by binding to soluble IL-15Rα. *Proc Natl Acad Sci U S A* **103**:9166–9171.
81. Xu W, Jones M, Liu B, *et al.* (2013) Efficacy and mechanism-of-action of a novel superagonist interleukin-15:Interleukin-15 receptor αSu/Fc fusion complex in syngeneic murine models of multiple myeloma. *Cancer Res* **73**:3075-86.
82. Mathios D, Park C-K, Marcus WD, *et al.* (2016) Therapeutic administration of IL-15 superagonist complex ALT-803 leads to long-term survival and durable antitumor immune response in a murine glioblastoma model. *Int J Cancer* **138**:187–194.
83. Kim PS, Kwilas AR, Xu W, *et al.* (2016) IL-15 superagonist/IL-15Rα–Sushi-Fc fusion complex (IL-15SA/IL-15RαSu-Fc; ALT-803) markedly enhances specific subpopulations of NK and memory CD8+ T cells, and mediates potent anti-tumor activity against murine breast and colon carcinomas. *Oncotarget* **7**:16130.
84. Felices M, Chu S, Kodal B, *et al.* (2017) IL-15 super-agonist (ALT-803) enhances natural killer (NK) cell function against ovarian cancer. *Gynecol Oncol* **145**:453–461.
85. Wrangle JM, Velcheti V, Patel MR, *et al.* (2018) ALT-803, an IL-15 super-agonist, in combination with nivolumab in patients with metastatic

non-small cell lung cancer: A non-randomised, open-label, phase 1b trial. *Lancet Oncol* **19**:694–704.

86. Margolin K, Morishima C, Velcheti V, *et al.* (2018) Phase I trial of ALT-803, a novel recombinant IL15 complex, in patients with advanced solid tumors. *Clin Cancer Res* **24**:5552–5561.

87. Romee R, Cooley S, Berrien-Elliott MM, *et al.* (2018) First-in-human phase 1 clinical study of the IL-15 superagonist complex ALT-803 to treat relapse after transplantation. *Blood* **131**:2515–2527.

88. Xiao R, Mansour AG, Huang W, *et al.* (2019) Adipocytes: A novel target for IL-15/IL-15Rα cancer gene therapy. *Mol Ther* **27**:922–932.

89. Donnelly ML, Hughes LE, Luke G, *et al.* (2001) The 'cleavage'activities of foot-and-mouth disease virus 2A site-directed mutants and naturally occurring '2A-like'sequences. *J Gen Virol* **82**:1027–1041.

90. Lewis JE, Brameld JM, Hill P, *et al.* (2015) The use of a viral 2A sequence for the simultaneous over-expression of both the vgf gene and enhanced green fluorescent protein (eGFP) in vitro and *in vivo*. *J Neurosci Methods* **256**:22–29.

91. Ryan MD, King AM, Thomas GP. (1991) Cleavage of foot-and-mouth disease virus polyprotein is mediated by residues located within a 19 amino acid sequence. *J Gen Virol* **72**:2727–2732.

92. Cha J, Roomi MW, Ivanov V, *et al.* (2013) Ascorbate supplementation inhibits growth and metastasis of B16FO melanoma and 4T1 breast cancer cells in vitamin C-deficient mice. *Int J Oncol* **42**:55–64.

93. Berger C, Berger M, Hackman RC, *et al.* (2009) Safety and immunologic effects of IL-15 administration in nonhuman primates. *Blood* **114**:2417–2426.

94. Waldmann TA, Lugli E, Roederer M, *et al.* (2011) Safety (toxicity), pharmacokinetics, immunogenicity, and impact on elements of the normal immune system of recombinant human IL-15 in rhesus macaques. *Blood* **117**:4787–95.

95. Guo Y, Luan L, Rabacal W, *et al.* (2015) IL-15 superagonist-mediated immunotoxicity: Role of NK cells and IFN-γ. *J Immunol* **195**:2353–2364.

96. Chang C-M, Lo C-H, Shih Y-M, *et al.* (2010) Treatment of hepatocellular carcinoma with adeno-associated virus encoding interleukin-15 superagonist. *Hum Gene Ther* **21**:611–621.

97. Baaten BJ, Li C-R, Deiro MF, *et al.* (2010) CD44 regulates survival and memory development in Th1 cells. *Immunity* **32**:104–115.

98. Wong KL, Tang LFM, Lew FC, *et al.* (2009) CD44high memory CD8 T cells synergize with CpG DNA to activate dendritic cell IL-12p70 production. *J Immunol* **183**:41–50.

99. Reeves GK, Pirie K, Beral V, *et al.* (2007) Cancer incidence and mortality in relation to body mass index in the Million Women Study: Cohort study. *BMJ* **335**:1134.

100. Renehan AG, Tyson M, Egger M, *et al.* (2008) Body-mass index and incidence of cancer: A systematic review and meta-analysis of prospective observational studies. *Lancet* **371**:569–578.

101. Whitlock G, Lewington S, P Sherliker S, *et al.* (2009) Body-mass index and cause-specific mortality in 900 000 adults: Collaborative analyses of 57 prospective studies. *Lancet* **373**:1083–1096.

102. Felices M, Lenvik AJ, McElmurry R, *et al.* (2018) Continuous treatment with IL-15 exhausts human NK cells via a metabolic defect. *JCI Insight* **3**:e96219.

103. Fehniger TA, Suzuki K, Ponnappan A, *et al.* (2001) Fatal leukemia in interleukin 15 transgenic mice follows early expansions in natural killer and memory phenotype CD8+ T cells. *J Exp Med* **193**:219–231.

104. Foglesong G, Queen N, Huang W, *et al.* (2019) Enriched environment inhibits breast cancer progression in obese models with intact leptin signaling. *Endocr Relat Cancer* **26**:483–495.

105. Queen NJ, Boardman AA, Patel RS, *et al.* (2020) Environmental enrichment improves metabolic and behavioral health in the BTBR mouse model of autism. *Psychoneuroendocrinology* **111**:104476.

106. Foglesong GD, Queen NJ, Huang W, *et al.* (2019) Enriched environment inhibits breast cancer progression in obese models with intact leptin signaling. *Endocr Relat Cancer* **26**:483–495.

107. Garofalo S, D'Alessandro G, Chece G, *et al.* (2015) Enriched environment reduces glioma growth through immune and non-immune mechanisms in mice. *Nat Commun* **6**:6623.

108. Xiao R, Bergin SM, Huang W, *et al.* (2016) Environmental and genetic activation of hypothalamic BDNF modulates T-cell immunity to exert an anticancer phenotype. *Cancer Immunol Res* **4**:488–497.

109. Garofalo S, Porzia A, Mainiero F, Di Angelantonio S. (2017) Environmental stimuli shape microglial plasticity in glioma. *Elife* **6**:e33415.

110. Arranz L, De Castro NM, Baeza I, *et al.* (2010) Environmental enrichment improves age-related immune system impairment: Long-term exposure since adulthood increases life span in mice. *Rejuvenation Res* **13**:415–428.

111. Perez-Perez A, Vilariño-García T, Fernández-Riejos P, *et al.* (2017) Role of leptin as a link between metabolism and the immune system. *Cytokine Growth Factor Rev* **35**:71–84.

112. Friedman J. (2016) The long road to leptin. *J Clin Invest* **126**:4727–4734.

113. Nicolas S, Veyssière J, Gandin C, *et al.* (2015) Neurogenesis-independent antidepressant-like effects of enriched environment is dependent on adiponectin. *Psychoneuroendocrinology* **57**:72–83.

114. Chabry J, Nicolas S, Cazareth J, *et al.* (2015) Enriched environment decreases microglia and brain macrophages inflammatory phenotypes through adiponectin-dependent mechanisms: Relevance to depressive-like behavior. *Brain Behav Immun* **50**:275–287.

115. Starr TK, Jameson SC, Hogquist KA. (2003) Positive and negative selection of T cells. *Annu Rev Immunol* **21**:139–176.

116. Klein L, Kyewski B, Allen PM, Hogquist KA. (2014) Positive and negative selection of the T cell repertoire: What thymocytes see (and don't see). *Nat Rev Immunol* **14**:377–391.

117. Xiao R, Bergin SM, Huang W, *et al.* (2019) Enriched environment regulates thymocyte development and alleviates experimental autoimmune encephalomyelitis in mice. *Brain Behav Immun* **75**:137–148.

118. Shiow LR, Rosen DB, Brdicková N, *et al.* (2006) CD69 acts downstream of interferon-α/β to inhibit S1P 1 and lymphocyte egress from lymphoid organs. *Nature* **440**:540–544.

119. Boursalian TE, Golob J, Soper DM, *et al.* (2004) Continued maturation of thymic emigrants in the periphery. *Nat Immunol* **5**:418–425.

120. Vale W, Spiess J, Rivier C, Rivier J. (1981) Characterization of a 41-residue ovine hypothalamic peptide that stimulates secretion of corticotropin and beta-endorphin. *Science* **213**:1394–1397.

121. Mittelstadt PR, Monteiro JP, Ashwell JD. (2012) Thymocyte responsiveness to endogenous glucocorticoids is required for immunological fitness. *J Clin Invest* **122**:2384–2394.

122. Goverman J. (2009) Autoimmune T cell responses in the central nervous system. *Nat Rev Immunol* **9**:393–407.

123. Fletcher JM, Lalor SJ, Sweeney CM, *et al.* (2010) T cells in multiple sclerosis and experimental autoimmune encephalomyelitis. *Clin Exp Immunol* **162**:1–11.

124. Domingues HS, Mues M, Lassmann H, *et al.* (2010) Functional and pathogenic differences of Th1 and Th17 cells in experimental autoimmune encephalomyelitis. *PLoS One* **5**:e15531.

125. McGeachy MJ, Stephens LA, Anderton SM. (2005) Natural recovery and protection from autoimmune encephalomyelitis: Contribution of CD4+CD25+ regulatory cells within the central nervous system. *J Immunol* **175**:3025–3032.

126. Lafaille JJ, Keere FV, Hsu AL, *et al.* (1997) Myelin basic protein-specific T helper 2 (Th2) cells cause experimental autoimmune encephalomyelitis in immunodeficient hosts rather than protect them from the disease. *J Exp Med* **186**:307–312.

127. Dooley J, Liston A. (2012) Molecular control over thymic involution: From cytokines and microRNA to aging and adipose tissue. *Eur J Immunol* **42**:1073–1079.

128. Ashwell JD, Lu FW, Vacchio MS. (2000) Glucocorticoids in T cell development and function*. *Annu Rev Immunol* **18**:309–345.

129. Shanley DP, Aw D, Manley NR, Palmer DB. (2009) An evolutionary perspective on the mechanisms of immunosenescence. *Trends Immunol* **30**:374–381.

130. Prelog M. (2006) Aging of the immune system: A risk factor for autoimmunity? *Autoimmun Rev* **5**:136–139.

131. Gui J, Mustachio LM, Su DM, Craig RW. (2012) Thymus size and age-related thymic involution: Early programming, sexual dimorphism, progenitors and stroma. *Aging Dis* **3**:280–290.

132. Chen JH, Tarry-Adkins JL, Heppolette CA, *et al.* (2010) Early-life nutrition influences thymic growth in male mice that may be related to the regulation of longevity. *Clin Sci (Lond)* **118**:429–438.

133. Cao L, During MJ. (2012) What is the brain-cancer connection? *Annu Rev Neurosci* **35**:331–345.

134. Hinrichs CS, Palmer DC, Rosenberg SA, Restifo NP. (2005) Glucocorticoids do not inhibit antitumor activity of activated CD8+ T cells. *J Immunother* **28**:517–524.

135. Knight JM, Lyness JM, Sahler OJ, *et al.* (2013) Psychosocial factors and hematopoietic stem cell transplantation: Potential biobehavioral pathways. *Psychoneuroendocrinology* **38**:2383–2393.

136. Heesen C, Gold SM, Huitinga I, Reul JM. (2007) Stress and hypothalamic-pituitary-adrenal axis function in experimental autoimmune encephalomyelitis and multiple sclerosis - A review. *Psychoneuroendocrinology* **32**:604–618.

137. Magalon K, Cantarella C, Monti G, *et al.* (2007) Enriched environment promotes adult neural progenitor cell mobilization in mouse demyelination models. *Eur J Neurosci* **25**:761–771.

138. Silva BA, Leal MC, Farías MI, *et al.* (2020) Environmental enrichment improves cognitive symptoms and pathological features in a focal model of cortical damage of multiple sclerosis. *Brain Res* **1727**:146520.

139. Pusic KM, Pusic AD, Kemme J, Kraig RP. (2014) Spreading depression requires microglia and is decreased by their M2a polarization from environmental enrichment. *Glia* **62**:1176–1194.

140. Pusic KM, Pusic AD, Kraig RP. (2016) Environmental enrichment stimulates immune cell secretion of exosomes that promote CNS myelination and may regulate inflammation. *Cell Mol Neurobiol* **36**:313–325.

141. Ziv Y, Ron N, Butovsky O, *et al.* (2006) Immune cells contribute to the maintenance of neurogenesis and spatial learning abilities in adulthood. *Nat Neurosci* **9**:268–275.

142. Loder BF, Mutschler B, Ray RJ, *et al.* (1999) B cell development in the spleen takes place in discrete steps and is determined by the quality of B cell receptor–derived signals. *J Exp Med* **190**:75–90.

143. Cooper MD. (2015) The early history of B cells. *Nat Rev Immunol* **15**:191–197.

144. Gurfein BT, Hasdemir B, Milush JM, *et al.* (2017) Enriched environment and stress exposure influence splenic B lymphocyte composition. *PLoS One* **12**:e0180771.

145. Kawamoto H, Minato N. (2004) Myeloid cells. *Int J Biochem Cell Biol* **36**:1374–1379.

146. Brod S, Gobbetti T, Gittens B, *et al.* (2017) The impact of environmental enrichment on the murine inflammatory immune response. *JCI Insight* **2**:e90723.

147. Herz J, Filiano AJ, Smith A, *et al.* (2017) Myeloid cells in the central nervous system. *Immunity* **46**:943–956.

148. Ali S, Liu X, Queen NJ, *et al.* (2019) Long-term environmental enrichment affects microglial morphology in middle age mice. *Aging (Albany NY)* **11**:2388–2402.

149. Ali S, Mansour AG, Huang W, *et al.* (2020) CSF1R inhibitor PLX5622 and environmental enrichment additively improve metabolic outcomes in middle-aged female mice. *Aging (Albany NY)* **12**:2101–2122.

150. Magalon K, Cantarella C, Monti G, *et al.* (2007) Enriched environment promotes adult neural progenitor cell mobilization in mouse demyelination models. *Eur J Neurosci* **25**:761–771.

151. Tauber SC, Bunkowski S, Ebert S, *et al.* (2009) Enriched environment fails to increase meningitis-induced neurogenesis and spatial memory in a mouse model of pneumococcal meningitis. *J Neurosci Res* **87**:1877–1883.

152. de Sousa AA, Reis R, Bento-Torres J, *et al.* (2011) Influence of enriched environment on viral encephalitis outcomes: Behavioral and neuropathological changes in albino Swiss mice. *PLoS One* **6**:e15597.

153. Gomes GF, da Fonseca Peixoto RD, Maciel BG, *et al.* (2019) Differential microglial morphological response, TNF α, and viral load in sedentary-like and active murine models after systemic non-neurotropic dengue virus infection. *J Histochem Cytochem* **67**:419–439.

154. Luo L, van Dixhoorn IDE, Reimert I, *et al.* (2017) Effect of enriched housing on levels of natural (auto-)antibodies in pigs co-infected with porcine reproductive and respiratory syndrome virus (PRRSV) and *Actinobacillus pleuropneumoniae. Vet Res* **48**:75.

155. van Dixhoorn ID, Reimert I, Middelkoop J, *et al.* (2016) Enriched housing reduces disease susceptibility to co-infection with porcine reproductive and respiratory virus (PRRSV) and actinobacillus pleuropneumoniae (A. pleuropneumoniae) in young pigs. *PLoS One* **11**:e0161832.

156. Jurgens HA, Johnson RW. (2012) Environmental enrichment attenuates hippocampal neuroinflammation and improves cognitive function during influenza infection. *Brain Behav Immun* **26**:1006–1016.

157. Pyter LM, Yang L, McKenzie C, *et al.* (2014) Contrasting mechanisms by which social isolation and restraint impair healing in male mice. *Stress* **17**:256–265.

158. Gurfein BT, Davidenko O, Premenko-Lanier M, *et al.* (2014) Environmental enrichment alters splenic immune cell composition and enhances secondary influenza vaccine responses in mice. *Mol Med* **20**:179–190.

159. Singhal G, Jaehne EJ, Corrigan F, Baune BT. (2014) Cellular and molecular mechanisms of immunomodulation in the brain through environmental enrichment. *Front Cell Neurosci* **8**:97.

160. Schapiro SJ. (2002) Effects of social manipulations and environmental enrichment on behavior and cell-mediated immune responses in rhesus macaques. *Pharmacol Biochem Behav* **73**:271–278.

161. De la Fuente M, Cruces J, Hernandez O, Ortega E. (2011) Strategies to improve the functions and redox state of the immune system in aged subjects. *Curr Pharm Des* **17**:3966–3993.

162. Cao X. (2020) COVID-19: Immunopathology and its implications for therapy. *Nat Rev Immunol* **20**:269–270.

7 Environmental Enrichment Promotes Healthy Aging

Lifespan and Healthspan

Our world is aging. According to United States Census Bureau 2019 Population Estimates by Demographic Characteristics, the nation's 65 and older population grew by over a third, or 13,787,044, during the past decade driven by the aging of Baby Boomers born between 1946 and 1964. Currently over 50 million Americans are over the age of 65,[1] and the number is projected to reach 73 million by 2030 when 1 in 5 Americans will be at the age of 65 or older.[2] The aging demographic shift of the United States mirrors the global phenomenon of increasing lifespan[3] that is expected to continue to grow.

To understand the aging process, we should first appreciate the nuances between lifespan, life expectancy, and healthspan. Lifespan is defined as the time between an organism's birth and death, whereas life expectancy is an estimate of the expected lifespan for an individual based on a statistical evaluation of the population. There have been debates about whether a maximum limit on human lifespan exist or what that limit is. The prevailing consensus is that the ultimate goal of extending lifespan is likely to be difficult to reach because the most significant improvements to life expectancy up to date have been achieved through reduction of childhood mortality. Further extension of life expectancy can only occur by prolonging the lives of elderly people, which has not been successful in spite of advances in medicine and technology.[4] What is more feasible and perhaps more important is to extend and enhance healthspan, the part of an organism's life during which they are in good health free from serious diseases. In 1987, Rowe and Kahn stated in one of the earliest references to healthspan in scientific literature, "[A substantial] increase in healthspan, the maintenance of full function as nearly as possible to the end of life, should be the next gerontological goal."[5] In other words, an ideally maximized healthspan allows an organism to live in perfect health until the exact moment of their death.

The reality has been far from ideal. Along with rising life expectancy, the incidence of deliberating diseases such as cancer, cardiovascular disorders, metabolic disorders, and neurodegeneration rises,[6–8] leading to poor quality of life and potential mortality. Depending on the onset and severity of late-life chronic disease, these increases in median lifespan may improve or worsen the lives of the elderly. Accordingly, framework of either an expansion or a compression of lifetime morbidity accompanying increased longevity has been proposed to conceptualize this phenomenon.[9–11]

With respect to morbidity-related disability, research has demonstrated a progressive reduction in functional impairment in older Americans toward the end of the 20th century.[12,13] Unfortunately, this positive population trend has staggered recently as the part of years free from disability has ceased to increase, despite the decrease in mortality.[10,14–16] These findings underscore the importance of determining when, where, and how age-related morbidities begin. Generally speaking, a prolonged lifespan without extension of healthspan is unlikely to be beneficial. From a personal perspective, a longer life might not be so desirable if one must suffer from diminished functionality, poor quality of life, and increased pain. On a population scale, the imperfect reconciliation between lifespan and healthspan can result in reduced societal productivity, and increased costs of healthcare. Hence, research and clinical efforts are now put on how to extend and improve healthspan.[4] The former is focused on increasing the "span," meaning the time someone spends healthy before declining. The latter is focused on improving "health." Health is a relative spectrum rather than a binary state of being. As individuals progress through life, they naturally experience a decline of physiological functions and general health due to the normal aging process. Thus, efforts to improve general health are equally valuable even without extending the duration of healthspan.

Brain Aging, Cognitive Decline and Reserve

Aging leads to the decline of certain cognitive functions such as reduced mental processing speed,[17,18] poor memory,[19,20] and impaired executive function.[21] These cognitive declines are associated with a variety of structural and functional changes in the brain including increased neuroinflammation,[22,23] subtle synapse loss[24,25] without global reductions,[26–29] reduced synaptic plasticity,[30] reduced spine density,[31] and dendritic regression.[31] The aging-related brain alterations can also influence behavior and emotionality in the elderly, resulting in higher risk for mental diseases, such as depression, anxiety, and schizophrenia. Of note, brain-derived neurotrophic factor (BDNF) plays an important role in brain aging. Decreased BDNF levels and mutations in genes involved in BDNF signaling are associated with memory impairment,[32] higher risk for depression,[33,34] schizophrenia,[35] and anxiety.[32–34] On the contrary, increasing physical activity can mitigate these pathologies and is linked to an increase in BDNF levels.[36,37]

Although aging-related cognitive decline is likely inevitable, the brain is resilient and capable of counteracting the natural aging process through multiple coping mechanisms and reserve factors. According to the cognitive reserve theory, the brain has an innate ability to cope with cerebral damage and thereby minimizing clinical manifestations of diseases like dementia and Alzheimer's disease.[38,39] Those who have a greater cognitive reserve can sustain more cerebral damage before symptomatic presentation. Stern and colleagues propose the concept of cognitive reserve and note that intellectual activities may increase the cognitive reserve capacity and therefore may lower risk for manifestation of neurodegenerative disease.[39,40] As a result, environmental and lifestyle factors are viewed as important modifiers of cognitive reserve.[40,41] Epidemiological evidence appears to support this notion[42] as education level,[43] occupational status,[44] smoking abstinence,[45] and regular physical activity[46] have been associated with increased cognitive reserve. These findings highlight the importance of maintaining healthy environmental stimuli, and should foster investigations whether and how environment-driven increases in cognitive reserve may extend "mind-span," defined as the length of an individual's healthy cognitive function.

Pathobiology of Adipose Tissue in Obesity and Aging

As aged populations rise worldwide, the prevalence of obesity is also increasing globally (also see Chapter 3). United States is among the most severely affected where obesity rate is estimated to be 42% in adults.[47] Without significant interventions, nearly one in two adults in the United States are projected to be obese by 2030.[48] Obesity disproportionally inflicts middle-aged and older adults, with the prevalence of obesity being highest in middle-aged adults, aged 40–59,[47] indicative of the convergence of aging and obesity. Obesity is a significant health concern because of its associated risk for other chronic diseases, including but not limited to hypertension, arteriosclerosis, stroke, diabetes, steatohepatitis, and certain types of cancer.[49,50] Above the age of 25, every 5-unit increment of body mass index (BMI) is associated with a 30% increase in all-cause mortality, a 40% higher vascular mortality, and an 120% increase in diabetes-related mortality.[51]

In addition to its role in energy storage, adipose tissues comprise a dynamic and adaptive organ system, responsive to immune, nervous, and nutritional signals. Dysfunction in adipose tissue during aging is thought to be a driver of systemic aging processes.[52] Aging is associated with alterations in the distribution and cellular composition of adipose tissue, and its immune and inflammatory signaling. With aging, both men and women display progressively increasing distribution of adipose tissue in the abdominal region and deposition in ectopic sites.[53] Visceral adipose tissue around abdominal viscera is strongly correlated with comorbidities of obesity, compared to adipose distribution in the rest of the body.[54–57]

Expansion of adipose tissue in obesity is associated with altered immune cell infiltration, which results in chronic low-grade inflammation.[58] Aging is also associated with a systemic pro-inflammatory state termed "inflammaging," related to reduced autophagy, increased oxidative stress, and subsequent activation of inflammasome proteins.[59] Adipocytes become senescent with advancing age and acquire a senescence-associated secretory phenotype (SASP). The "old" adipocytes can release high levels of IL-6 (Interlukin-6), IL-1β, monocyte chemoattractant protein-1 (MCP-1, also known as CCL2), and other chemokines and matrix metalloproteases.[60] IL-6 from adipose tissue is a major contributor to systemic inflammation in old age.[61] These chronic inflammation states are closely linked to the health hazards of obesity, including the development of insulin resistance and cardiovascular disease.[62–64]

Hence, interventions to reduce adiposity may be beneficial in addressing this pathophysiology. Accumulating clinical evidence supports this notion. Meta-analyses demonstrate exercise is an effective intervention for reducing visceral adiposity in overweight adults.[65] Obese patients undergoing gastric bypass surgery display significantly reduced premature aging markers following dramatical weight loss.[66] Reductions in plasma concentrations of CRP, IL6, and PAI-1 all point to reduced circulating SASP load 2 years after surgery. Since resolving obesity may reduce health risks and address the adipose drivers of aging, we have put efforts on the exploration of anti-obesity mechanisms, as well as environmental and genetic approaches to preventing and treating obesity, and promoting healthy aging.

Environmental Enrichment as an Antiaging Intervention?

In order to develop effective ways to prevent, diagnose, and treat age-related diseases, as well as to improve healthspan, it is vital to understand more about the dynamics of aging, how they interact with various environmental and lifestyle factors, and the connections between disease processes and aging. Research on model organisms has demonstrated an interaction between genes and environment in determining lifespan and healthspan.[67,68] Calorie restriction (CR) without malnutrition remains the most robust and reproducible intervention able to extend lifespan and delay the onset of age-related disorders in a wide range of model organisms from yeast to monkeys.[67] Intermittent fasting, a diet regime based on timed periods of fasting (e.g., alternative-day feeding, time-restricted eating) also increases resistance to toxicity and stress, and extends lifespan.[69,70] The metabolic and physiological effects of CR including a reduction in adiposity, higher insulin sensitivity, improved lipid profiles, reduced inflammation and oxidative stress, may contribute to its antiaging ability.[71–75]

Our studies on environmental enrichment (EE) and the hypothalamic-sympathoneural-adipocyte (HSA) axis demonstrate beneficial effects on health in young animals (Chapters 2–6), and some of the features overlap with CR and/or several transgenic mouse models with prolonged lifespan such as Pten transgenic mice (Pten[tg]) and fat-specific insulin receptor knockout (FIRKO) mice[76–78] (**Table 7.1**). These shared features intrigued us to propose that EE, via the activation of the HSA axis, may regulate systemic aging and age-related diseases.[79]

HSA axis activation is highly effective to lower adiposity with little change in body weight.[80,81] Studies in several genetically modified mouse models have linked reduction in adiposity to longevity, including the translational inhibitor 4E-BP1 (Eif4ebp1-/-) knockout,[82]

Table 7.1 Comparison of Phenotypic Characteristics of Models of HSA Axis Activation (EE/BDNF Overexpression) to Models for Extended Longevity (CR, Pten[tg], and FIRKO Mice)

Parameter	EE/BDNF	CR	Pten[tg]	FIRKO
BMI	↓	↓	↓	↓
Body fat content	↓	↓	↓	↓
Insulin sensitivity	↑	↑	↑	↑
Food intake	↑(→)	↓	↑	↑
IGF-1	↓	↓	↓	↓
Leptin	↓	↓	↓	↓
Adiponectin	↑	↑	↑	↑
Corticosterone	↑	↑	NA	NA
BDNF	↑	↑	NA	NA
Immune functions	↑	↑	NA	NA
Cancer	↓	↓	↓	NA
Energy expenditure	↑	↓	↑	↑
Mitochondrial activity	↑	→	↑	↑
Brown fat function	↑	NA	↑	NA
Longevity	?	↑	↑	↑

NA: no data available.

C/EBPß knock-in (ß/ß),[83] c-Cbl knockout,[84] and FIRKO.[77,85] The FIRKO mice with fat-specific deletion of the insulin receptor gene have reduced fat mass by 50%, improved whole-body insulin sensitivity, and an extended lifespan by 18%.[77,85] EE initiated in young mice results in over 60% reduction of intra-abdominal fat when maintained on normal diet although body weight identical to the mice living in standard environment (SE).[86] An increase of muscle mass is observed in EE mice as well as mice overexpressing BDNF in the hypothalamus. These data suggest that the HSA axis stimulation is particularly efficient in decreasing adiposity and therefore allows the dissociation of fat loss from weight loss which is difficult to achieve with other interventions.[87] This specific fat loss induced by the HSA axis can provide a new model to clarify the controversy between weight loss and mortality.[88]

In young animals, the HSA axis activation is associated with increased whole-body metabolic rate, increased oxygen consumption in fat, increased mitochondrial content, and upregulation of genes involved in mitochondrial biogenesis and activity such as PGC-1α,[86] resembling FIRKO and Pten[tg] mice. Moreover, the HSA axis activation alleviates obesity-associated insulin resistance, hyperglycemia, and dyslipidemia,[81,86] mimicking CR.

HSA axis activation leads to reduced serum IGF-1 levels, also mirroring CR. The IGF-1/growth hormone pathway is one of the most conserved pathways implicated in aging.[89] Both spontaneous and genetically engineered IGF-1 deficiency leads to smaller body size, delayed age-related pathology, and an extended lifespan.[89]

HSA axis activation alters adipokine levels with higher adiponectin and lower leptin expression in adipose tissue as well as in the circulation,[80,81] again mimicking CR. Adiponectin, an abundant protein secreted from fat, has insulin-sensitizing, anti-inflammatory, and anti-atherogenic properties in both rodents and humans. Transgenic expression of human adiponectin inhibits diet-induced obesity (DIO) and reduces the morbidity and mortality in DIO models.[90] Adiponectin may also suppress carcinogenesis and inhibit angiogenesis in cancer models.[91]

Numerous epidemiological studies have revealed that lifestyle and environmental factors can profoundly influence cancer initiation and progression, suggesting that many cancers are preventable. Among the key players are excessive adiposity, decreased physical activity, and unhealthy diet.[92,93] CR has been shown to be broadly effective in cancer prevention in rodents and monkeys, and the metabolic adaptations to CR are thought to be responsible for CR-mediated cancer inhibition.[72,94,95] Our studies have shown that HSA axis activation via EE or BDNF overexpression markedly suppresses tumor growth in young animals.[80,96,97]

EE is associated with enhanced immunocompetence that is mediated at least in part, by the hypothalamic BDNF (see Chapter 6). Immune dysfunction associated with aging exerts a strong influence on age-related morbidity and mortality.[98] Several age-related changes in immunity have been correlated with increased mortality including low lymphoproliferative response to mitogens and low natural killer (NK) cytotoxicity.[99–101] We and others have shown that EE and BDNF overexpression in young mice increase lymphocyte proliferation in response to the mitogen Concavalin A, enhance NK cell activity, promote NK cell maturation,[80,102,103] and boost antitumor T cell immunity.[80,104]

EE leads to a modest increase in serum corticosterone consistent with a mild stress. The exposure to the mild, nonaversive challenges within EE may lead to a more agile and adaptive stress system and may therefore buffer the reaction to subsequent major external stressors.[80,102,105] Similarly, animals maintained on dietary restriction regimens exhibit increased glucocorticoid levels and yet their health is improved and lifespan is prolonged.[106] Additionally, both regular physical exercise and cognitive stimulation are beneficial on health, and they also increase cortisol levels,[107,108] suggesting that eustress may increase resistance to disease and be beneficial for health and longevity (also see Chapter 8).

To date, the majority of studies on EE and aging focus on the effects on cognitive decline and neurodegenerative diseases. A growing body of research suggests that EE can mitigate age-related neural, cognitive, and behavioral impairments.[109–114] However, scarce evidence is available with respect to whether or not EE can affect peripheral systems and healthspan or lifespan under conditions of normal aging. We have been fortunately funded by the National Institute on Aging (NIA) to fill in this gap by investigating EE on healthy aging and lifespan from a unique perspective of the HSA axis. The following sections summarize our recent work in this field to which talented graduate students Travis McMurphy, Seemaab Ali, and Nicholas Queen have made most contributions.[115–119]

Implementing Environmental Enrichment After Middle Age Improves Healthy Aging

Mice are the preferred mammalian model for longitudinal aging research due to their relatively short lifespan, genetic homology, small size, and ease of rearing. Laboratory mice have mean lifespan of 2–3 years in appropriately controlled housing conditions.[120] The murine aging process mirrors that of humans so that investigators can conduct research on the biology of aging in a shorter time frame. It is important to note that certain mouse strain- and resource-dependent observations have been found in aging research. Hence, these factors must be taken into consideration for experimental design, data interpretation, and comparison among results from different labs.[120,121] We have been using aged C57BL/6 mice supplied by NIA Aged Rodent Colonies. To prevent the risk of fighting in group housed older male mice, we only used females in these aging studies.

Because age-related metabolic decline starts to occur at middle-age, we chose to investigate EE effects in mice at middle age of 10 months (https://www.jax.org/research-and-faculty/research-labs/the-harrison-lab/gerontology/life-span-as-a-biomarker). Many of the EE studies on cognition and behavior use young mice because it is thought young brains are more plastic than in old age and therefore more susceptible to EE. Prior to a long-term EE study, we first tested whether EE could activate the HSA axis in middle-age female mice in a similar way to young mice after a short-term 6-week EE. Some changes in serum biomarkers associated with EE in young male mice such as a decrease of IGF-1, an increase of adiponectin, and an increase of corticosterone were not observed in the middle-age female mice. But importantly, we found a significant upregulation of hypothalamic *Bdnf* expression together with core features of the HSA axis activation, namely robust reduction of adiposity (visceral WAT [white adipose tissue] reduced by ~60%) and drop of leptin (~60%) in middle-age female mice compared to their counterparts in SE.[115] These encouraging results suggest that older animals are highly responsive to EE with regard to metabolic outcomes.

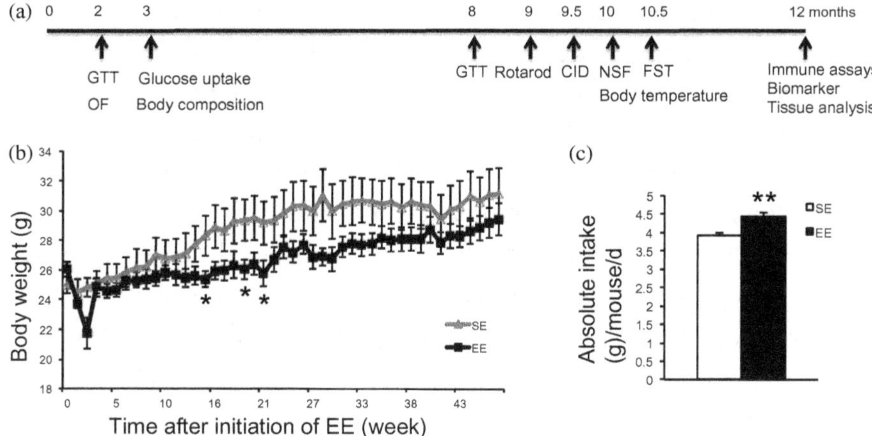

Fig. 7.1. Long-term EE initiated at middle age. (a) Timeline. Female 10-month-old mice were randomized to live in EE or SE for 12 months and subjected to metabolic and behavioral assessments at times indicated above the line. (b) Body weight. (c) Food intake measured 8~10.5 months in EE. Data are mean ± SEM, $n = 10$ per group. *$P < 0.05$, **$P < 0.01$. GTT, glucose tolerance test; OF, open field test; CID, cold-induced defecation; NSF, novelty-suppressed feeding; FST, forced swim test. Reprinted from McMurphy *et al.* Implementation of environmental enrichment after middle age promotes healthy aging. Aging (Albany NY). 2018, 10(7), 1698–1721.

Then, we conducted a long-term EE study to assess whether implementing EE at middle age could exert lasting benefits and therefore improve healthspan. We enrolled female mice with no history of EE at 10 months of age to live in SE or EE for an additional 12 months. Mice were subjected to a battery of metabolic measurements and behavioral tests during the 12-month EE study **(Fig. 7.1(a))**.

Metabolic Improvements of Long-Term EE

EE had a temporary effect on body weight, significant weight reduction only observed between 14 and 21 weeks while no difference was found by the end of the study. Food intake was monitored for 10 weeks and showed a significant increase in absolute intake and relative intake calibrated to per gram body weight (**Fig. 7.1(b), (c)**). EE significantly improved glucose tolerance. At the end of the 12-month study, EE mice showed a robust reduction of adiposity and significant decrease of circulating leptin (~50%) and serum glucose levels.[115]

To test reproducibility and explore additional metabolic outcomes, we repeated the EE study in a separate cohort of mice. Body composition measurement by EchoMRI showed 40% of reduction of fat mass and a significant increase of lean mass without change of body weight at 3-month EE exposure (**Fig. 7.2(a), (b)**). Then we performed *in vivo* glucose uptake during a glucose tolerance test

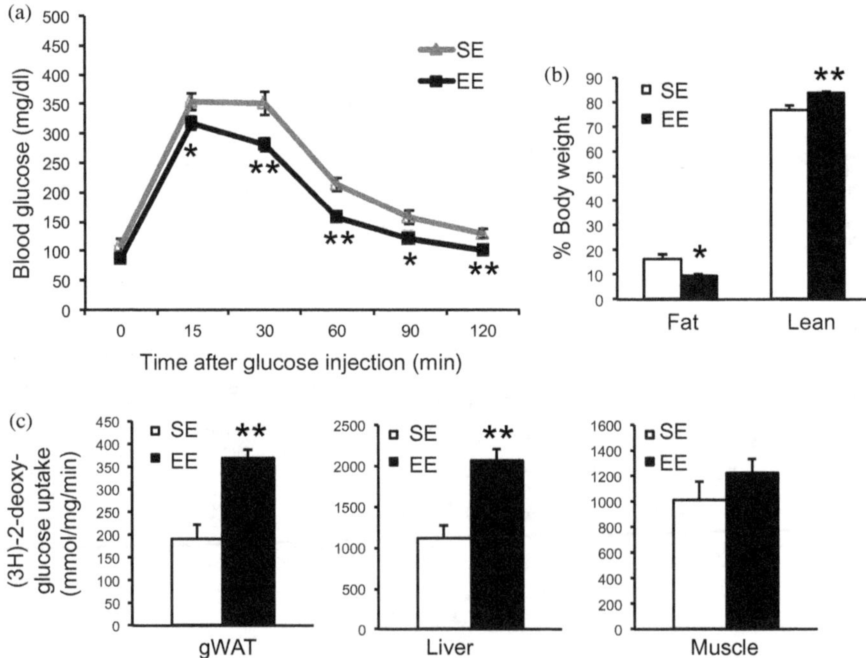

Fig. 7.2. EE improves glycemic control in middle-age mice. (a) Glucose tolerance test at 8 weeks in EE (n = 10 per group). (b) EchoMRI measurement of body composition (n = 5 per group). (c) Glucose uptake assay at 12 weeks in EE (n = 5 per group). Data are mean ± SEM. *P < 0.05, **P < 0.01. Reprinted from McMurphy *et al*. Implementation of environmental enrichment after middle age promotes healthy aging. Aging (Albany NY). 2018, 10(7), 1698–1721.

(GTT) using glucose analog tracer 2-[³H] deoxyglucose (2-DG). EE significantly increased the glucose uptake by WAT and liver but not by skeletal muscle (**Fig. 7.2(c)**).[115]

There has been a controversy in aging research: whether weight loss is beneficial to lifespan and whether fat loss with no loss of lean mass is required.[88] EE could offer a physiological model to tackle this question as EE robustly reduces adiposity with little or no effect on body weight in mice of normal body weight. EE increases muscle mass in aged animals, which may contribute to the improvement of health. In fact, frailty is a great health concern for elder populations.[122] We are currently collaborating with neuromuscular experts to explore and characterize the muscle phenotypes induced by EE.

Behavioral Effects of Long-Term EE

Studies have shown that EE can alleviate motor dysfunction in disease models.[123–125] To evaluate whether EE could mitigate aging-related motor function decline, we conducted a Rotarod treadmill test that measures motor abilities such as balance, coordination, physical condition, and motor planning.[126] After living in EE for 9 months, EE mice were able to remain on the rod for a prolonged period of time and for a faster rotating speed before the first fall (**Fig. 7.3(a)**) indicating significant improvement in motor abilities.[115]

Moreover, we examined a series of anxiety and depression behavioral tests, and found that EE significantly reduced anxiety-like behaviors in both the open field test classically used to assess exploratory behavior, general locomotion, and anxiety[127,128] and the novelty suppressed feeding test[129] (**Fig. 7.3(b), (c)**). No significant effect was found in the forced swimming test often used for screening antidepressant drugs.[115,130] This anxiolytic effect of EE is consistent with previous reports.[131,132]

The anxiolytic mechanisms of EE could be multifactorial and worthy of further investigations. It is well documented that EE can modulate the limbic system in animal models of affective disorder.[133]

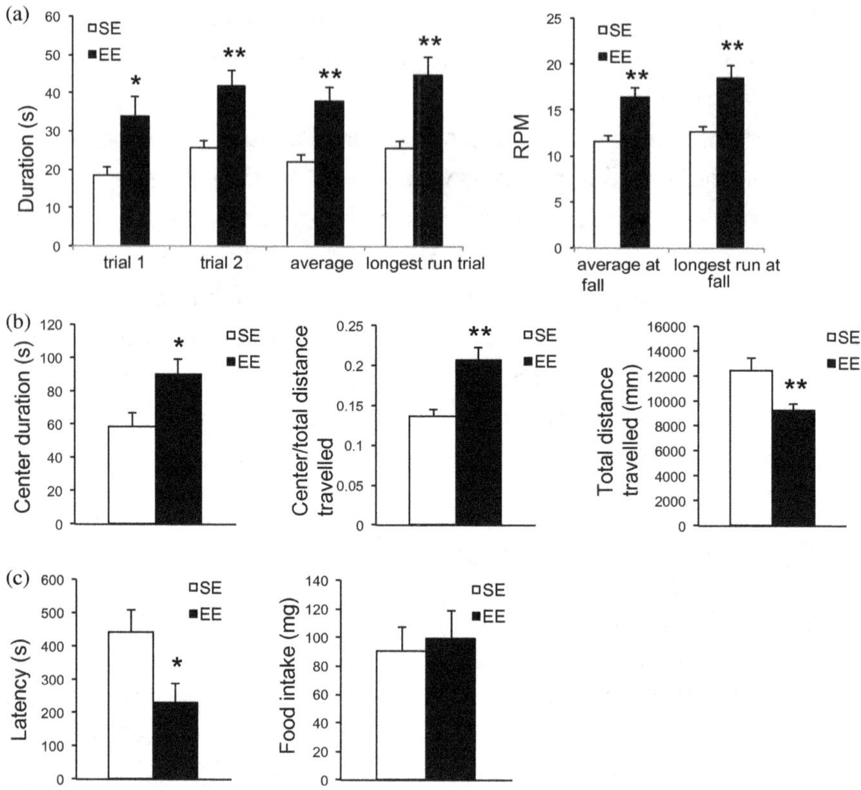

Fig. 7.3. EE improves motor behavior and reduces anxiety in aged mice. (a) Rotarod treadmill test at the age of 19 months after 9-month EE (n = 9 per group). (b) Open field test at the age of 12 months after 2-month EE (n = 10 per group). (c) Novelty suppressed feeding test at the age of 20 months after 10-month EE (n = 10 for SE, n = 9 for EE). Data are mean ± SEM. *P < 0.05, **P < 0.01. Reprinted from McMurphy *et al.* Implementation of environmental enrichment after middle age promotes healthy aging. Aging (Albany NY). 2018, 10(7), 1698–1721.

Limbic structures include hippocampus, prefrontal cortex, nucleus accumbens, ventral striatum, amygdala, and hypothalamus.[134] The hypothalamus integrates metabolic, stress, and immune signals and functions. The hypothalamus is highly responsive to EE independent of age, and could contribute to the anxiolytic effect in addition to the extensively investigated hippocampus. Our research in young animals demonstrates that EE stimulates BDNF expression in the arcuate nucleus, ventromedial hypothalamic nucleus (VMH) and dorsomedial hypothalamic nucleus (DMH).[80] The DMH is critically involved in behavioral regulation, particularly fear, anxiety, and panic-like disorders in addition to physiological functions such as metabolism and environmental threats.[135–137] On the other hand, obesity has been linked to neuropsychiatric and anxiety disorders including generalized anxiety disorder, panic disorder, post-traumatic stress disorder, emotional reactivity, and cognitive dysfunctions.[138,139] Given the concomitant anti-obesity and anxiolytic effects of EE, the DMH could be a target to investigate whether or not the anti-obesity and anxiolytic effects are linked, and driven by a shared molecular pathway. Beside the DMH, paraventricular hypothalamus (PVH) could be involved as well. Loss of *Crh* in the PVH leads to reduced anxiety behaviors.[140] Study in young animals finds that EE downregulates *Crh* expression in the PVH,[86] which might contribute to the anxiolytic effect of EE. It is also possible that systemic metabolic improvement induced by activating the HSA axis indirectly influences brain functions and behaviors including anxiety.

Adipose Remodeling of Long-Term EE

Aging-related decline of brown adipose tissue (BAT) activity has been reported.[141] At the age of 22 months, the BAT of mice living in SE was visibly pale. In contrast, the BAT in EE mice appeared darker and maintained typical BAT morphology of younger mice devoid of white adipocyte infiltration often linked with aging (**Fig. 7.4(a, b)**). Consistent with the morphological changes, long-term EE robustly modulated BAT gene expression with an over 80% downregulation of leptin expression and an increasing trend of adiponectin expression. Some genes involved in glucose metabolism (*Glut4*, *Insr*), lipolysis (*Lpl*), and lipogenesis (*Gpat*) were upregulated in BAT of EE mice. UCP1 is a specific BAT marker and mediates BAT's thermogenic

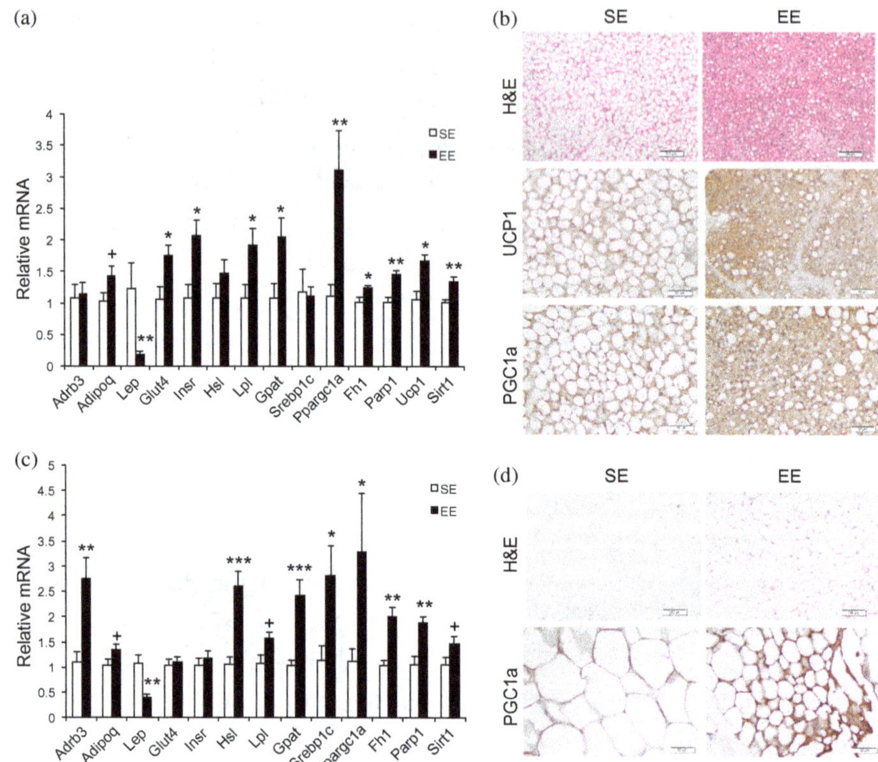

Fig. 7.4. EE remodels adipose tissue. Tissue analyses at the age of 22 months after 12-month EE. (a) Gene expression profile of BAT ($n = 6$ per group). (b) Immunohistochemistry of BAT. (c) Gene expression profile of rWAT ($n = 6$ per group). (d) Immunohistochemistry of rWAT. Data are mean ± SEM. $*P < 0.05$, $**P < 0.01$, $***P < 0.001$. Reprinted from McMurphy *et al.* Implementation of environmental enrichment after middle age promotes healthy aging. Aging (Albany NY). 2018, 10(7), 1698–1721.

activity to dissipate energy via releasing chemical energy from mitochondria in the form of heat.[142] EE significantly enhanced the expression of *Ucp1* at both messenger RNA (mRNA) and protein levels, indicative of preventing aging-related loss of BAT functions (**Fig. 7.4(a), (b)**). This finding is further supported by an over 3-fold increase of PGC-1α, the transcriptional coactivator switching cells from energy storage to energy expenditure by inducing mitochondrial biogenesis and genes involved in thermogenesis.[143]

The size of white adipocyte in EE mice was markedly smaller than that in SE mice (**Fig. 7.4(d)**). *Ppargc1a* (encoding PGC-1α) was also induced by EE in intra-abdominal WAT depots (rWAT: retroperitoneal WAT; gWAT: gonadal WAT) but not in liver. Consistent with the upregulation of mitochondrial genes transcription (**Fig. 7.4(c)**), EE mice showed higher mitochondrial DNA contents in adipose tissue and liver indicating increased mitochondrial biogenesis.[115] Sirtuins are linked to longevity.[144] EE upregulated *Sirt1* expression in BAT, rWAT, and liver.

These data suggest that EE induces adipose remodeling to reverse aging-related decline of adipose tissue functions, which may contribute to the improvements of general health in aged mice by EE.

EE Ameliorates Liver Steatosis and Suppresses Hepatic Glucose Production

Aging is associated with liver steatosis.[145] To further investigate the liver effects of EE, we performed another short-term EE (8 weeks) experiment in 10-month-old female mice. The reduction of fat mass, increase of lean mass, and improved performance in GTT were confirmed and appeared highly reproducible. Because hepatic glucose production (HGP) is a key aspect of glycemic control, we conducted a pyruvate tolerance test (PTT) at 7-week EE after fasting. EE mice displayed a significantly lower blood glucose level during PTT, indicative of lower hepatic glucose output (**Fig. 7.5(a)**).[115]

At the end of the 8-week EE study, neither nonfast serum glucagon level nor liver glycogen content were different between the two groups. EE resulted in a significant reduction of hepatic triglyceride level (**Fig. 7.5(b)**) while had no effect on circulating triglyceride level. Lipid accumulation in the livers were observed in SE mice at 12 months of age. Notably, EE potently diminished liver steatosis.[115]

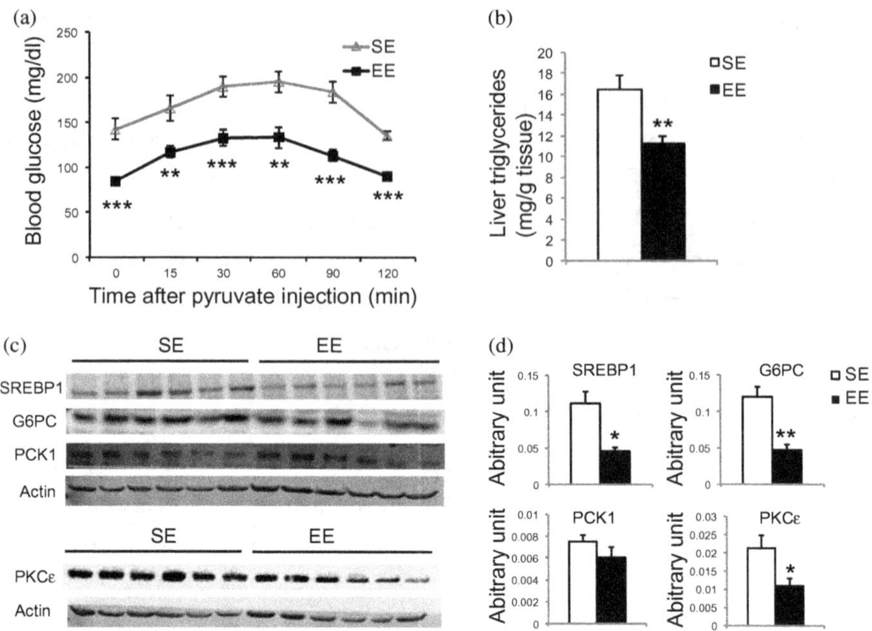

Fig. 7.5.   Short-term EE regulates liver phenotypes in middle-age mice. (a) Pyruvate tolerance test at 7 weeks in EE (n = 10 per group). (b) Liver triglycerides level (n = 10 per group). (c) Western blotting of livers. (d) Quantification of western blotting of livers (n = 6 per group). Data are mean ± SEM. *P < 0.05, **P < 0.01, ***P < 0.001. Reprinted from McMurphy *et al.* Implementation of environmental enrichment after middle age promotes healthy aging. Aging (Albany NY). 2018, 10(7), 1698–1721.

Immunoblotting revealed an over 50% reduction of SREBP1, the major transcription factor regulating *de novo* lipogenesis enzymes,[146,147] consistent with attenuation of hepatic steatosis. Moreover, we examined the mRNA and protein levels of two major gluconeogenic enzymes, phosphoenolpyruvate carboxykinase 1 (PCK1) and glucose-6-phosphatase (G6PC), and found suppression of G6PC at both protein and mRNA levels in EE livers (**Fig. 7.5(c), (d)**). Protein kinase Cε (PKCε) is implicated in lipid-induced hepatic insulin resistance and the resulting impaired insulin-induced suppression of hepatic gluconeogenesis.[148,149] Interestingly, EE decreased hepatic PKCε level by approximately 50% (**Fig. 7.5(c), (d)**).[115]

It is worth noting that short-term EE does not change GTT in young female mice although their adiposity is markedly reduced. One explanation of this age-dependent effect is that the aging-related hepatic functional decline allows revealing the liver modulation by EE. The EE regulation of liver is characterized as reversing aging-related hepatosteatosis, increasing glucose uptake during GTT, and suppressing HGP. These phenotypic changes of liver likely contribute to the improved glycemic control in aged EE mice.

HGP, crucial for systemic glucose homeostasis, is regulated through diverse mechanisms.[149] Nonalcoholic fatty liver disease is associated with impaired suppression of HGP. And the activation of PKCε is thought to mediate hepatic insulin resistance and hepatosteatosis in metabolic disease models.[150] EE lowered the liver PKCε level by approximately 50%, suggesting hepatic PKCε linking EE's hepatic effects to the improved systemic glucose homeostasis.[115] It will be interesting to further investigate signaling pathways and liver metabolites in aged EE mice.

It is not known whether EE regulates liver phenotypes through a brain-liver axis, or through the cross talk between liver and the HSA axis–remodeled adipose tissue. Leptin suppresses HGP[151] whereas lipolysis stimulates HGP.[152] EE results in a sharp drop of circulating leptin level and an increase of adipose tissue lipolysis, both contradictory to the lowering of HGP in EE. Consequently, the EE-induced adipose remodeling is unlikely a key mechanism of HGP suppression. Future studies are required to identify the central and/or peripheral circuits through which EE modulates HGP.[153–155]

Physical Exercise Does not Account for EE Effects

Physical exercise can lower adiposity and increase energy expenditure, and has positive effects on healthy aging but unable to extend maximum lifespan.[156] As offering an opportunity of physical exercise is a component of EE, whether EE equals to exercise has been the most frequently asked question. Our studies in young mice have

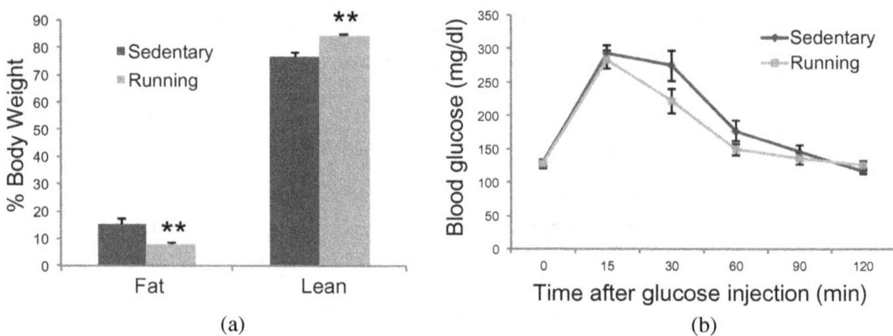

Fig. 7.6. Metabolic effects of voluntary wheel running in middle age mice. (a) EchoMRI analysis of body composition after 7-week running (n = 12 for Running, n = 8 for Sedentary). (b) Glucose tolerance test after 5-week running initiated at 10 months of age (n = 11 for Running, n = 7 for Sedantary). Data are mean ± SEM. **P < 0.01. Reprinted from McMurphy *et al.* Implementation of environmental enrichment after middle age promotes healthy aging. Aging (Albany NY). 2018, 10(7), 1698–1721.

repeatedly shown that the answer is no (see Chapters 2 and 3). In the aging project, we once again compared the phenotypes induced by EE versus by physical exercise alone. We subjected another cohort of 10-month-old mice to voluntary wheel running.[115] Running had no effect on body weight but reduced adiposity and increased lean mass similarly to EE (**Fig. 7.6(a)**). However, differing from EE, running did not significantly alter GTT (**Fig. 7.6(b)**) or hepatic G6PC level.

We examined gene expression of the major organs involved in systemic glucose homeostasis (liver, fat, and muscle), and found distinct patterns between EE and running. Specifically, short-term EE altered expression of genes involved in gluconeogenesis, glycolysis, lipogenesis, and inflammation in liver (**Fig. 7.7(a)**). Running resulted in fewer changes among this hepatic gene expression panel (**Fig. 7.7(b)**). Consistent with the HSA axis activation, EE upregulated *Adrb3*, *Srebp1c*, and *Ppargc1a* while sharply downregulated *Lep* in visceral fat (**Fig. 7.8(a)**). This adipose gene signature associated with EE was not observed in running mice (**Fig. 7.8(b)**). On the contrary, EE

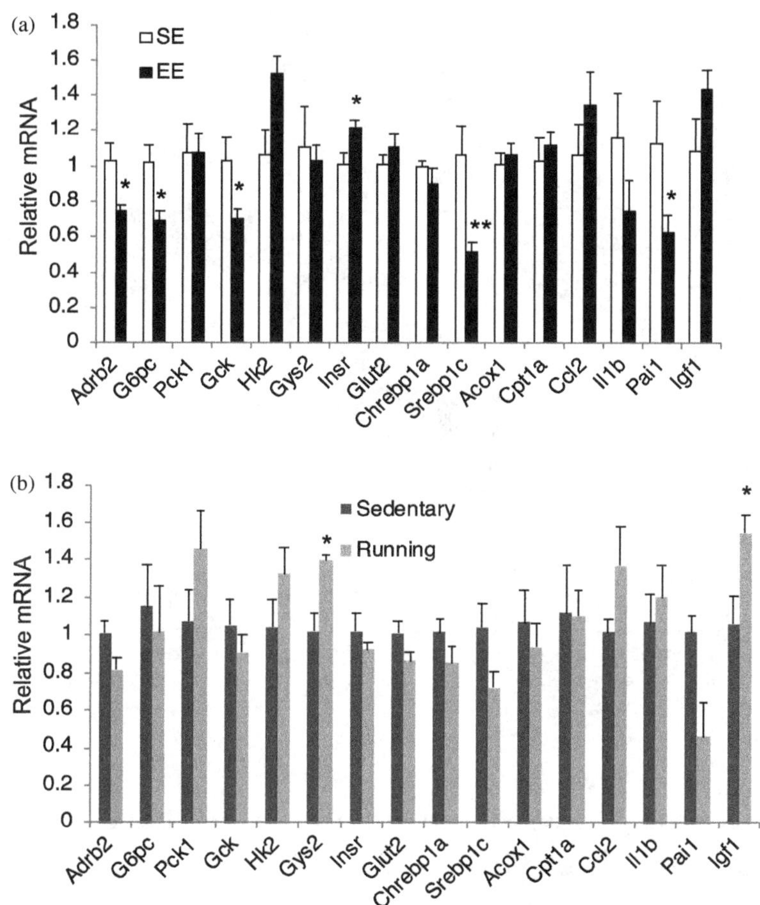

Fig. 7.7. Liver gene expression profile of short-term EE (a) and voluntary running (b) in middle-age mice. n = 6 per group for EE study. n = 7 for Running, n = 5 for Sedentary. Data are mean ± SEM. *P < 0.05, **P < 0.01. Reprinted from McMurphy *et al.* Implementation of environmental enrichment after middle age promotes healthy aging. Aging (Albany NY). 2018, 10(7), 1698–1721.

had minimal effect on muscle gene expression (**Fig. 7.8(c)**) whereas running potently upregulated genes involved in glucose metabolism, fatty acid oxidation, and mitochondrial biogenesis in gastrocnemius muscle (**Fig. 7.8(d)**). These data suggest that voluntary running fails to reproduce several key metabolic effects of EE in aged mice, and

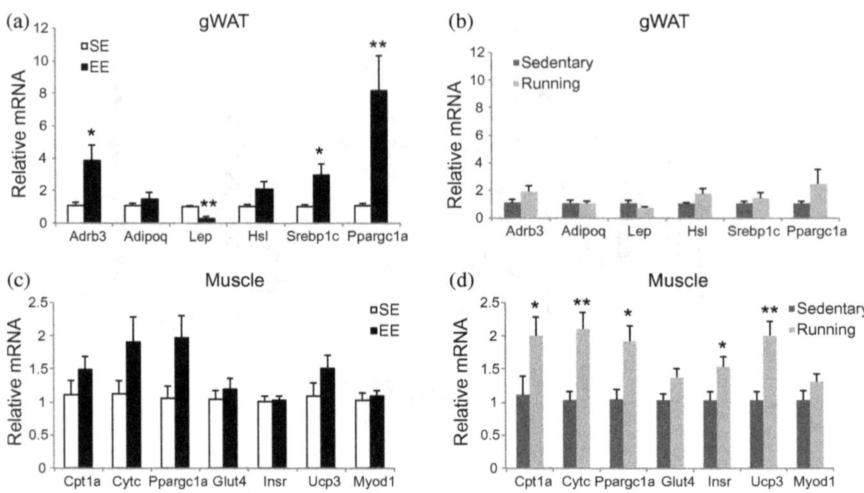

Fig. 7.8. Gene expression profile of short-term EE and voluntary running in middle age mice. (a) and (b) Gene expression profile of gWAT. (c) and (d) Gene expression profile of gastrocnemius muscle. n = 6 per group for EE study. n = 7 for Running, n = 5 for Sedentary. Data are mean ± SEM. *P < 0.05, **P < 0.01. Reprinted from McMurphy *et al.* Implementation of environmental enrichment after middle age promotes healthy aging. Aging (Albany NY). 2018, 10(7), 1698–1721.

certain phenotypic changes shared between EE and running might be regulated through distinct mechanisms.

Implementing EE at Old Age Results in Upward Trend of Mean Lifespan

To investigate whether old animals respond to EE intervention, we initiated EE to mice at 18-month of age. Glucose tolerance is an important indicator for frailty in old age in humans.[157] Three-month EE living resulted in significant improvement of glycemic control in old mice, much like what was observed in middle-aged mice (**Fig. 7.9(a)**). For a lifespan study, 18-month-old mice were randomized to live in EE or SE, and maintained in their respective housing till

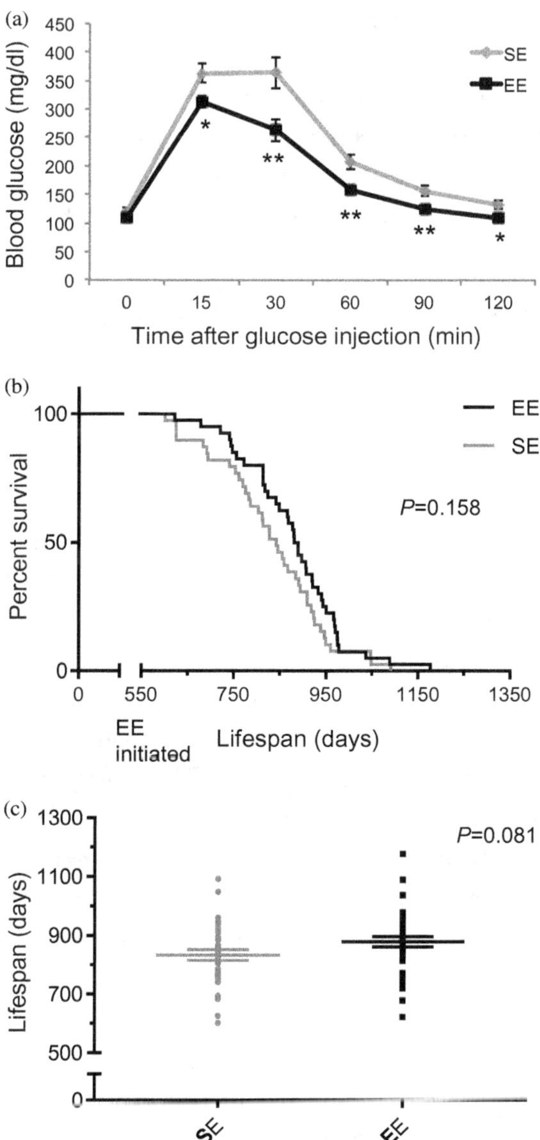

Fig. 7.9. EE effects on lifespan initiated at 18-month of age. (a) Glucose tolerance test after 3-month EE. $n = 10$ per group, $*P < 0.05$, $**P < 0.01$. (b) Kaplan-Meier survival curves of combined data of 4 cohorts. $n = 39$ for SE, $n = 40$ for EE. Log-rank test P value shown in figure. (c) Means of lifespan. Individual value plot of lifespan. Two-sample T test P value shown in figure. Reprinted from McMurphy *et al*. Implementation of environmental enrichment after middle age promotes healthy aging. Aging (Albany NY). 2018, 10(7), 1698–1721.

death. EE showed an increasing trend of means of lifespan (~45 days) (**Fig. 7.9(b), (c)**). These data are encouraging because mice as old as 18 months are still readily responsive to EE. Although EE did not significantly extend maximum lifespan when initiated at the age of 18 months, it remains to be seen whether implementing EE at earlier age might impact more positively on lifespan.

EE Inhibits Neuroinflammatory Markers

Chronic inflammation is implicated in the etiology of disease across lifespan.[158] A conceptual model has been proposed in which hypothalamic microinflammation is a common basis of metabolic syndrome and aging.[159] Chronic overnutrition induces inflammation-like changes in the hypothalamus (including TNF-α and interleukins, ILs), and interrupt the central regulation of energy balance, glucose homeostasis, and core features of metabolic syndromes.[160–164] Notably, low-grade inflammation is also a hallmark of aging, and systemic inflammation is negatively correlated with human longevity.[165–167] Recent studies have demonstrated that hypothalamic microinflammation promotes systemic aging.[168,169] The underlying mechanisms involve numerous neural signaling pathways and neural cell types. The activated neuroinflammatory axis and related proinflammatory cytokines, collectively mediate and propagate the development of metabolic dysfunction and aging-related disorders.[159]

To examine whether EE could modulate microinflammation, particularly in the hypothalamus, we profiled hypothalamic gene expression in mice after a long-term EE of 12 months, and a short-term EE of 6 weeks, both initiated at the age of 10 months.[115] Different patterns of gene expression were found in the two cohorts. EE of 6 weeks (endpoint age of 11.5 months) upregulated *Bdnf* and other genes involved in energy homeostasis such as *Npy*, *Pomc*, and *Lepr*. These changes were not detected in mice after EE of 12 months. Instead, a cluster of genes involved in inflammation including *Il1b*, *Il6*, *Ccl2* (encoding MCP-1), *Nfkbia* (encoding nuclear factor of κ light polypeptide gene enhance in B cells inhibitor α), and *Socs3* (encoding suppressor cytokine signaling 3) were collectively down-regulated in long-term EE mice at older age (endpoint age of 22 months) (**Fig. 7.10(a)**). *Ccl2* and *Nfkbia* were also downregulated in the amygdala, a brain area critically involved in emotionality including anxiety (**Fig. 7.10(b)**). Experimental evidence suggests neuroinflammation in the aging hypothalamus may contribute to

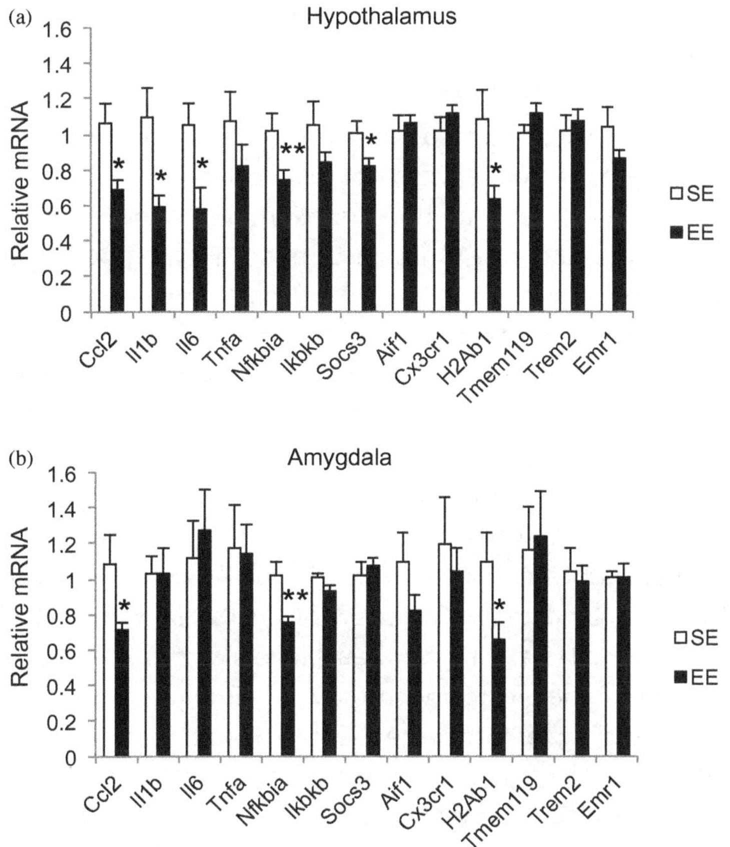

Fig. 7.10.   Gene expression profiles after 12-month EE initiated at 10 months of age (a) Hypothalamus. (b) Amygdala. *n* = 8 per group. Data are mean ± SEM. *P* < 0.05, **P* < 0.01. Reprinted from McMurphy *et al.* Implementation of environmental enrichment after middle age promotes healthy aging. Aging (Albany NY). 2018, 10(7), 1698–1721.

metabolic disorders through induction of hypothalamic NFκB or variable *Socs3* signaling in microglia.[159] Hence, these findings drew our attention to microglial cells. We went on to study how EE affects microglial cell morphology and function in aged mice.

Long-Term Environmental Enrichment Initiated at Middle Age Modulates Microglial Morphology

Microglial cells are the resident immune cells of the central nervous system (CNS). In their "quiescent" (or baseline) state in absence of CNS insult, microglial cells are highly ramified and continuously survey their territory using thin processes with multiple branches.[170,171] In this surveilling state, microglial cells not only monitor for CNS injury, but also contribute to the formation, function, and removal of synapse. This plasticity-facilitating function of microglia is thought partially through the expression of BDNF.[172,173] Microglia can be activated to undergo phenotypic and morphological changes when homeostatic disturbance is detected. Sensing of immunogenic stimuli or tissue injury activates microglia to produce proinflammatory molecules, to phagocytose cellular debris, and to present antigens to the immune system.[23] These so-called "reactive" microglial cells acquire a bushy morphology characterized as short, retracted processes and cellular hypertrophy, associated with reduced surveilling process motility.[174]

Aging can trigger dysfunction of microglia.[168,175,176] Microglia from aged animals have higher basal levels of cytokine expression, and are hyper-reactive to inflammatory stimuli.[177] Aged microglia exhibit shortening of processes, slower process movement, and enlarged soma volumes compared to young microglia.[178] One hypothesis postulate that microglia experience progressively functional decline over the lifespan, due to the accumulation of deleterious changes to these cells such as oxidative DNA damage and accumulation of nondegradable protein and lipid aggregates. For example, myelin breakdown in the CNS over time can cause lipofuscin accumulation in microglia.[179] Studies have shown that this inflamed and dysfunctional microglial profile plays a role in the development of age-related neurodegenerative diseases.[22,180]

Recent studies have revealed a role of microglia in orchestrating hypothalamic inflammatory response to dietary excess (e.g., high-fat diet feeding) and mediating obesity susceptibility.[181–183] Our previous studies demonstrate that EE suppresses the expression of a cluster of cytokines and inflammatory molecules in the hypothalamus of obese mice (young and old) as well as old mice of normal weight,[97,115] including the cytokine IL-1β and molecules in the NFκB signaling pathway, which is a key pro-inflammatory pathway of hypothalamic microinflammation.[159,168]

We then examined the expression of a group of genes related to microglia identity and function in the hypothalamus and amygdala microdissection from the aforementioned 12-month EE study (end-point age of 22 months).[117] Among the six genes profiled, including *Aif1* (encoding allograft inflammatory factor 1, also known as Iba1), *Tmem119* (encoding transmembrane protein 119), *Cx3cr1* (encoding C-X3-C motif chemokine receptor 1), *H2Ab1* (encoding histocompatibility 2, class II antigen A, β1, or MHC-II), *Trem2* (encoding triggering receptor expressed on myeloid cells 2), and *Emr1* (encoding EGF-like module-containing mucin-like hormone receptor-like 1, also known as F4/80),[184] only *H2Ab1* expression was significantly altered at transcription level in both the hypothalamus and the amygdala (**Fig. 7.10**). Studies have linked chronic expression of MHC-II to brain aging, as ~25% of microglia in mice at 18–20 months of age expressing MHC-II, in contrast to <3% of MHC-II positive microglia in mice at 3–4 months of age.[185,186] This study is limited to transcription profiling of a set of selected genes. Unfortunately, we no longer have hypothalamic or amygdala samples from this long-term 12-month EE study sufficient for nonbiased transcriptome analysis. Another limitation is that microglial cells were not isolated from these brain regions.[117] Future studies are required to address these weaknesses.

Nevertheless, the gene expression data point to a plausible phenotypic difference in microglia between EE and SE. We reasoned that the microglial changes associated with EE would be detectable at an age when age-related microglia changes start to emerge. Thus, we subjected 10-month-old mice to EE or SE housing for 7.5 months so that the mice entered early old age at the end of the experiment. Once again, EE initiated at middle age reduced adiposity and improved GTT.[117]

We examined the immunoreactivity of Iba1, a microglial marker, across the brain to assess the microglial changes after long-term EE of 7.5 months. Relative to SE mice, Iba1 staining appeared prominent in the hypothalamus, amygdala, and hippocampus of EE mice (**Fig. 7.11**).[117] SE microglia in these regions had fewer and shorter

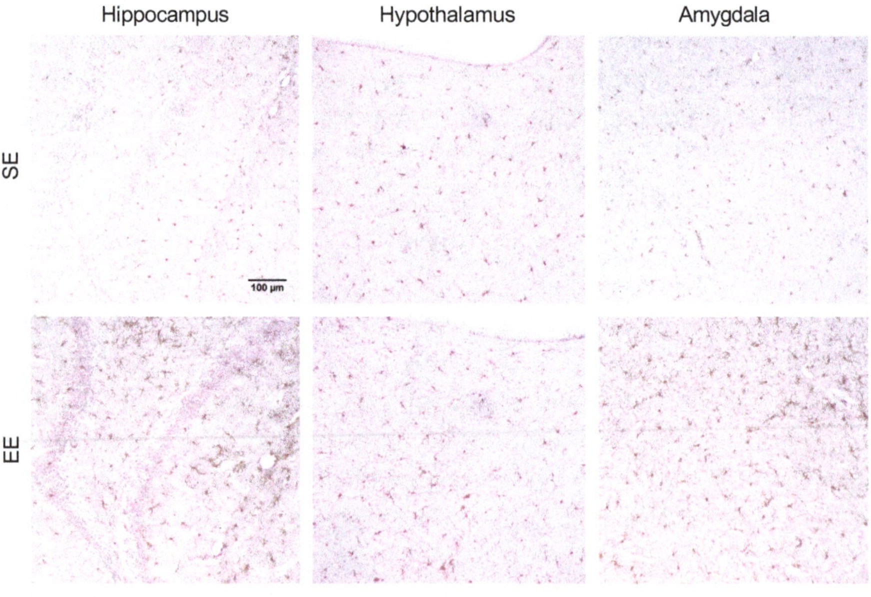

Fig. 7.11. Microglial morphological changes after 7.5-month EE initiated at 10-month of age. Representative fields of Iba1 staining in the hippocampus, hypothalamus, and amygdala. Scale bar: 100 µm. Reprinted from Ali *et al*. Long-term environmental enrichment affects microglial morphology in middle age mice. Aging (Albany NY). 2019, 11(8), 2388–2402.

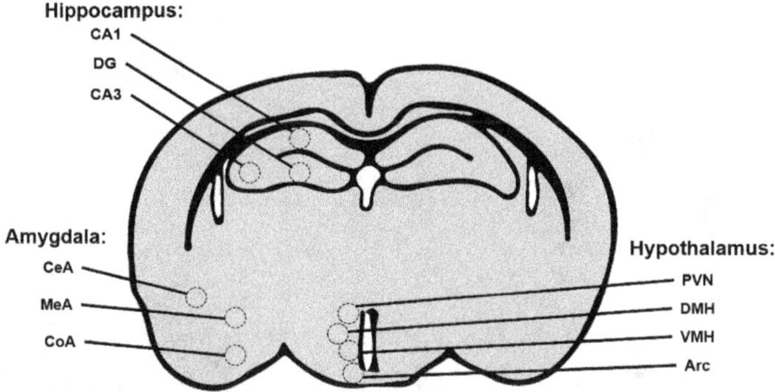

Fig. 7.12. Selected subfields within the hippocampus, hypothalamus, and amygdala for microglial morphology survey. CA1, cornu ammonis 1; CA3, cornus ammonis 3; DG, dentate gyrus; Arc, arcuate nucleus; DMH, dorsomedial hypothalamic nucleus; PVN, paraventricular nucleus; VMH, ventromedial hypothalamic nucleus; CeA, central nucleus of the amygdala; MeA, medial nucleus of the amygdala; CoA, cortical nucleus of the amygdala. Reprinted from Ali *et al*. Long-term environmental enrichment affects microglial morphology in middle age mice. Aging (Albany NY). 2019, 11(8), 2388–2402.

processes.[117] It is reported that aged microglia display deramified morphology compared to young microglia.[187] In contrast, EE microglia showed a highly ramified morphology, resembling young adult microglia. We noted no gross differences in astrocytic reactivity or morphology.[117]

We quantified the microglia morphological changes in a total of 10 subfields or nuclei within hypothalamus (Arc, DMH, PVN, VMH), amygdala (CeA, CoA, MeA), and hippocampus (CA1, CA3, DG) (**Fig. 7.12**).[117] First, EE had unremarkable impact on microglial cell counts among the brain nuclei examined. Microglial cell count was decreased by long-term EE only in two nuclei Arc and CeA, important for feeding behavior and fear response, respectively. Second, Iba1 positive area was increased in many regions of EE mice (CA3, DG, PVH, VMH, CeA, CoA, MeA), indicative of microglia cellular hypertrophy given the absence of increases in cell density (indicator of cellular proliferation or infiltration). Finally, we directly measured microglial ramification by analyzing microglial branching

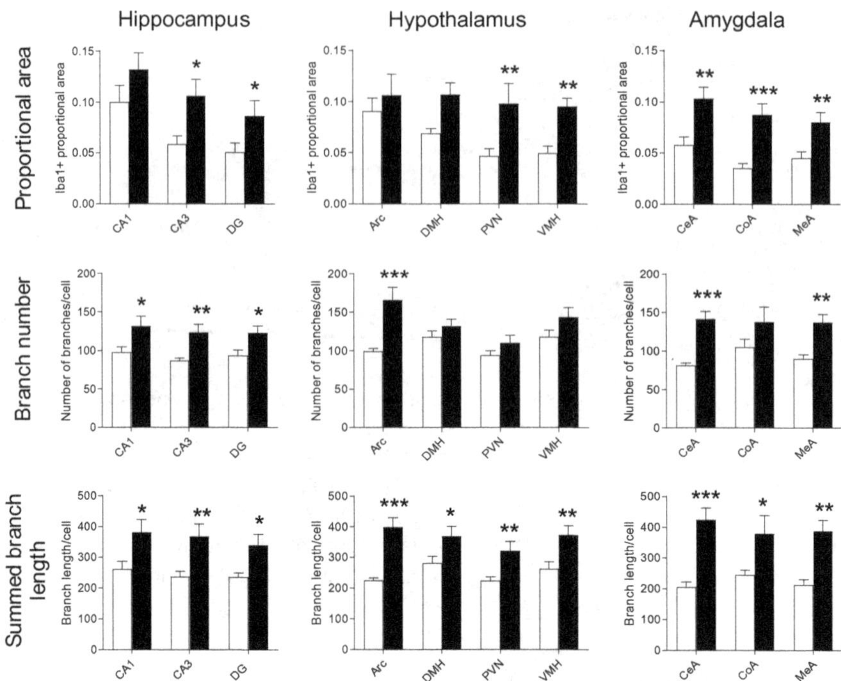

Fig. 7.13. Quantification of microglial morphology across hippocampus, hypothalamus, and amygdala. $n = 4$ for SE mice, $n = 5$ for EE mice. Data are mean ± SEM. *$P < 0.05$, **$P < 0.01$, ***$P < 0.001$. Reprinted from Ali *et al.* Long-term environmental enrichment affects microglial morphology in middle age mice. Aging (Albany NY). 2019, 11(8), 2388–2402.

metrics including branch number and branch length.[188] EE resulted in higher branch numbers in CA1, CA3, DG, Arc, CeA, and MeA (**Fig. 7.13**). More prominently, EE led to longer microglial process per microglia in all of the 10 brain nuclei examined, revealing a robust difference in microglial branching phenotype across all three brain regions (**Fig. 7.13**). This is not the regular hypertrophy seen in aged microglia associated with inflammatory responses, but rather represents a possible reversal of the deramified morphology of old microglia by EE.

Taken together, compared to aged morphologies from SE housing, long-term EE initiated at middle age leads to hypertrophied microglia with more numerous branches and longer branches, indicative of mitigation of the deramified morphology associated with aged microglia. This observation is consistent with a previous report that long-term EE of 16–20 months increases microglial branch number and branch length in CA3 in female albino Swiss mice.[189] Because most studies have focused on hippocampus, there is sparse information on hypothalamic and amygdala microglia response to EE. We are particularly interested in the hypothalamus because it serves as a key CNS regulator of metabolic homeostasis, immune function, and stress response. Our data suggest that EE impacts microglia morphology in aged mice preserving a morphology similar to that of microglia in young mice. The morphologic features characterized as hypertrophy and ramification without increases in microglial cell density are accompanied by downregulation of MHC-II together with a cluster of pro-inflammatory genes in hypothalamus, as well as improved systemic metabolic outcome. These findings brought about the question whether microglia are important for either the hypothalamic alterations (e.g., upregulation of BDNF) or the systemic metabolic effects associated with EE. To answer this question, we conducted a microglial depletion study described in the following section.

CSF1R Inhibitor and Environmental Enrichment Additively Improve Metabolic Outcomes

In order to understand the role of microglia in the metabolic improvements induced by EE, we used PLX5622 (PLX), a highly potent and selective inhibitor of the receptor tyrosine kinase activity of CSF1R.[190,191] Studies have shown that CSF1R inhibitors deplete the microglia in the CNS without causing behavioral or cognitive deficits.[192,193] We treated female mice aged 10–11 months with PLX5622 supplied in diet (PLX5622 provided by Plexxikon, Inc., and formulated at 1200 ppm into rodent diet AIN-76A by Research Diets) or a normal chow diet AIN-76A. Three days later, mice were

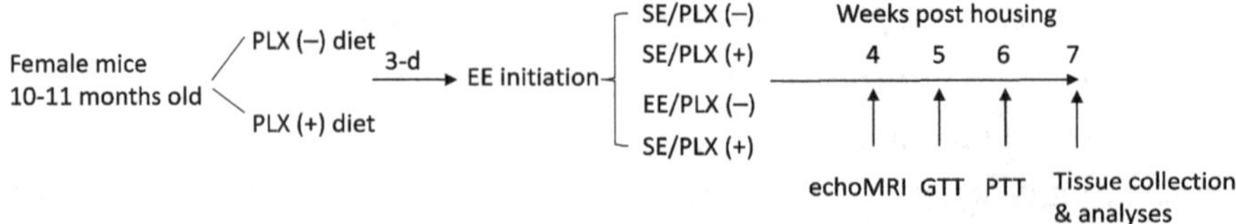

Fig. 7.14. Timeline and study design of combining EE and CSF1R inhibitor. PLX5622 (PLX) was formulated into rodent diet AIN-76A.

randomly assigned to live in either EE or SE housing for 7 weeks. We examined *in vivo* metabolic outcomes and analyzed central and peripheral tissues to investigate whether CSF1R inhibition interferes with the EE-induced metabolic outcomes in middle-aged mice. This study yielded several interesting findings (**Figs. 7.14, 7.15**).[118]

(1) PLX5622 treatment in SE housing elicited limited metabolic effects in middle-aged mice — lower body weight and lower fasting blood glucose level, PLX(+)/SE compared to PLX(–)/SE. These changes were not observed in young adults. This finding supports the notion that aged microglia contribute to age-related metabolic decline.[159,194] However, our new evidence suggests that in addition to acting on microglia removal, PLX5622 may also improve metabolic homeostasis via peripheral immune modulation.

(2) Microglia depletion by PLX5622 did not attenuate the metabolic phenotypes associated with EE (**Fig. 7.15(a)–(c)**), suggesting microglia not essential for the metabolic benefits.

(3) PLX5622 treatment had no effect on EE-induced hypothalamic gene expression central to the HSA axis. Hypothalamic BDNF is a master regulator of EE's metabolic and immune effects. PLX5622-induced microglia depletion did not attenuate the upregulation of hypothalamic BDNF induced by EE (**Fig. 7.15(f)**), indicating microglia not the major source of BDNF.

(4) Chronic PLX5622 treatment reduced hypothalamic microglia by ~75% (**Fig. 7.15(d), (e)**). Of note, EE increased ramification

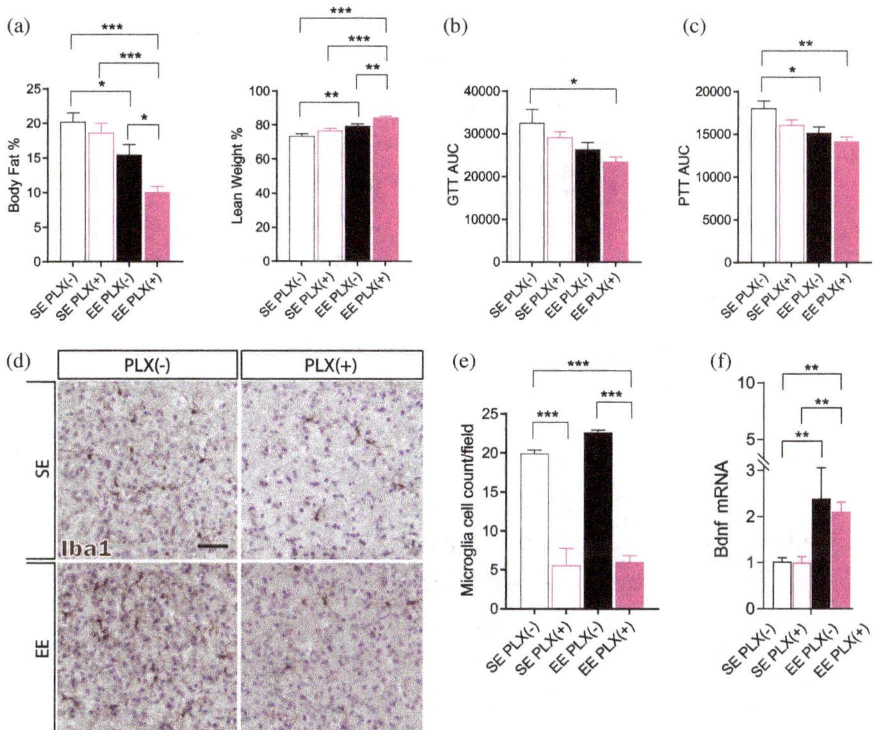

Fig. 7.15. CSF1R inhibitor PLX5622 and EE additively improve metabolic outcomes in middle-age female mice. (a) Body composition. (b) Area under the curve of glucose tolerance test. (c) Area under the curve of pyruvate tolerance test. (d) Representative Iba1 immunohistochemistry of medial hypothalamus. (e) Microglia cell count within hypothalamus. $n = 4$ per group. (f) Hypothalamic *Bdnf* gene expression, $n = 6$ per group. $n = 10$–12 per group for a–d. $*P < 0.05$, $**P < 0.01$, $***P < 0.001$. Reprinted from Ali *et al*. CSF1R inhibitor PLX5622 and environmental enrichment additively improve metabolic outcomes in middle-aged female mice. Aging (Albany NY). 2020, 12(3), 2101–2122.

of microglia regardless of PLX5622 treatment, which suggests short-term EE (7 weeks) sufficient to affect microglia morphology and this modulation sustains in the remaining (surviving) microglia in PLX-treated mice.

(5) EE and longitudinal PLX5622 additively improved metabolic outcomes, in cases where PLX5622 alone and EE alone had

weaker effects or no effect, including decrease in adiposity, increase in lean mass, and improved GTT (**Fig. 7.15(a)–(c)**). The mechanisms of the surprisingly additive benefits of PLX5622 plus EE are not known. We speculate two potential hypotheses if the combined effect is primarily mediated by CNS changes.[118] First, aged microglia in the hypothalamus might inhibit EE-induced signals downstream of or parallel to BDNF locally in the hypothalamus. If so, removal of microglia by PLX5622 would allow full display of EE metabolic benefits without altering BDNF levels. Second, our data show that both EE without PLX5622 and partial microglial depletion by PLX5622 alone suppress hypothalamic inflammatory gene expression. Hence, EE may improve the function of the remaining microglia in PLX-treated mice and thereby further mitigating age-related metabolic decline. These two hypotheses may not be mutually exclusive but rather acting synergistically.

(6) PLX5622 modulated adipose tissue macrophages (ATMs) (**Fig. 7.16**). ATMs have been implicated in the development and maintenance of obese states, and age-related ATM alterations inhibit lipolysis and fat loss. One mechanism is that aged ATMs uptake and metabolize catecholamines. As a result, aged ATMs weaken sympathetic nervous system (SNS) signals to adipose tissue and thereby inhibiting norepinephrine-induced lipolysis of adipocytes.[195–198] Although most studies report PLX5622 primarily affect CNS microglial cells, with substantially smaller peripheral immune effects,[183,199,200] we examined its effect on ATMs with or without EE exposure.

We isolated stromal vascular fraction (SVF) from visceral fat and identified macrophages by flow cytometry (defined as F4/80$^+$, CD11b$^+$ cells as a subset of CD45$^+$, CD19$^-$ live cells). Macrophages are highly plastic cells that change their phenotype in response to microenvironment conditions. Classically activated "M1" macrophage (defined as CD11c$^+$, CD206$^-$) accumulate in obese adipose tissue and are thought to contribute

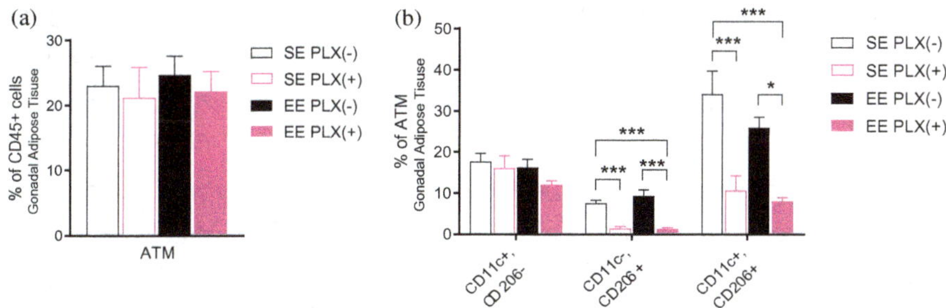

Fig. 7.16. EE and PLX5622 modulate adipose tissue macrophages (ATM) in middle age female mice. (a) ATM from gonadal WAT. (b) ATM polarization. n = 5–6 per group. Data are mean ± SEM. *P < 0.05, ***P < 0.001. Reprinted from Ali *et al.* CSF1R inhibitor PLX5622 and environmental enrichment additively improve metabolic outcomes in middle-aged female mice. Aging (Albany NY). 2020, 12(3), 2101–2122.

to systemic inflammation and insulin resistance, whereas alternatively activated "M2" macrophages (defined as CD11c⁻, CD206⁺) are present in leaner adipose tissue and associated with insulin-sensitive state.[196] Neither PLX5622 nor EE altered the abundance of ATM despite the significant reduction in visceral fat mass compared to SE/PLX(−) (**Fig. 7.16(a)**).

In terms of macrophage subpopulations, we identified CD11c⁺, CD206⁺ ATMs as the most abundant subtypes in middle-aged mice without PLX5622 treatment. In humans, CD11c⁺, CD206⁺ ATMs have been implicated as a source of proinflammatory cytokines and a driver of insulin resistance, with a mix of M1 and M2 features.[201] PLX5622 treatment regardless of housing condition, potently depleted both M2 (CD11c⁻, CD206⁺) and double positive (CD11c⁺, CD206⁺) ATMs, while had no effect on M1 (CD11c⁺, CD206⁻) ATMs (**Fig. 7.16(b)**). Remarkably, CD206⁺ ATMs regardless of CD11c status were nearly eliminated in PLX-treated animals, with a small population of CD11c⁺, CD206⁺ ATMs remaining. Furthermore, we also identified a subpopulation of F4/80ˡᵒʷ, CD11bˡᵒʷ immune cells residing in visceral fat which were eliminated by PLX5622 treatment. However, these cells were not the primary ATM population. Of note, EE had no effect on ATM polarization despite inducing leanness in middle-aged mice.[118]

(7) PLX5622 treatment regulated adipose gene expression. In order to search for adipose changes following PLX5622 treatment that might account for the additive treatment effect, we examined rWAT gene expression because rWAT mass was reduced to a greater degree by PLX5622 than by EE. We first assessed the adipose gene expression signature associated with EE by quantitative reverse transcription polymerase chain reaction (qRT-PCR). Interestingly, PLX5622 treatment showed significant effects across genes involved with sympathetic response — increased expression levels of *Adrb3*, the responsive receptor to sympathetic norepinephrine release onto adipose tissue; *Hsl*, mobilizing lipids in response to sympathetic tone; lipogenic transcription factor *Srebp1c*; thermogenic regulator *Ppargc1a*; whereas decreased expression level of *Lep*.[118]

The gene expression data together with ATM results suggest that PLX5622 treatment enables a sympathetic-sensitive phenotype in adipose tissue of middle-aged animals. It is possible that the combined metabolic benefits of PLX5622 and EE are peripherally driven, at least in part. Moreover, the peripheral mechanisms may apply to other metabolic active organs such as liver and muscle, which are worthy of further investigation.

Our study demonstrates a robust drug–environment additive effect that was previously unknown. These new findings intrigue us to ask several questions for future studies. One is the interplay between PLX5622 and EE on sympathetic sensitivity of aged adipose tissue. Chronic sympathetic overactivity is a shared hallmark of obesity and aging,[202] which can desensitize β-adrenergic signaling in adipocytes.[203] Inflammasome-activated ATMs in aged animals exhibit elevated catecholamine catabolism and abrogate lipolysis signals from the SNS.[197] Our data show that PLX5622 treatment alone in middle-aged mice leads to the ATM phenotypic shifts consistent with increased sympathetic responsiveness of visceral fat, and this change is associated with reduction of visceral fat mass. EE is known to act through preferential elevation of sympathetic tone to induce lean phenotypes. Thus, the significant combined benefits of PLX5622 with EE support the hypothesis that adipose sympathetic resistance contributes to age-related metabolic decline, which can be mitigated by treatments acting on sympathetic efficacy.[118] We intend to delineate pathway-overlapping interactions between PLX5622 and EE in adipose tissue and other metabolic active tissues in future research.

A major safety concern for long-term use of microglia-depleting drugs is interference in microglial capacity of debris clearance and synaptic maintenance in the healthy brain. Yet, it is not clear that these drugs deplete microglia in humans. Our study suggests that peripheral targets of CSF1R antagonists should not be ignored. For example, targeting adipose tissue via directed delivery or reformulation to prevent crossing blood–brain barrier might potentially be effective. Moreover, our data suggest that combining a short course of CSF1R inhibitor with lifestyle interventions could be therapeutic. This combination regime may avoid the side effects of chronic use of this class of drugs. Other strategies have been investigated such as "refreshing" microglia or macrophages depleted by CSF1R antagonists and then allowing repopulation after a short treatment course.[204,205] A caveat of this strategy is that the repopulated microglia may adopt a pro-inflammatory profile in the aged brain possibly influenced by aged brain microenvironment.[204] Thus, we propose a hypothesis that EE improves brain microenvironment and through which modulates the morphology and function of aged microglia, and furthermore prevents pro-inflammatory states of repopulated microglia. Studies to test this hypothesis are underway.

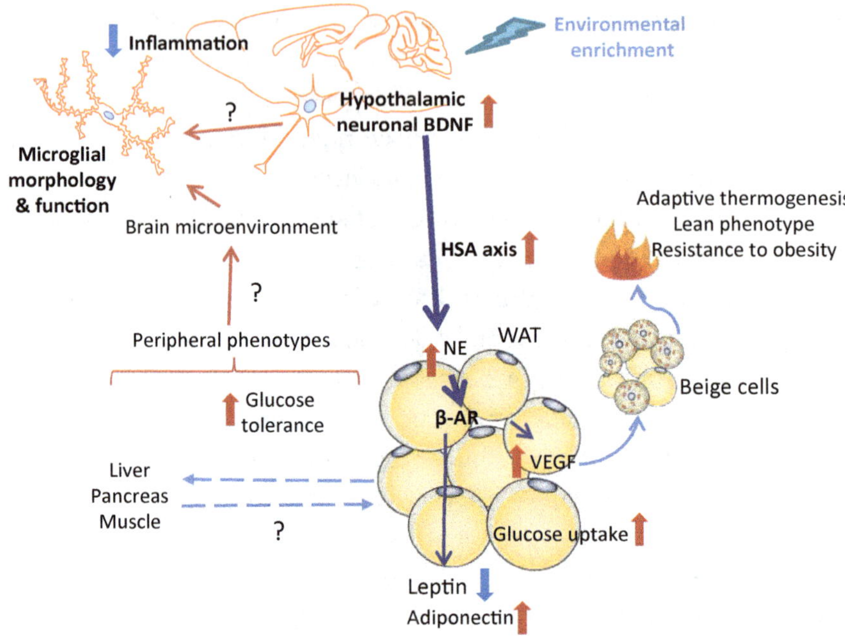

Fig. 7.17.   Proposed mechanisms of EE-induced microglial modulation. EE stimulates hypothalamic neuronal BDNF signaling and subsequently activates the HSA axis leading to systemic metabolic benefits. The improved brain microenvironment, through either peripheral feedback and/or interaction with local neuronal BDNF, modulates microglial morphology and function, which in turn contributing to reduced CNS inflammation.

We are also interested in elucidating the role of neuronal BDNF signaling in EE-induced microglial regulation. Moreover, we will assess whether this microglia regulation is mediated via local BDNF-microglia interaction or feedback from BDNF-driven systemic metabolic changes (**Fig. 7.17**).

Hypothalamic BDNF Gene Transfer Promotes Healthy Aging

Our studies in young animals have collectively identified hypothalamic BDNF as a key driver of multifaceted peripheral benefits of EE including improvements of metabolic and immune functions, as well as protection against obesity and cancer (Chapters 2–6). Naturally we posited that hypothalamic BDNF would mediate the positive impact of EE on healthspan. In fact, evidence from literature supports BDNF as a target for antiaging research. Mattson and colleagues propose BDNF signaling, insulin, IGF-1, and serotonin to be the important determinants of healthy aging due to their cooperative influence on energy metabolism, stress response, and cardiovascular function.[206] Impaired BDNF signaling has been documented during normal aging. In addition, reduced BDNF levels are associated with vulnerable neuronal populations in various neurodegenerative diseases such as Alzheimer's, Parkinson's, and Huntington's diseases, highlighting the need for further therapeutic research on components of the BDNF signaling pathway.[207] Administrating exogenous BDNF and/or stimulating its receptor expression can mitigate certain physiologic or pathologic age-related alterations in the CNS.[207] Furthermore, brain BDNF signaling is thought to mediate at least some of the antiaging effects of an intermittent fasting regimen.[208,209] However, little is known regarding BDNF signaling in the hypothalamus during normal aging. Moreover, it remains unclear how BDNF signaling in neurons is relayed to the periphery to improve the healthspan of many different organ systems.

Hence, we sought to examine whether overexpressing BDNF in the hypothalamus can reproduce the positive impact on healthspan induced by EE initiated after middle age.[116] As described in Chapter 4, we have developed an autoregulatory system to control BDNF transgene expression in order to prevent serious side effects. Several studies have demonstrated the impressive efficacy and safety profile of this autoregulatory adeno-associated virus (AAV)-BDNF gene therapy in obesity and diabetes models in young mice.[81,210] Thus, we conducted a gene therapy study using this autoregulatory AAV-BDNF vector in middle-aged mice with a study design largely mirroring the EE study described earlier in this chapter. Briefly, female C57BL/6 mice, age of 12 months, were randomized to receive autoregulatory BDNF vector or yellow fluorescent protein (YFP) vector by bilateral stereotaxic surgery. All mice were maintained in SE and fed with normal chow diet. A battery of metabolic and behavioral measurements was conducted across the 7-month duration of the study with endpoint age of 19 months (**Fig. 7.18(a)**).[116]

AAV-mediated BDNF overexpression was sustained at the end of the study, 193 days after AAV injection. Similar to the observation of long-term EE, inflammation-modulatory genes were collectively downregulated in BDNF-overexpressing hypothalamus including *Il1b, Il6, Il2rg* (encoding interkeukin-2 receptor γ), *Ly6d* (encoding lymphocyte antigen 6 family member D), *Cxcl10* (encoding C-X-C motif chemokine 10), and *Nfkbia* (encoding NFκB inhibitor α). It is worth noting that these changes were not observed in the amygdala or hippocampus, unlike the findings in EE. These results demonstrate that local stimulation of BDNF suppresses hypothalamic microin-flammation but the resulting systemic metabolic alterations are insufficient to affect neuroinflammation in brain regions other than hypothalamus. Along the same vein, this interpretation appears to support the hypothesis that the EE modulation of neuroinflamma-tion in extrahypothalamic regions is disassociated from its systemic metabolic/immune outcomes.

Hypothalamic BDNF gene transfer largely replicated the met-abolic benefits induced by EE (**Table 7.2**). Some metabolic effects were more pronounced in BDNF-overexpressing mice compared to EE mice. For instance, EE had little effect on body weight. In contrast, BDNF gene transfer completely prevented age-related weight gain, and the stable body weight was maintained throughout the 7-month duration of the study (**Fig. 7.18(b)**). BDNF-treated mice performed better in a GTT. Indirect calorimetry was used to measure energy expenditure (**Fig. 7.18(c)**). This approach is hardly applicable to EE mice because singly housing in the metabolic chamber distorts the metabolic status in a complex housing of EE. As such, we think

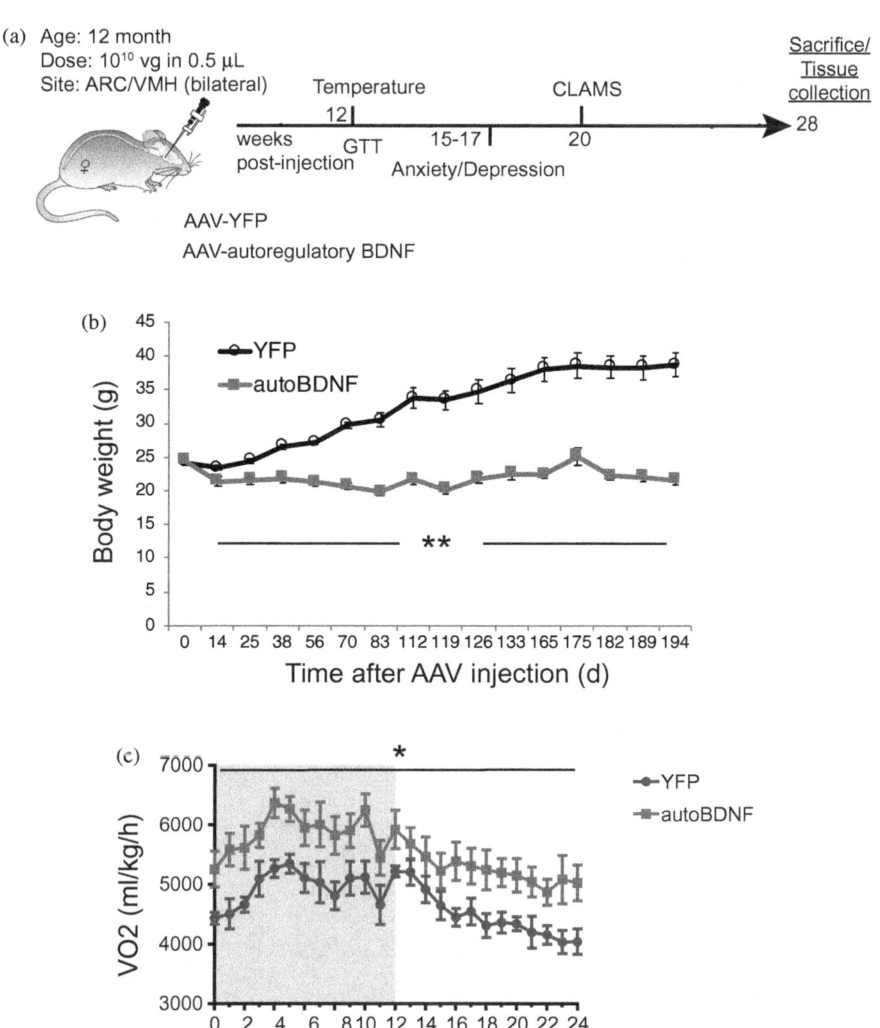

Fig. 7.18. Hypothalamic BDNF gene transfer promotes healthy aging. (a) Experimental design. (b) Body weight. n = 9–10 per group. (c) Oxygen consumption at 20-week post AAV injection. Shaded area, dark phase. n = 6 per group. Data are mean ± SEM. *P < 0.05, **P < 0.01. Reprinted from McMurphy *et al.* Hypothalamic gene transfer of BDNF promotes healthy aging in mice. Aging Cell 2019, 18(2): e12846.

Table 7.2   Comparison of Phenotypic Changes Induced by Environmental Enrichment and Hypothalamic Gene Transfer of BDNF in Middle Age Mice

Phenotypic Changes	Environmental Enrichment	Hypothalamic BDNF Gene Transfer
Hypothalamic BDNF expression	↑	↑
Body weight	N.S.	↓
Relative food intake	↑	N.S.
Adiposity	↓	↓
Glucose tolerance	↑	↑
Energy expenditure	N.A.	↑
Serum leptin	↓	↓
Serum adiponectin	N.S.	↑
Liver steatosis	↓	↓
Hepatic triglycerides	↓	↓
Brown adipose tissue functional decline	↓	↓
Beige cell gene program	↑	↑
Adipose mitochondrial biogenesis/function	↑	↑
Hypothalamic pro-inflammatory gene expression	↓	↓
Anxiety-like behaviors	↓	↓
Depression-like behaviors	N.S.	↓

N.S.: not significant; N.A.: no data available.

hypothalamic overexpressing BDNF could serve as a surrogate for assessment of systemic energy expenditure in EE mice. Compared to YFP control mice, BDNF-treated mice showed higher oxygen consumption in both dark and light phases, lower physical activity, and no difference in food intake within the metabolic chambers.[116] The increased oxygen consumption concurrent with lower physical activity strongly indicates that BDNF overexpression raises the resting metabolic rate.

BDNF overexpression resulted in a lean phenotype and profound adipose remodeling, resembling the long-term EE (**Table 7.2**).

BDNF treatment diminished liver steatosis, and reduced the hepatic triglyceride levels by approximately 80% compared to YFP mice. This mitigation of age-related fatty liver by BDNF gene transfer appears to be more effective than EE.

Besides metabolic improvements, BDNF treatment reduced anxiety-like behaviors as measured during cold-induced defecation and novelty suppressed feeding tests, and decreased depression-like behaviors as measured during tail suspension and forced swimming tests.[116] Taken together, these results suggest long-term hypothalamic BDNF overexpression does not elicit adverse behavioral changes. In fact, the anxiolytic and anti-depressant effects of hypothalamic BDNF gene transfer are alike those associated with long-term EE, which points to the possibility that hypothalamic BDNF plays a role in certain behavioral effects of EE.

Discussions on Hypothalamic BDNF Gene Transfer and Aging

Our physiological autoregulatory BDNF expression vector achieves a sustainable plateau of weight loss and leanness in aged mice maintained on a normal diet.[116] Hypothalamic BDNF gene transfer largely reproduces many metabolic benefits of EE, indicating a specific brain-fat axis — the HSA axis — as one mechanism linking a socially, physically, and cognitively active lifestyle to enhanced healthy aging.[115] These results also bring about more questions to tackle in future research. We have recently discussed these topics in a book chapter[211] and will revisit them in the following sections.

Neuroinflammation

Our data have shown that hypothalamic BDNF gene transfer leads to a suppression of NFκB pathway genes in young obese mice and in aged mice of normal weight. Because AAV1 vectors predominantly transduce neurons,[212] BDNF was primarily overexpressed in neurons in this study.[116] However, this study is unable to distinguish between the autocrine and paracrine effects of BDNF, because BDNF can be secreted from transduced neurons and act on other cell types such as microglial cells and astrocytes. To solve this problem, we are currently using AAV1 to deliver a dominant-negative form of the TrkB receptor[86] to the hypothalamus of aged mice. This approach will antagonize BDNF signaling specifically in the hypothalamic neurons and therefore help to elucidate the roles of neuronal BDNF signaling in hypothalamic microinflammation and systemic aging.

Microglial Modulation

Long-term EE results in morphological changes of microglia featured as hypertrophy and ramification without increase in microglial cell density.[117] CSF1R inhibitor PLX5622 in combination with EE additively improves metabolic outcomes in middle-aged mice over PLX5622 or EE alone. Interestingly, chronic PLX5622 treatment depletes 75% of microglia within the hypothalamus and reduces inflammatory markers but not interfering the upregulation of BDNF by EE.[118] These results intrigue us to test the hypothesis that EE modulates microglia function via hypothalamic BDNF signaling and subsequently contributing to the metabolic adaptations in aging.

Glucose Homeostasis and Multiorgan Cross Talk

Hypothalamic BDNF overexpression improves glycemic control in aged mice on a normal diet, concurrent with reduced adiposity, a favorable adipokine profile (lower leptin, higher adiponectin), and prevention of fatty liver in aged mice. Similar to the conditions of EE, adipose remodeling may contribute to the better performance of glucose tolerance either directly by elevation of adipose glucose uptake or indirectly by cross talk to the liver. Notably, BDNF-treated mice had drastic fat loss and hypoleptinemia but they did not display symptoms of lipodystrophy such as ectopic deposit of lipid in vital organs. On the contrary, the age-related fatty liver was almost diminished, accompanied by a 5-fold reduction of hepatic triglyceride content and downregulation of the transcription factors critical for *de novo* lipogenesis in the livers of BDNF-treated mice.[116] A previous study reports that infusion of BDNF to either the lateral cerebral ventricle or the VMH attenuates hyperglycemia in an uncontrolled insulin-deficient diabetes model through inhibition of HGP independent of insulin.[213] Our study shows EE reduces HGP possibly through suppression of PKCε level in liver.[115] Future studies are required to elucidate whether a hypothalamus-liver axis exists through which hypothalamic BDNF directly regulates liver glucose and lipid metabolism, thereby contributing to systemic glycemic control in aged animals. Alike questions regarding EE and healthy aging, how hypothalamic BDNF may influence the complex cross talk among metabolic active tissues such as fat, liver, muscle, and pancreas warrants investigation (**Fig. 7.19**).

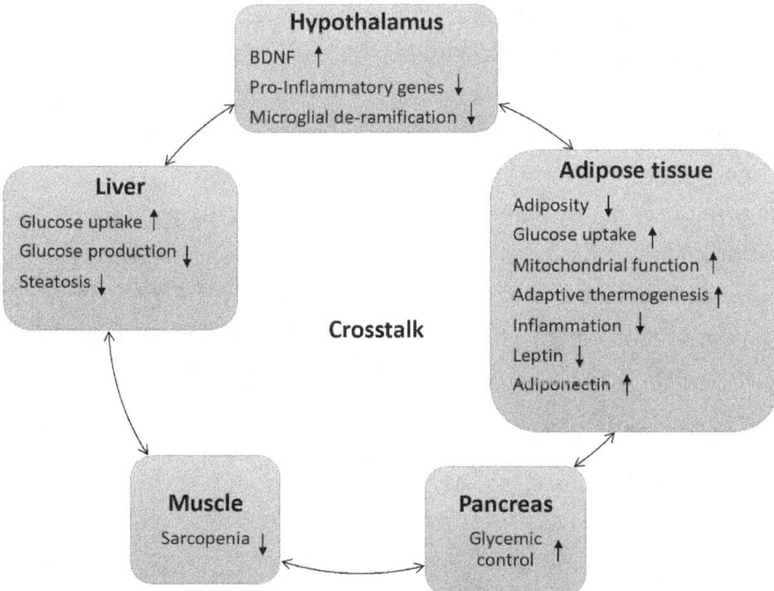

Fig. 7.19.   EE and hypothalamic gene transfer of BDNF promote healthy aging.

Behavioral Outcomes

Many studies demonstrate a link between reduction in BDNF with anxiety,[214] depression,[215,216] or impairment in spatial learning and discrimination.[217] However, the role of hypothalamic BDNF in emotionality is poorly understood. Our study may be the first to determine how hypothalamic BDNF induces behavioral adaptations during aging, revealing reduced anxiety-like and depression-like behaviors.[116] The underlying mechanisms are not clear. In this study, BDNF was overexpressed mainly in the ARC and VMH nuclei of the hypothalamus, from which BDNF protein could be secreted and diffused to the adjacent DMH. As DMH is a brain region important for behavioral regulation, particularly fear, anxiety, and panic-like disorders,[135,136] it is possible that higher BDNF protein level in DMH mediates the anxiolytic and/or the antidepressant effects. An alternative is through the HPA axis. In young animals, we have demonstrated that hypothalamic BDNF regulates T cell immunity in thymus and spleen through the HPA axis.[104,218] With advanced age, the body's stress response system becomes dysfunctional. It will be interesting to investigate whether hypothalamic BDNF renders the HPA axis more agile and functional appropriately, subsequently leading to reduction of depression-like behaviors in aged animals. Another possibility is that the global metabolic improvement induced by overexpressing BDNF in the hypothalamus may in turn indirectly influence functions of other limbic structures, such as the prefrontal cortex, hippocampus, nucleus accumbens, ventral striatum, and amygdala, all involved in the pathogenesis of affective disorders.[134,139]

Immune Outcomes

Another limitation of the published study is the lack of immune profiling. We have identified hypothalamic BDNF as the key brain mediator orchestrating EE-induced diverse immunomodulatory effects on innate and adaptive immune systems in normal mice as well as in conditions of cancer and autoimmune disease (Chapter 6).

In light of the link between aging process and decline of immune function,[194,219–221] it is highly relevant to study how hypothalamic BDNF may affect the aging-immune interplay.

Potential Adverse Effects

Even though the currently available data indicate benefits of hypothalamic BDNF gene transfer in middle-aged mice, we recognize that potential adverse effects are yet adequately assessed. For instance, leanness is not always associated with better health, and the concept of "obesity paradox" remains controversial while the underlying mechanisms are hotly debated. In times of stress, fat stores help organisms to sustain metabolic function. In this sense, a drastic loss of fat stores in advanced age might be contraindicated. Indeed, contrary to the increased risks in younger patients, morbidity and mortality are reduced for older adults with overweight and mildly obese BMIs.[222,223] Many studies attribute this contradictory phenomenon to BMI as a misleading metric, which is especially true for the elderly. Rather than BMI, adiposity, body fat distribution, and preservation of lean mass are better predictors of survival.[222,224,225] We are mindful that sustained low adiposity and elevated basal metabolic rate resulting from BDNF overexpression might not be beneficial at old age. How hypothalamic BDNF gene transfer affects lean mass and bones remain to be determined. On the other hand, since implementing EE at old age of 18 months positively impacts mean lifespan,[115] it will be interesting to explore antiaging mechanisms independent of hypothalamic BDNF.

Environmental Enrichment Mitigates Age-Related Metabolic Decline and Tumor Progression

According to "Age and Cancer Risk" published by the National Cancer Institute (NCI), advancing age is the most important risk factor for cancer overall and for many individual cancer types (cancer.gov/

about-cancer/causes-prevention/risk/age). Overall cancer incidence rate rises steadily along age increases — cases per 100,000 people from fewer than 25 in age groups under age 20, to ~350 aged 45–49, to over 1000 among people 60 and older. This age-related increase of cancer incidence is far greater than any known risk factors. The most recent statistical data from NCI's Surveillance, Epidemiology, and End Results (SEER) Program finds the median age of a cancer diagnosis is 66 years. Many common cancer types have similar pattern of median age at diagnosis: 62 years for breast cancer, 66 years for prostate cancer, 67 years for colorectal cancer, and 71 years for lung cancer. Of note, certain types of cancer can occur at young age. For instance, although only 1% of cancer overall is diagnosed in age group under 20, about 25% of bone cancer and 12% of brain and other nervous system cancers are diagnosed in this age group.

Aging, metabolic dysfunction, and cancer risk are inextricably connected. With age, many individuals lose lean mass and experience increases in total adiposity. Fat becomes dysfunctional and is redistributed from subcutaneous and visceral adipose depots to ectopic sites, including liver, skeletal muscle, heart, and the pancreas.[226] Accordingly, age is considered as a risk factor for the development of metabolic syndrome, obesity, insulin resistance, and related inflammation of adipose tissue.[227] Obesity-driven chronic inflammatory states, dyslipidemia, insulin resistance, hyperglycemia, and adipokine aberrations can promote cancer initiation, proliferation, and cancer-favorable microenvironments.[228,229] Hence, it is utterly important to characterize multifaceted therapeutics and interventions that are effective for all three actors. Animal studies suggest EE, which recapitulates aspects of healthy lifestyle, can be such an intervention for aging, metabolic dysfunction, and cancer.

Based on the positive impact of EE on healthspan, we sought to test the idea that implementing EE in aged mice can "rejuvenize" the body systems and mitigate the age-related functional decline thereby leading to inhibition of cancer progression. For the first attempt in this area, we chose to use a murine cancer cell line syngeneic to the C57BL/6 mice and its progression would be affected by host age. Beheshti and colleagues report that host age has a significant impact on the progression of implanted Lewis lung carcinoma (LLC), revealing a link between LLC progression and age-related dysregulation in apoptosis, angiogenesis, and metabolism of tumor.[230] As such, we enrolled young (3 months of age) and middle age (14 months of age) female mice to an experiment of 2 × 2 design (housing × age). Mice were randomized to EE or SE and maintained on normal chow diet. At week 8 post EE housing, 2.5×10^5 LLC cells were implanted subcutaneously to mice (**Fig. 7.20**).[30]

Along the duration of the study, we examined various metabolic parameters. Middle-aged EE mice exhibited significant reduction in body weight when compared to middle-age SE mice whereas young EE mice showed no difference in weight compared to young SE mice. Because middle-age SE mice weighed heavier compared to young SE mice, EE appears to attenuate this age-related weight

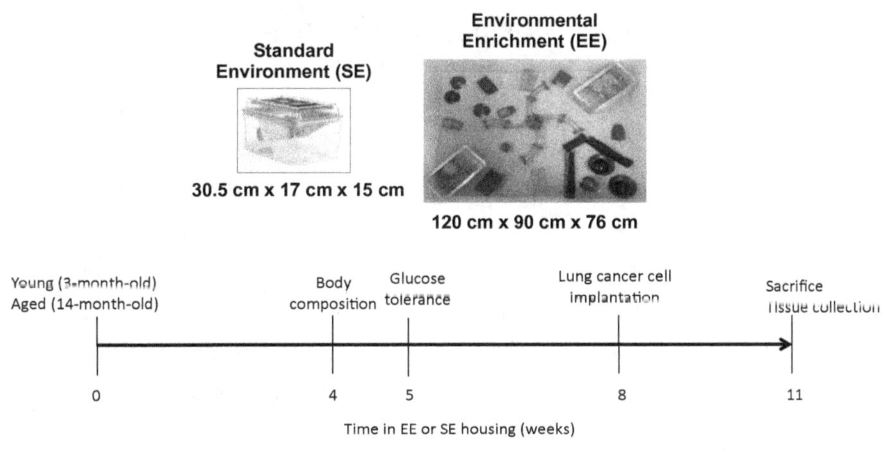

Fig. 7.20. Timeline of the study to investigate whether implementing EE in aged mice can mitigate the age-related metabolic decline and inhibit tumor growth.

gain. EE reduced fat mass and increased lean mass in both young and middle-aged mice. The effect on body composition by EE was more robust in middle-aged mice when comparing the difference between EE and SE for respective age groups: Middle-age (EE–SE) versus Young (EE–SE). Middle-age SE mice exhibited impaired glucose tolerance compared to young SE mice. EE completely prevented this age-related functional decline. In summary, exposure to EE of 2 months was sufficient to mitigate several age-related metabolic alterations.

LLC tumor growth was not affected by EE in young mice. In contrast, EE significantly reduced the growth rate of LLC in middle-aged mice. Notably, the tumor burden in middle-age SE mice was substantially higher than that in young SE mice. And this age-related faster tumor growth was completed abolished by EE. Pathological examination of tumors from middle-aged groups found less obvious tumor necrosis and apoptosis in middle-age EE mice. Tumors from middle-age EE mice exhibited signs of slow growth and lower malignancy compared to tumors from middle-age SE mice.

To examine the molecular changes in LLC tumors, we profiled several markers of apoptosis, angiogenesis, inflammation, and immune response at mRNA and protein levels. Most notable change was Cox2 (encoding cyclelxygenase-2) that expresses in many cancer types and promotes apoptotic resistance, proliferation, angiogenesis, inflammation, invasion, and metastasis of cancer cells.[232] Tumor levels of Cox2 were significantly higher in middle-age SE mice versus young SE mice: a 2-fold increase in mRNA and a 5-fold increase in protein. This age-related increase of tumor Cox2 level was diminished by EE housing as no difference was found between middle-age EE mice and young mice. Moreover, tumors from middle-age EE mice showed a significant decrease in Ki-67 staining, consistent with the tumor volume and weight observations.

Additionally, we examined serum biomarkers, and gene expression signatures of adipose tissue and hypothalamus known to be associated with EE. Both age and housing had significant impacts on serum leptin level. EE led to a robust drop of serum leptin level in both young and middle-aged mice while the reduction was larger in middle-aged mice. It is worth noting that serum leptin level in middle-age SE mice was almost 3 folds higher than that of young SE mice. Living in EE completely prevented this age-related increase of leptin. Leptin expression in adipose tissue showed similar pattern of change characterized as mitigation of age-related alteration by EE. Importantly, an age-related downregulation of hypothalamic *Bdnf* expression was observed (middle-age SE versus young SE), and EE exposure not only robustly upregulated hypothalamic *Bdnf* expression (middle-age EE versus middle-age SE) but also brought the *Bdnf* level above that of young SE mice.

In this study, we observed several changes associated with advancing age including higher weight, higher adiposity, lower lean mass, worsened glucose tolerance, higher circulating leptin, decreased hypothalamic *Bdnf* expression, accelerated LLC growth, and increased level of Cox2 in tumors. A short-term EE (8 weeks) almost completely abolished these age-related alterations. In other words, implementing EE at the age of 14 months could turn back the clock to the age of 3 months, at least regarding these parameters (**Fig. 7.21**).[231] These findings support the notion that lifestyle interventions favorable for healthy aging can have positive impact on cancer. We are fully aware that the phenotypic assessments in the current study are narrow and limited. New study is underway to generate samples for nonbiased screening of age- and environment-related phenotypic and molecular changes.

Beheshti *et al.* report that host age has a substantial impact on the progression of implanted LLC tumors, higher growth rate of LLC in young male mice (4.8 months) than in old male mice (18.4 months).[230] On the contrary, we observed higher growth rate and increased final tumor mass in older female mice (16 months at tumor implantation, aged SE) as compared to that in young female

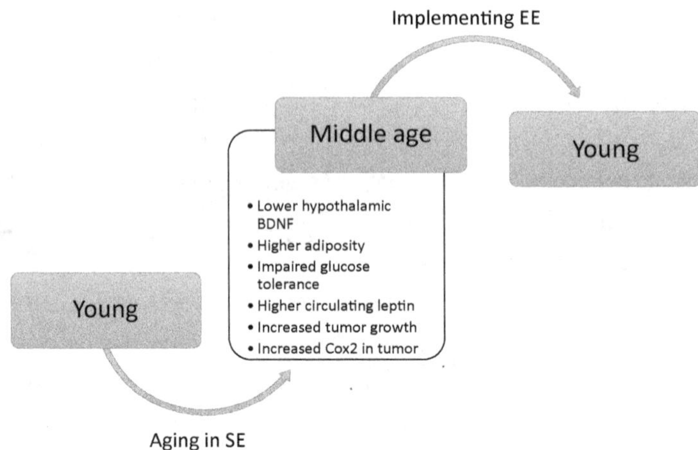

Fig. 7.21. Environmental enrichment inhibits aging associated phenotypic changes.

mice (5 months at tumor implantation, young SE). We think this inconsistency of tumor growth between the two studies is unlikely attributable to the age discrepancies, but rather sex is a more crucial biological variable.

For mice, menopause is thought to occur between 12 and 14 months of age.[233] Menopause has been linked to increased risk of weight gain and central obesity, as well as associated metabolic dysfunctions such as insulin resistance, glucose intolerance, and dyslipidemia,[234] all risk factors for certain types of cancer. The natural drop of estrogen levels is clearly a major cause of the propensity to postmenopausal obesity and associated metabolic syndromes.[235] Our study suggests postmenopausal female mice manifest metabolic declines concomitant with faster LLC tumor growth, as compared to young adults. These deleterious features can be reversed by implementing EE during menopause. As postmenopausal obesity is associated with a 50% higher risk of breast cancer,[236] we predict that EE is more effective at mitigating postmenopausal metabolic dysfunction and breast cancer than other cancer types. We will conduct a study using both estrogen receptor (ER)-positive and triple negative breast cancer models.

It is worth noting that EE had no effect on LLC progression in young female mice, unlike previous data in various tumor models[80,96,104] (see Chapter 2). It is possible that the ineffectiveness of EE is inherent to the LLC model. However, in a preliminary experiment, we saw a trend of reduced LLC burden in male mice living in EE. An alternative explanation is the sexual dimorphism that has been documented. Overall, young males exhibit more pronounced metabolic effects responding to EE exposure relative to young females[237] (an unpublished data). As discussed in Chapters 2 and 3, we speculate mechanisms overlapping ERα and BDNF signaling[238] in the context of EE. Premenopausal females may have a fitter baseline because female brain is more sensitive to signaling molecules crucial to metabolic homeostasis such as leptin and BDNF. This might partially explain the more modest metabolic effects and cancer effects by EE in young females.

Our data in this study are promising but short of mechanistic interrogation. Future research should address whether the concept of EE as an intervention for aging and cancer is applicable to other cancer types and spontaneous cancer models, and moreover identify the underlying regulatory pathways.

Summary

Our research has shown that implementing EE after middle age promotes healthy aging characterized as mitigation of age-related metabolic decline, enhanced motor abilities, and reduced anxiety. Hypothalamic gene transfer of BDNF reproduces EE-induced metabolic adaptations including reduced adiposity, improved systemic glycemic control, increased mitochondrial biogenesis/function, decreased leptin, adipose remodeling, and prevention of age-related hepatosteatosis. Moreover, overexpressing BDNF in the hypothalamus results in reduced anxiety-like and depression-like behaviors in aged mice as well as suppression of neuroinflammation, also resembling EE. These data suggest that a physically, mentally, and socially active environment can positively impact healthspan and a specific brain-fat axis may be one of the underlying mechanisms. Furthermore, recent research suggests EE can "rejuvenize" middle-aged mice to mitigate age-related tumor growth.

Although some metabolic adaptations induced by EE overlap with CR that improves healthspan and extends lifespan in a wide range of species, there are notable differences. CR requires sustained reduction of food consumption that is difficult to achieve outside the laboratory. EE leads to leanness without suppression of food intake and instead largely via elevating basal metabolic rate that is contrary to the reduced metabolic rate of CR. Up to date, EE has yet to be investigated sufficiently as an antiaging intervention. The studies described here only provide a glimpse to the interplay between an active and engaging lifestyle with normal aging, healthspan, and lifespan. Our future research will focus on identifying cellular and molecular effectors mediating the benefits of EE on healthy aging.

References

1. U. C. Bureau (2018) *US Census Bureau Projected Age Groups and Sex Composition of the Population: Main Projections Series for the United States, 2017–2060*. US Census Bureau, Population Division, Washington, DC.
2. Colby SL, Ortman JM. (2014) *Projections of the Size and Composition of the U.S. Population: 2014 to 2060*. U. S. D. o. Commerce (ed), United States Census Bureau, Current Population Reports, pp. P25–1143.
3. He W, Goodkind D, Kowal P. (2016) *An Aging World: 2015*. U. S. D. o. Commerce (eds), U.S. Census Bureau, International Population Reports, pp. P95/16–91.
4. Olshansky SJ. (2018) From lifespan to healthspan. *JAMA* **320**:1323–1324.
5. Rowe JW, Kahn RL. (1987) Human aging: Usual and successful. *Science* **237**:143–149.

6. Mather M, Jacobsen LA, Pollard KM. (2015) Aging in the United States. *Popul Bull* **70**(2):1–23.

7. Ferrucci L, Giallauria F, Guralnik JM. (2008) Epidemiology of aging. *Radiol Clin North Am* **46**:643–652, v.

8. Needham SL. (2014) Toward priorities for aging research. *Rejuvenation Res* **17**:154–156.

9. Fries JF. (1980) Aging, natural death, and the compression of morbidity. *N Engl J Med* **303**:130–135.

10. Crimmins EM. (2015) Lifespan and healthspan: Past, present, and promise. *Gerontologist* **55**:901–911.

11. Gore PG, Kingston A, Johnson GR, *et al.* (2018) New horizons in the compression of functional decline. *Age Ageing* **47**:764–768.

12. Schoeni RF, Freedman VA, Martin LG. (2008) Why is late-life disability declining? *Milbank Q* **86**:47–89.

13. Freedman VA, Crimmins E, Schoeni RF, *et al.* (2004) Resolving inconsistencies in trends in old-age disability: Report from a technical working group. *Demography* **41**:417–441.

14. Seeman I. (2010) Data on disability. *Am J Public Health* **100**:1367.

15. Crimmins EM, Beltran-Sanchez H. (2011) Mortality and morbidity trends: Is there compression of morbidity? *J Gerontol B Psychol Sci Soc Sci* **66**:75–86.

16. Zhang YS, Saito Y, Crimmins EM. (2019) Changing impact of obesity on active life expectancy of older Americans. *J Gerontol A Biol Sci Med Sci* **74**:1944–1951.

17. Verhaeghen P, Salthouse TA. (1997) Meta-analyses of age–cognition relations in adulthood: Estimates of linear and nonlinear age effects and structural models. *Psychol Bull* **122**:231.

18. Salthouse TA. (2000) Aging and measures of processing speed. *Biol Psychol* **54**:35–54.

19. Spencer WD, Raz N. (1995) Differential effects of aging on memory for content and context: A meta-analysis. *Psychol Aging* **10**:527.

20. Zacks RT, Hasher L, Li KZH. (2000) Human memory. In: *The Handbook of Aging and Cognition*, 2nd ed. ELawrence rlbaum Associates Publishers, Mahwah, NJ, pp. 293–357.

21. Buckner RL. (2004) Memory and executive function in aging and AD: Multiple factors that cause decline and reserve factors that compensate. *Neuron* **44**:195–208.
22. Chen WW, Zhang X, Huang WJ. (2016) Role of neuroinflammation in neurodegenerative diseases. *Mol Med Rep* **13**:3391–3396.
23. Guillemot-Legris O, Muccioli GG. (2017) Obesity-induced neuroinflammation: Beyond the hypothalamus. *Trends Neurosci* **40**:237–253.
24. Smith TD, Adams MM, Gallagher M, *et al.* (2000) Circuit-specific alterations in hippocampal synaptophysin immunoreactivity predict spatial learning impairment in aged rats. *J Neurosci* **20**:6587–6593.
25. Adams MM, Donohue HS, Linville MC, *et al.* (2010) Age-related synapse loss in hippocampal CA3 is not reversed by caloric restriction. *Neuroscience* **171**:373–382.
26. Calhoun ME, Kurth D, Phinney AL, *et al.* (1998) Hippocampal neuron and synaptophysin-positive bouton number in aging C57BL/6 mice. *Neurobiol Aging* **19**:599–606.
27. Newton IG, Forbes ME, Linville MC, *et al.* (2008) Effects of aging and caloric restriction on dentate gyrus synapses and glutamate receptor subunits. *Neurobiol Aging* **29**:1308–1318.
28. Poe BH, Linville C, Riddle DR, *et al.* (2001) Effects of age and insulin-like growth factor-1 on neuron and synapse numbers in area CA3 of hippocampus. *Neuroscience* **107**:231–238.
29. Shi L, Adams MM, Linville MC, *et al.* (2007) Caloric restriction eliminates the aging-related decline in NMDA and AMPA receptor subunits in the rat hippocampus and induces homeostasis. *Exp Neurol* **206**:70–79.
30. Hatanpää K, Isaacs KR, Shirao T, *et al.* (1999) Loss of proteins regulating synaptic plasticity in normal aging of the human brain and in Alzheimer disease. *J Neuropathol Exp Neurol* **58**:637–643.
31. Dickstein DL, Weaver CM, Luebke JI, Hof PR. (2013) Dendritic spine changes associated with normal aging. *Neuroscience* **251**:21–32.
32. Egan MF, Kojima M, Callicott JH, *et al.* (2003) The BDNF val66met polymorphism affects activity-dependent secretion of BDNF and human memory and hippocampal function. *Cell* **112**:257–269.
33. Erickson KI, Miller DL, Roecklein KA. (2012) The aging hippocampus: Interactions between exercise, depression, and BDNF. *Neuroscientist* **18**:82–97.

34. Martinowich K, Manji H, Lu B. (2007) New insights into BDNF function in depression and anxiety. *Nat Neurosci* **10**:1089–1093.
35. Angelucci F, Brenè S, Mathé AA. (2005) BDNF in schizophrenia, depression and corresponding animal models. *Mol Psychiatry* **10**:345–352.
36. Laske C, Stellos K, Hoffmann N, *et al.* (2011) Higher BDNF serum levels predict slower cognitive decline in Alzheimer's disease patients. *Int J Neuropsychopharmacol* **14**:399–404.
37. Lampinen P, Heikkinen RL, Ruoppila I. (2000) Changes in intensity of physical exercise as predictors of depressive symptoms among older adults: An eight-year follow-up. *Prev Med* **30**:371–380.
38. Solé-Padullés C, Bartrés-Faz D, Junqué C, *et al.* (2009) Brain structure and function related to cognitive reserve variables in normal aging, mild cognitive impairment and Alzheimer's disease. *Neurobiol Aging* **30**:1114–1124.
39. Stern Y. (2002) What is cognitive reserve? Theory and research application of the reserve concept. *J Int Neuropsychol Soc* **8**:448–460.
40. Scarmeas N, Stern Y. (2003) Cognitive reserve and lifestyle. *J Clin Exp Neuropsychol* **25**:625–633.
41. Gelfo F. (2019) Does experience enhance cognitive flexibility? An overview of the evidence provided by the environmental enrichment studies. *Front Behav Neurosci* **13**:150.
42. Stern Y, Barulli D. (2019) Chapter 11 — Cognitive reserve. In: ST Dekosky, S Asthana (eds), *Handbook of Clinical Neurology*, vol. 167. Elsevier, pp. 181–190.
43. Meng X, D'arcy C. (2012) Education and dementia in the context of the cognitive reserve hypothesis: A systematic review with meta-analyses and qualitative analyses. *PLoS One* **7**:e38268.
44. Stern Y, Gurland B, Tatemichi TK, *et al.* (1994) Influence of education and occupation on the incidence of Alzheimer's disease. *JAMA* **271**:1004–1010.
45. Flicker L, Liu-Ambrose T, Kramer AF. (2011) Why so negative about preventing cognitive decline and dementia? The jury has already come to the verdict for physical activity and smoking cessation. *British J Sports Med* **45**:465–467.
46. Rovio S, Kåreholt I, Helkala E-L, *et al.* (2005) Leisure-time physical activity at midlife and the risk of dementia and Alzheimer's disease. *Lancet Neurol* **4**:705–711.

47. Hales C, Carroll M, Fryar C, Ogden C. (2020) *Prevalence of Obesity and Severe Obesity Among Adults: United States, 2017–2018*. U. S. D. o. H. H. Services (ed), Centers for Disease Control and Prevention, National Center for Health Statistics, NCHS Data Brief, no 360.

48. Ward ZJ, Bleich SN, Cradock AL, *et al.* (2019) Projected U.S. state-level prevalence of adult obesity and severe obesity. *N Engl J Med* **381**:2440–2450.

49. Pi-Sunyer X. (2009) The medical risks of obesity. *Postgrad Med* **121**:21–33.

50. Attlee A, Kassem H, Hashim M, Obaid RS. (2015) Physical status and feeding behavior of children with autism. *Indian J Pediatr* **82**:682–687.

51. Prospective Studies Collaboration, Whitlock G, Lewington S, *et al.* (2009) Body-mass index and cause-specific mortality in 900 000 adults: Collaborative analyses of 57 prospective studies. *Lancet* **373**:1083–1096.

52. Palmer AK, Kirkland JL. (2016) Aging and adipose tissue: Potential interventions for diabetes and regenerative medicine. *Exp Gerontol* **86**:97–105.

53. Kuk JL, Saunders TJ, Davidson LE, Ross R. (2009) Age-related changes in total and regional fat distribution. *Ageing Res Rev* **8**:339–348.

54. Kissebah AH, Krakower GR. (1994) Regional adiposity and morbidity. *Physiol Rev* **74**:761–811.

55. Matsuzawa Y. (2008) The role of fat topology in the risk of disease. *Int J Obes (Lond)* **32 Suppl 7**:S83–92.

56. Ibrahim MM. (2010) Subcutaneous and visceral adipose tissue: Structural and functional differences. *Obes Rev* **11**:11–18.

57. Tchernof A, Despres JP. (2013) Pathophysiology of human visceral obesity: An update. *Physiol Rev* **93**:359–404.

58. Choe SS, Huh JY, Hwang IJ, *et al.* (2016) Adipose tissue remodeling: Its role in energy metabolism and metabolic disorders. *Front Endocrinol (Lausanne)* **7**:30.

59. Salminen A, Kaarniranta K, Kauppinen A. (2012) Inflammaging: Disturbed interplay between autophagy and inflammasomes. *Aging (Albany NY)* **4**:166–175.

60. Stout MB, Justice JN, Nicklas BJ, Kirkland JL. (2017) Physiological aging: Links among adipose tissue dysfunction, diabetes, and frailty. *Physiology (Bethesda)* **32**:9–19.

61. Starr ME, Evers BM, Saito H. (2009) Age-associated increase in cytokine production during systemic inflammation: Adipose tissue as a major source of IL-6. *J Gerontol A Biol Sci Med Sci* **64**:723–730.

62. Rodriguez-Hernandez H, Simental-Mendia LE, Rodriguez-Ramirez G, Reyes-Romero MA. (2013) Obesity and inflammation: Epidemiology, risk factors, and markers of inflammation. *Int J Endocrinol* **2013**:678159.

63. Ellulu MS, Patimah I, Khaza'ai H, *et al.* (2017) Obesity and inflammation: The linking mechanism and the complications. *Arch Med Sci* **13**:851–863.

64. Ferrucci L, Fabbri E. (2018) Inflammageing: Chronic inflammation in ageing, cardiovascular disease, and frailty. *Nat Rev Cardiol* **15**:505–522.

65. Vissers D, Hens W, Taeymans J, *et al.* (2013) The effect of exercise on visceral adipose tissue in overweight adults: A systematic review and meta-analysis. *PLoS One* **8**:e56415.

66. Hohensinner PJ, Kaun C, Ebenbauer B, *et al.* (2018) Reduction of premature aging markers after gastric bypass surgery in morbidly obese patients. *Obes Surg* **28**:2804–2810.

67. Fontana L, Partridge L, Longo VD. (2010) Extending healthy lifespan–from yeast to humans. *Science* **328**:321–326.

68. Smith DL Jr, Nagy TR, Allison DB. (2010) Calorie restriction: What recent results suggest for the future of ageing research. *Eur J Clin Invest* **40**:440–450.

69. Mattson MP. (2005) Energy intake, meal frequency, and health: A neurobiological perspective. *Annu Rev Nutr* **25**:237–260.

70. de Cabo R, Mattson MP. (2019) Effects of Intermittent Fasting on Health, Aging, and Disease. *N Engl J Med* **381**:2541–2551.

71. Anderson RM, Shanmuganayagam D, Weindruch R. (2009) Caloric restriction and aging: Studies in mice and monkeys. *Toxicol Pathol* **37**:47–51.

72. Colman RJ, Anderson RM, Johnson SC, *et al.* (2009) Caloric restriction delays disease onset and mortality in rhesus monkeys. *Science* **325**:201–204.

73. Fontana L, Klein S. (2007) Aging, adiposity, and calorie restriction. *JAMA* **297**:986–994.

74. Fontana L, Meyer TE, Klein S, Holloszy JO. (2004) Long-term calorie restriction is highly effective in reducing the risk for atherosclerosis in humans. *Proc Natl Acad Sci U S A* **101**:6659–6663.

75. Heilbronn LK, de Jonge L, Frisard MI, *et al.* (2006) Effect of 6-month calorie restriction on biomarkers of longevity, metabolic adaptation, and oxidative stress in overweight individuals: A randomized controlled trial. *JAMA* **295**:1539–1548.

76. Katic M, Kennedy AR, Leykin I, *et al.* (2007) Mitochondrial gene expression and increased oxidative metabolism: Role in increased lifespan of fat-specific insulin receptor knock-out mice. *Aging Cell* **6**:827–839.

77. Bluher M, Michael MD, Peroni OD, *et al.* (2002) Adipose tissue selective insulin receptor knockout protects against obesity and obesity-related glucose intolerance. *Dev Cell* **3**:25–38.

78. Ortega-Molina A, Efeyan A, Lopez-Guadamillas E, *et al.* (2012) Pten positively regulates brown adipose function, energy expenditure, and longevity. *Cell Metab* **15**:382–394.

79. Cao L, During MJ. (2012) What is the brain-cancer connection? *Annu Rev Neurosci* **35**:331–345.

80. Cao L, Liu X, Lin E-JD, *et al.* (2010) Environmental and genetic activation of a brain-adipocyte BDNF/leptin axis causes cancer remission and inhibition. *Cell* **142**:52–64.

81. Cao L, Lin E-JD, Cahill MC, *et al.* (2009) Molecular therapy of obesity and diabetes by a physiological autoregulatory approach. *Nat Med* **15**:447–454.

82. Tsukiyama-Kohara K, Poulin F, Kohara M, *et al.* (2001) Adipose tissue reduction in mice lacking the translational inhibitor 4E-BP1. *Nat Med* **7**:1128–1132.

83. Chiu CH, Lin WD, Huang SY, Lee YH. (2004) Effect of a C/EBP gene replacement on mitochondrial biogenesis in fat cells. *Genes Dev* **18**:1970–1975.

84. Molero JC, Jensen TE, Withers PC, *et al.* (2004) c-Cbl-deficient mice have reduced adiposity, higher energy expenditure, and improved peripheral insulin action. *J Clin Invest* **114**:1326–1333.

85. Bluher M, Kahn BB, Kahn CR. (2003) Extended longevity in mice lacking the insulin receptor in adipose tissue. *Science* **299**:572–574.

86. Cao L, Choi EY, Liu X, *et al.* (2011) White to brown fat phenotypic switch induced by genetic and environmental activation of a hypothalamic-adipocyte axis. *Cell Metab* **14**:324–338.

87. Heitmann BL, Garby L. (2002) Composition (lean and fat tissue) of weight changes in adult Danes. *Am J Clin Nutr* **75**:840–847.

88. Allison DB, Zannolli R, Faith MS, *et al.* (1999) Weight loss increases and fat loss decreases all-cause mortality rate: Results from two independent cohort studies. *Int J Obes Relat Metab Disord* **23**:603–611.

89. Brown-Borg HM. (2009) Hormonal control of aging in rodents: The somatotropic axis. *Mol Cell Endocrinol* **299**:64–71.

90. Otabe S, Yuan X, Fukutani T, *et al.* (2007) Overexpression of human adiponectin in transgenic mice results in suppression of fat accumulation and prevention of premature death by high-calorie diet. *Am J Physiol Endocrinol Metab* **293**:E210–E218.

91. Fujisawa T, Endo H, Tomimoto A, *et al.* (2008) Adiponectin suppresses colorectal carcinogenesis under the high-fat diet condition. *Gut* **57**:1531–1538.

92. Calle EE, Kaaks R. (2004) Overweight, obesity and cancer: Epidemiological evidence and proposed mechanisms. *Nat Rev Cancer* **4**:579–591.

93. Hursting SD, Slaga TJ, Fischer SM, *et al.* (1999) Mechanism-based cancer prevention approaches: Targets, examples, and the use of transgenic mice. *J Natl Cancer Inst* **91**:215–225.

94. Albanes D. (1987) Total calories, body weight, and tumor incidence in mice. *Cancer Res* **47**:1987–1992.

95. Longo VD, Fontana L. (2010) Calorie restriction and cancer prevention: Metabolic and molecular mechanisms. *Trends Pharmacol Sci* **31**:89–98.

96. Foglesong GD, Queen NJ, Huang W, *et al.* (2019) Enriched environment inhibits breast cancer progression in obese models with intact leptin signaling. *Endocr Relat Cancer* **26**:483–495.

97. Liu X, McMurphy T, Xiao R, *et al.* (2014) Hypothalamic gene transfer of BDNF inhibits breast cancer progression and metastasis in middle age obese mice. *Mol Ther* **22**:1275–1284.

98. Wayne SJ, Rhyne RL, Garry PJ, Goodwin JS. (1990) Cell-mediated immunity as a predictor of morbidity and mortality in subjects over 60. *J Gerontol* **45**:M45–M48.

99. DelaRosa O, Pawelec G, Peralbo E, *et al.* (2006) Immunological bio-markers of ageing in man: Changes in both innate and adaptive immunity are associated with health and longevity. *Biogerontology* **7**:471–481.

100. De la Fuente M, Miquel J. (2009) An update of the oxidation-inflammation theory of aging: The involvement of the immune system in oxi-inflamm-aging. *Curr Pharm Des* **15**:3003–3026.

101. Guayerbas N, De La Fuente M. (2003) An impairment of phagocytic function is linked to a shorter lifespan in two strains of prematurely aging mice. *Dev Comp Immunol* **27**:339–350.

102. Benaroya-Milshtein N, Hollander N, Apter A, *et al.* (2004) Environmental enrichment in mice decreases anxiety, attenuates stress responses and enhances natural killer cell activity. *Eur J Neurosci* **20**:1341–1347.

103. Mansour AG, Xiao R, Bergin SM, *et al.* (2020) Enriched environment enhances NK cell maturation through hypothalamic BDNF in male mice. *Eur J Immunol* **51**:557–566.

104. Xiao R, Bergin SM, Huang W, *et al.* (2016) Environmental and genetic activation of hypothalamic BDNF modulates T-cell immunity to exert an anticancer phenotype. *Cancer Immunol Res* **4**:488–497.

105. Larsson F, Winblad B, Mohammed AH. (2002) Psychological stress and environmental adaptation in enriched vs. impoverished housed rats. *Pharmacol Biochem Behav* **73**:193–207.

106. Patel NV, Finch CE. (2002) The glucocorticoid paradox of caloric restriction in slowing brain aging. *Neurobiol Aging* **23**:707–717.

107. Gotthardt U, Schweiger U, Fahrenberg J, *et al.* (1995) Cortisol, ACTH, and cardiovascular response to a cognitive challenge paradigm in aging and depression. *Am J Physiol* **268**:R865–R873.

108. Witt KA, Snook JT, O'Dorisio TM, *et al.* (1993) Exercise training and dietary carbohydrate: Effects on selected hormones and the thermic effect of feeding. *Int J Sport Nutr* **3**:272–289.

109. Goldberg NR, Haack AK, Meshul CK. (2011) Enriched environment promotes similar neuronal and behavioral recovery in a young and

aged mouse model of Parkinson's disease. *Neuroscience* **172**:443–452.

110. Harburger LL, Lambert TJ, Frick KM. (2007) Age-dependent effects of environmental enrichment on spatial reference memory in male mice. *Behav Brain Res* **185**:43–48.

111. Segovia G, del Arco A, Mora F. (2009) Environmental enrichment, prefrontal cortex, stress, and aging of the brain. *J Neural Transm* **116**:1007–1016.

112. Mattson MP, Duan W, Lee J, Guo Z. (2001) Suppression of brain aging and neurodegenerative disorders by dietary restriction and environmental enrichment: Molecular mechanisms. *Mech Ageing Dev* **122**:757–778.

113. Leon M, Woo C. (2018) Environmental enrichment and successful aging. *Front Behav Neurosci* **12**:155.

114. Sampedro-Piquero P, Begega A. (2017) Environmental enrichment as a positive behavioral intervention across the lifespan. *Curr Neuropharmacol* **15**:459–470.

115. McMurphy T, Huang W, Queen NJ, *et al.* (2018) Implementation of environmental enrichment after middle age promotes healthy aging. *Aging (Albany NY)* **10**:1698–1721.

116. McMurphy T, Huang W, Liu X, *et al.* (2019) Hypothalamic gene transfer of BDNF promotes healthy aging in mice. *Aging Cell* **18**:e12846.

117. Ali S, Liu X, Queen NJ, *et al.* (2019) Long-term environmental enrichment affects microglial morphology in middle age mice. *Aging (Albany NY)* **11**:2388–2402.

118. Ali S, Mansour AG, Huang W, *et al.* (2020) CSF1R inhibitor PLX5622 and environmental enrichment additively improve metabolic outcomes in middle-aged female mice. *Aging (Albany NY)* **12**:2101–2122.

119. Queen NJ, Hassan QN 2nd, Cao L. (2020) Improvements to healthspan through environmental enrichment and lifestyle interventions: Where are we now? *Front Neurosci* **14**:605.

120. Turturro A, Witt WW, Lewis S, *et al.* (1999) Growth curves and survival characteristics of the animals used in the Biomarkers of Aging Program. *J Gerontol A Biol Sci Med Sci* **54**:B492–B501.

121. Brayton C, Treuting P, Ward J. (2012) Pathobiology of aging mice and GEM: Background strains and experimental design. *J Vet Pathol* **49**:85–105.

122. Dent E, Martin FC, Bergman H, *et al.* (2019) Management of frailty: Opportunities, challenges, and future directions. *Lancet* **394**:1376–1386.

123. Kreilaus F, Spiro AS, Hannan AJ, *et al.* (2016) Therapeutic effects of anthocyanins and environmental enrichment in R6/1 Huntington's disease Mice. *J Huntingtons Dis* **5**:285–296.

124. Mazarakis NK, Mo C, Renoir T, *et al.* (2014) 'Super-Enrichment' reveals dose-dependent therapeutic effects of environmental stimulation in a transgenic mouse model of Huntington's disease. *J Huntingtons Dis* **3**:299–309.

125. Kondo M, Gray LJ, Pelka GJ, *et al.* (2008) Environmental enrichment ameliorates a motor coordination deficit in a mouse model of Rett syndrome–Mecp2 gene dosage effects and BDNF expression. *Eur J Neurosci* **27**:3342–3350.

126. Jones BJ, Roberts DJ. (1968) The quantiative measurement of motor inco-ordination in naive mice using an acelerating rotarod. *J Pharm Pharmacol* **20**:302–304.

127. Ramos A. (2008) Animal models of anxiety: Do I need multiple tests? *Trends Pharmacol Sci* **29**:493–498.

128. Stanford SC. (2007) The open field test: Reinventing the wheel. *J Psychopharmacol* **21**:134–135.

129. Samuels BA, Hen R. (2011) Neurogenesis and affective disorders. *Eur J Neurosci* **33**:1152–1159.

130. Cryan JF, Mombereau C. (2004) In search of a depressed mouse: Utility of models for studying depression-related behavior in genetically modified mice. *Mol Psychiatry* **9**:326–357.

131. Huttenrauch M, Salinas G, Wirths O. (2016) Effects of long-term environmental enrichment on anxiety, memory, hippocampal plasticity and overall brain gene expression in C57BL6 mice. *Front Mol Neurosci* **9**:62.

132. Tomiga Y, Ito A, Sudo M, *et al.* (2016) Effects of environmental enrichment in aged mice on anxiety-like behaviors and neuronal nitric oxide synthase expression in the brain. *Biochem Biophys Res Commun* **476**:635–640.

133. Renoir T, Pang TY, Hannan AJ. (2013) Effects of environmental manipulations in genetically targeted animal models of affective disorders. *Neurobiol Dis* **57**:12–27.

134. Russo SJ, Murrough JW, Han MH, *et al.* (2012) Neurobiology of resilience. *Nat Neurosci* **15**:1475–1484.

135. Shekhar A, Sims LS, Bowsher RR. (1993) GABA receptors in the region of the dorsomedial hypothalamus of rats regulate anxiety in the elevated plus-maze test. II. Physiological measures. *Brain Res* **627**:17–24.

136. Silva MS, Pereira BA, Céspedes IC, *et al.* (2014) Dorsomedial hypothalamus CRF type 1 receptors selectively modulate inhibitory avoidance responses in the elevated T-maze. *Behav Brain Res* **271**:249–257.

137. Canteras NS. (2002) The medial hypothalamic defensive system: Hodological organization and functional implications. *Pharmacol Biochem Behav* **71**:481–491.

138. Gariepy G, Nitka D, Schmitz N. (2010) The association between obesity and anxiety disorders in the population: A systematic review and meta-analysis. *Int J Obes (Lond)* **34**:407–419.

139. de Noronha SR, Campos GV, Abreu AR, *et al.* (2016) High fat diet induced obesity facilitates anxiety-like behaviors due to GABAergic impairment within the dorsomedial hypothalamus in rats. *Behav Brain Res* **316**:38–46.

140. Zhang R, Asai M, Mahoney CE, *et al.* (2017) Loss of hypothalamic corticotropin-releasing hormone markedly reduces anxiety behaviors in mice. *Mol Psychiatry* **22**:733–744.

141. Enerback S. (2010) Human brown adipose tissue. *Cell Metab* **11**:248–252.

142. Enerback S, Jacobsson A, Simpson EM, *et al.* (1997) Mice lacking mitochondrial uncoupling protein are cold-sensitive but not obese. *Nature* **387**:90–94.

143. Puigserver P, Wu Z, Park CW, *et al.* (1998) A cold-inducible coactivator of nuclear receptors linked to adaptive thermogenesis. *Cell* **92**:829–839.

144. Giblin W, Skinner ME, Lombard DB. (2014) Sirtuins: Guardians of mammalian healthspan. *Trends Genet* **30**:271–286.

145. Sheedfar F, Di Biase S, Koonen D, Vinciguerra M. (2013) Liver diseases and aging: Friends or foes? *Aging Cell* **12**:950–954.

146. Horton JD, Goldstein JL, Brown MS. (2002) SREBPs: Activators of the complete program of cholesterol and fatty acid synthesis in the liver. *J Clin Invest* **109**:1125–1131.

147. Iizuka K, Bruick RK, Liang G, *et al.* (2004) Deficiency of carbohydrate response element-binding protein (ChREBP) reduces lipogenesis as well as glycolysis. *Proc Natl Acad Sci U S A* **101**:7281–7286.

148. Petersen MC, Madiraju AK, Gassaway BM, *et al.* (2016) Insulin receptor Thr1160 phosphorylation mediates lipid-induced hepatic insulin resistance. *J Clin Invest* **126**:4361–4371.

149. Petersen MC, Vatner DF, Shulman GI. (2017) Regulation of hepatic glucose metabolism in health and disease. *Nat Rev Endocrinol* **13**:572–587.

150. Samuel VT, Liu Z-X, Wang A, *et al.* (2007) Inhibition of protein kinase Cepsilon prevents hepatic insulin resistance in nonalcoholic fatty liver disease. *J Clin Invest* **117**:739–745.

151. Perry RJ, Petersen KF, Shulman GI. (2016) Pleotropic effects of leptin to reverse insulin resistance and diabetic ketoacidosis. *Diabetologia* **59**:933–937.

152. Perry RJ, Camporez J-PG, Kursawe R, *et al.* (2015) Hepatic acetyl CoA links adipose tissue inflammation to hepatic insulin resistance and type 2 diabetes. *Cell* **160**:745–758.

153. Myers MG Jr, Olson DP. (2012) Central nervous system control of metabolism. *Nature* **491**:357–363.

154. Pocai A, Obici S, Schwartz GJ, Rossetti L. (2005) A brain-liver circuit regulates glucose homeostasis. *Cell Metab* **1**:53–61.

155. Obici S, Zhang BB, Karkanias G, Rossetti L. (2002) Hypothalamic insulin signaling is required for inhibition of glucose production. *Nat Med* **8**:1376–1382.

156. Huffman DM. (2010) Exercise as a calorie restriction mimetic: Implications for improving healthy aging and longevity. *Interdiscip Top Gerontol* **37**:157–174.

157. Walston J, McBurnie MA, Newman A, *et al.* (2002) Frailty and activation of the inflammation and coagulation systems with and without

clinical comorbidities: Results from the Cardiovascular Health Study. *Arch Intern Med* **162**:2333–2341.

158. Furman D, Campisi J, Verdin E, *et al.* (2019) Chronic inflammation in the etiology of disease across the lifespan. *Nat Med* **25**:1822–1832.

159. Tang Y, Purkayastha S, Cai D. (2015) Hypothalamic microinflammation: A common basis of metabolic syndrome and aging. *Trends Neurosci* **38**:36–44.

160. Zhang X, Zhang G, Zhang H, *et al.* (2008) Hypothalamic IKKbeta/NF-kappaB and ER stress link overnutrition to energy imbalance and obesity. *Cell* **135**:61–73.

161. De Souza CT, Araujo EP, Bordin S, *et al.* (2005) Consumption of a fat-rich diet activates a proinflammatory response and induces insulin resistance in the hypothalamus. *Endocrinology* **146**:4192–4199.

162. Kleinridders A, Schenten D, Könner AC, *et al.* (2009) MyD88 signaling in the CNS is required for development of fatty acid-induced leptin resistance and diet-induced obesity. *Cell Metab* **10**:249–259.

163. Thaler JP, Yi C-X, Schur EA, *et al.* (2012) Obesity is associated with hypothalamic injury in rodents and humans. *J Clin Invest* **122**:153–162.

164. Purkayastha S, Zhang G, Cai D. (2011) Uncoupling the mechanisms of obesity and hypertension by targeting hypothalamic IKK-beta and NF-kappaB. *Nat Med* **17**:883–887.

165. Khabour OF, Barnawi JM. (2010) Association of longevity with IL-10 -1082 G/A and TNF-alpha-308 G/A polymorphisms. *Int J Immunogenet* **37**:293–298.

166. Harris TB, Ferrucci L, Tracy RP, *et al.* (1999) Associations of elevated interleukin-6 and C-reactive protein levels with mortality in the elderly. *Am J Med* **106**:506–512.

167. Franceschi C, Olivieri F, Marchegiani F, *et al.* (2005) Genes involved in immune response/inflammation, IGF1/insulin pathway and response to oxidative stress play a major role in the genetics of human longevity: The lesson of centenarians. *Mech Ageing Dev* **126**:351–361.

168. Zhang G, Li J, Purkayastha S, *et al.* (2013) Hypothalamic programming of systemic ageing involving IKK-beta, NF-kappaB and GnRH. *Nature* **497**:211–216.
169. Tang Y, Cai D. (2013) Hypothalamic inflammation and GnRH in aging development. *Cell Cycle* **12**:2711–2712.
170. Nimmerjahn A, Kirchhoff F, Helmchen F. (2005) Resting microglial cells are highly dynamic surveillants of brain parenchyma in vivo. *Science* **308**:1314–1318.
171. Hanisch UK, Kettenmann H. (2007) Microglia: Active sensor and versatile effector cells in the normal and pathologic brain. *Nat Neurosci* **10**:1387–1394.
172. Ferrini F, De Koninck Y. (2013) Microglia control neuronal network excitability via BDNF signalling. *Neural Plast* **2013**:429815.
173. Parkhurst CN, Yang G, Ninan I, *et al.* (2013) Microglia promote learning-dependent synapse formation through BDNF. *Cell* **155**:1596–1609.
174. Ziebell JM, Adelson PD, Lifshitz J. (2015) Microglia: Dismantling and rebuilding circuits after acute neurological injury. *Metab Brain Dis* **30**:393–400.
175. Perry VH, Nicoll JA, Holmes C. (2010) Microglia in neurodegenerative disease. *Nat Rev Neurol* **6**:193–201.
176. Streit WJ, Xue QS, Tischer J, Bechmann I. (2014) Microglial pathology. *Acta Neuropathol Commun* **2**:142.
177. Norden DM, Muccigrosso MM, Godbout JP. (2015) Microglial priming and enhanced reactivity to secondary insult in aging, and traumatic CNS injury, and neurodegenerative disease. *Neuropharmacology* **96**:29–41.
178. Hefendehl JK, Neher JJ, Sühs RB, *et al.* (2014) Homeostatic and injury-induced microglia behavior in the aging brain. *Aging Cell* **13**:60–69.
179. Safaiyan S, Kannaiyan N, Snaidero N, *et al.* (2016) Age-related myelin degradation burdens the clearance function of microglia during aging. *Nat Neurosci* **19**:995–998.
180. Spittau B. (2017) Aging microglia-phenotypes, functions and implications for age-related neurodegenerative diseases. *Front Aging Neurosci* **9**:194.
181. Valdearcos M, Douglass JD, Robblee MM, *et al.* (2017) Microglial inflammatory signaling orchestrates the hypothalamic immune

response to dietary excess and mediates obesity susceptibility. *Cell Metab* **26**:185–197 e3.

182. Aguzzi A, Barres BA, Bennett ML. (2013) Microglia: Scapegoat, saboteur, or something else? *Science* **339**:156–161.

183. Valdearcos M, Robblee MM, Benjamin DI, *et al.* (2014) Microglia dictate the impact of saturated fat consumption on hypothalamic inflammation and neuronal function. *Cell Rep* **9**:2124–2138.

184. Hickman S, Izzy S, Sen P, *et al.* (2018) Microglia in neurodegeneration. *Nat Neurosci* **21**:1359–1369.

185. Henry CJ, Huang Y, Wynne AM, Godbout JP. (2009) Peripheral lipopolysaccharide (LPS) challenge promotes microglial hyperactivity in aged mice that is associated with exaggerated induction of both pro-inflammatory IL-1beta and anti-inflammatory IL-10 cytokines. *Brain Behav Immun* **23**:309–317.

186. Satoh A, Imai SI, Guarente L. (2017) The brain, sirtuins, and ageing. *Nat Rev Neurosci* **18**:362–374.

187. Rawji KS, Mishra MK, Michaels NJ, *et al.* (2016) Immunosenescence of microglia and macrophages: Impact on the ageing central nervous system. *Brain* **139**:653–661.

188. Young K, Morrison H. (2018) Quantifying microglia morphology from photomicrographs of immunohistochemistry prepared tissue using ImageJ. *J Vis Exp* **136**:57648.

189. de Sousa AA, Dos Reis RR, de Lima CM, *et al.* (2015) Three-dimensional morphometric analysis of microglial changes in a mouse model of virus encephalitis: Age and environmental influences. *Eur J Neurosci* **42**:2036–2050.

190. Yu W, Chen J, Xiong Y, *et al.* (2012) Macrophage proliferation is regulated through CSF-1 receptor tyrosines 544, 559, and 807. *J Biol Chem* **287**:13694–13704.

191. Coniglio SJ, Eugenin E, Dobrenis K, *et al.* (2012) Microglial stimulation of glioblastoma invasion involves epidermal growth factor receptor (EGFR) and colony stimulating factor 1 receptor (CSF-1R) signaling. *Mol Med* **18**:519–527.

192. Elmore MRP, Najafi AR, Koike MA, *et al.* (2014) Colony-stimulating factor 1 receptor signaling is necessary for microglia viability, unmasking a microglia progenitor cell in the adult brain. *Neuron* **82**:380–397.

193. Acharya MM, Green KN, Allen BD, *et al.* (2016) Elimination of microglia improves cognitive function following cranial irradiation. *Sci Rep* **6**:31545.

194. Cai D, Khor S. (2019) "Hypothalamic Microinflammation" paradigm in aging and metabolic diseases. *Cell Metab* **30**:19–35.

195. Thomas D, Apovian C. (2017) Macrophage functions in lean and obese adipose tissue. *Metabolism* **72**:120–143.

196. Boutens L, Stienstra R. (2016) Adipose tissue macrophages: Going off track during obesity. *Diabetologia* **59**:879–894.

197. Camell CD, Sander J, Spadaro O, *et al.* (2017) Inflammasome-driven catecholamine catabolism in macrophages blunts lipolysis during ageing. *Nature* **550**:119–123.

198. Pirzgalska RM, Seixas E, Seidman JS, *et al.* (2017) Sympathetic neuron-associated macrophages contribute to obesity by importing and metabolizing norepinephrine. *Nat Med* **23**:1309–1318.

199. Cavnar MJ, Zeng S, Kim TS, *et al.* (2013) KIT oncogene inhibition drives intratumoral macrophage M2 polarization. *J Exp Med* **210**:2873–2886.

200. Hilla AM, Diekmann H, Fischer D. (2017) Microglia are irrelevant for neuronal degeneration and axon regeneration after acute injury. *J Neurosci* **37**:6113–6124.

201. Wentworth JM, Naselli G, Brown WA, *et al.* (2010) Pro-inflammatory CD11c+CD206+ adipose tissue macrophages are associated with insulin resistance in human obesity. *Diabetes* **59**:1648–1656.

202. Balasubramanian P, Hall D, Subramanian M. (2019) Sympathetic nervous system as a target for aging and obesity-related cardiovascular diseases. *Geroscience* **41**:13–24.

203. Mori S, Nojiri H, Yoshizuka N, Takema Y. (2007) Rapid desensitization of lipolysis in the visceral and subcutaneous adipocytes of rats. *Lipids* **42**:307–314.

204. O'Neil SM, Witcher KG, McKim DB, Godbout JP. (2018) Forced turnover of aged microglia induces an intermediate phenotype but does not rebalance CNS environmental cues driving priming to immune challenge. *Acta Neuropathol Commun* **6**:129.

205. Elmore MRP, Hohsfield LA, Kramár EA, *et al.* (2018) Replacement of microglia in the aged brain reverses cognitive, synaptic, and neuronal deficits in mice. *Aging Cell* **17**:e12832.

206. Mattson MP, Maudsley S, Martin B. (2004) A neural signaling triumvirate that influences ageing and age-related disease: Insulin/IGF-1, BDNF and serotonin. *Ageing Res Rev* **3**:445–464.

207. Tapia-Arancibia L, Aliaga E, Silhol M, Arancibia S. (2008) New insights into brain BDNF function in normal aging and Alzheimer disease. *Brain Res Rev* **59**:201–220.

208. Lee J, Duan W, Mattson MP. (2002) Evidence that brain-derived neurotrophic factor is required for basal neurogenesis and mediates, in part, the enhancement of neurogenesis by dietary restriction in the hippocampus of adult mice. *J Neurochem* **82**:1367–1375.

209. Duan W, Guo Z, Jiang H, *et al.* (2003) Dietary restriction normalizes glucose metabolism and BDNF levels, slows disease progression, and increases survival in huntingtin mutant mice. *Proc Natl Acad Sci U S A* **100**:2911–2916.

210. Siu JJ, Queen NJ, Liu X, *et al.* (2017) Molecular therapy of melanocortin-4-receptor obesity by an autoregulatory BDNF vector. *Mol Ther Methods Clin Dev* **7**:83–95.

211. Cao L, Ali S, Queen NJ. (2021) Hypothalamic gene transfer of BDNF promotes healthy aging. *Vitam Horm* **115**:39–66.

212. Wang C, Wang CM, Clark KR, Sferra TJ. (2003) Recombinant AAV serotype 1 transduction efficiency and tropism in the murine brain. *Gene Ther* **10**:1528–1534.

213. Meek TH, Wisse BE, Thaler JP, *et al.* (2013) BDNF action in the brain attenuates diabetic hyperglycemia via insulin-independent inhibition of hepatic glucose production. *Diabetes* **62**:1512–1518.

214. Rios M, Fan G, Fekete C, *et al.* (2001) Conditional deletion of brain-derived neurotrophic factor in the postnatal brain leads to obesity and hyperactivity. *Mol Endocrinol* **15**:1748–1757.

215. Karege F, Bondolfi G, Gervasoni N, *et al.* (2005) Low brain-derived neurotrophic factor (BDNF) levels in serum of depressed patients probably results from lowered platelet BDNF release unrelated to platelet reactivity. *Biol Psychiatry* **57**:1068–1072.

216. Shimizu E, Hashimoto K, Okamura N, *et al.* (2003) Alterations of serum levels of brain-derived neurotrophic factor (BDNF) in depressed patients with or without antidepressants. *Biol Psychiatry* **54**:70–75.

217. Gorski JA, Balogh SA, Wehner JM, Jones KR. (2003) Learning deficits in forebrain-restricted brain-derived neurotrophic factor mutant mice. *Neuroscience* **121**:341–354.

218. Xiao R, Bergin SM, Huang W, *et al.* (2019) Enriched environment regulates thymocyte development and alleviates experimental autoimmune encephalomyelitis in mice. *Brain Behav Immun* **75**:137–148.

219. Weiskopf D, Weinberger B, Grubeck-Loebenstein B. (2009) The aging of the immune system. *Transpl Int* **22**:1041–1050.

220. Pereira BI, Akbar AN. (2016) Convergence of innate and adaptive immunity during human aging. *Front Immunol* **7**:445.

221. Nikolich-Žugich J. (2018) The twilight of immunity: Emerging concepts in aging of the immune system. *Nat Immunol* **19**:10–19.

222. Chang SH, Beason TS, Hunleth JM, Colditz GA. (2012) A systematic review of body fat distribution and mortality in older people. *Maturitas* **72**:175–191.

223. Hainer V, Aldhoon-Hainerova I. (2013) Obesity paradox does exist. *Diabetes Care* **36 Suppl 2**:S276–281.

224. Lee DH, Keum N, Hu FB, *et al.* (2018) Predicted lean body mass, fat mass, and all cause and cause specific mortality in men: Prospective US cohort study. *BMJ* **362**:k2575.

225. Abramowitz MK, Hall CB, Amodu A, *et al.* (2018) Muscle mass, BMI, and mortality among adults in the United States: A population-based cohort study. *PLoS One* **13**:e0194697.

226. Sepe A, Tchkonia T, Thomou T, *et al.* (2011) Aging and regional differences in fat cell progenitors — A mini-review. *Gerontology* **57**:66–75.

227. De Pergola G, Silvestris F. (2013) Obesity as a major risk factor for cancer. *J Obes* **2013**:291546.

228. Avgerinos KI, Spyrou N, Mantzoros CS, Dalamaga M. (2019) Obesity and cancer risk: Emerging biological mechanisms and perspectives. *Metabolism* **92**:121–135.

229. Deng T, Lyon CJ, Bergin S, *et al.* (2016) Obesity, inflammation, and cancer. *Annu Rev Pathol* **11**:421–449.

230. Beheshti A, Benzekry S, Tyson McDonald J, *et al.* (2015) Host age is a systemic regulator of gene expression impacting cancer progression. *Cancer Res* **75**:1134–1143.

231. Queen NJ, Deng H, Huang W, *et al.* (2021) Environmental enrichment mitigates age-related metabolic decline and lewis lung carcinoma growth in aged female mice. *Cancer Prev Res* **14**:1075–1088.

232. Hashemi Goradel N, Najafi M, Salehi E, *et al.* (2019) Cyclooxygenase-2 in cancer: A review. *J Cell Physiol* **234**:5683–5699.

233. Siler LM. (1995) *Mouse Genetics: Concepts and Applications.* Oxford University Press, New York.

234. Kwasniewska M, Pikala M, Kaczmarczyk-Chałas K, *et al.* (2012) Smoking status, the menopausal transition, and metabolic syndrome in women. *Menopause* **19**:194–201.

235. Palmer BF, Clegg DJ. (2015) The sexual dimorphism of obesity. *Mol Cell Endocrinol* **402**:113–119.

236. Trentham-Dietz A, Newcomb PA, Egan KM, *et al.* (2000) Weight change and risk of postmenopausal breast cancer (United States). *Cancer Causes Control* **11**:533–542.

237. Queen NJ, Boardman AA, Patel RS, *et al.* (2020) Environmental enrichment improves metabolic and behavioral health in the BTBR mouse model of autism. *Psychoneuroendocrinology* **111**:104476.

238. Solum DT, Handa RJ. (2002) Estrogen regulates the development of brain-derived neurotrophic factor mRNA and protein in the rat hippocampus. *J Neurosci* **22**:2650–2659.

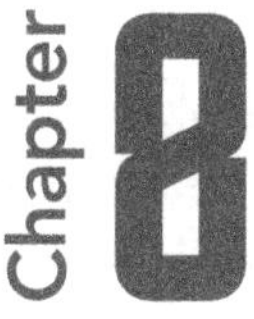

Environmental Enrichment as a Eustress Model: Identifying Brain Mediators Distinguishing Eustress and Distress Impact on Cancer

Introduction

In a review article "What is the brain-cancer connection?" published in *Annual Review of Neuroscience* in 2012,[1] we put forward some thoughts of environmental enrichment (EE) as a model of eustress and potential regulatory mechanisms distinguishing eustress and distress impact on cancer. During the following years, we have attempted to test these ideas and the results suggest adjustment of the hypothesis. This chapter will revisit the original ideas,[1] summarize experimental data for and against the hypothesis, and propose a revised hypothesis.

Social Determinant of Health and Survival

The notion that social relationship strongly influences human health has been recognized for a long time. Three decades ago, House and colleagues published a review article, summarizing five prospective studies published in the 1970–80s, noting a causal impact of social relationships on health.[2] With regard to influence on human longevity, the effect size of social relationships is on par with or greater than that of more appreciated risk factors, such as cigarette smoking, obesity, sedentary lifestyle, and hypertension. Prospective studies consistently show increased mortality in people with low quantity, and in some cases low quality, of social relationships.[2] This seminal report in 1988 has drawn intensive attention to the field of social determinant of health and longevity. In 2010, Holt-Lunstad and colleagues published a meta-analysis review of 148 studies on social relationships and mortality risk.[3] This meta-analysis shows a mean odds ratio (OR) = 1.50, meaning a 50% increased likelihood of survival for participants with stronger social relationships. Of note, the effect size appears to be affected by the approaches used to assess social relationships. Studies simply discriminating between people who lived alone versus those who did not show the weakest effect (OR = 1.13), whereas studies employing a more complex assessment to determine social integration revealed the strongest effect (OR = 1.91). This meta-analysis[3] confirms and strengthens the conclusion of the 1988 report[2] by providing compelling prospective epidemiological support of the link between social integration and all-cause mortality, including cancer.

The strength of this relationship between social integration and mortality appears as robust as that of cigarette smoking. Cacioppo and Patrick have advocated the subjective feeling of loneliness as a better predictor than many objective measurements of social integration such as the size of social networks. Accumulating evidence supports this notion. For example, perceived loneliness is associated with a specific pattern of and brain activation on functional magnetic resonance imaging (fMRI),[4] and loneliness activates the hypothalamic-pituitary-adrenal (HPA) axis,[5] moreover, circulating dendritic cells and monocytes, typical antigen-presenting cells, display gene expression patterns suggestive of altered immune function responsive to the state of loneliness.[6] Holt-Lunstad published another review in 2018 summarizing recent progress in the field and proposed a framework through which to bring social connection into the realm of public health.[7]

Although many of these studies did not specifically address cancer, evidence is increasingly compelling that an individual's perception of their social integration is an important risk factor for overall morbidity and mortality, including cancer. As social stimulation is an integral component of EE, EE can serve as a valuable paradigm to investigate how social environments influence health and disease including cancer. In an EE, animals often live with more peers. Even the number of mice in EE does not differ from the standard environment (SE), the presence of novel objects, toys, and running wheels can promote social engagement. As such, EE may serve as a model to study the quality of social relationships instead of simply the number of social contacts. Our work in the past decade has shown that EE exerts multiple benefits on metabolic and immune health, aging, and cancer resistance (Chapters 2, 3, 4, 6, and 7). Interestingly, EE is associated with a mild but significant increase of circulating corticosterone, the main glucocorticoid in mice, in absence of any experimentally imposed stress. Moreover, these EE-induced benefits are mediated by either the sympathetic nervous system (SNS) or HPA axis, or sometimes both arms of stress responses, in a tissue- and organ-dependent manner. This finding brought about the idea of EE as a model for eustress.

Flavors of Stress

Stress bears a bad taste to general public. However, the term "stress" is rather ambiguous. The concept of stress originated with the pioneering work of Walter Cannon purporting to show that physiological regulation primarily concerns maintaining each internal parameter at a set point and using feedback to defend this set point against deviation. He coined the term "homeostasis" to describe this theory of "stability through constancy" — body-centered, error-correcting theory of regulation.[8] Broadly speaking, stress relates general concepts associated with external and/or internal changes that induce an adaptive response in the organism. Any actual or potential disturbance of an organism's internal or external environment (stressor) is recognized or perceived by specific brain regions. The subjective state of sensing potentially adverse changes in the environment is defined as stress, which activates the HPA axis and/or the autonomic nervous system (ANS) in order to mitigate a threat.[9] Stress is most commonly used to describe a negative or excessive maladaptive state harmful to health and well-being. But as McEwen and Gianaros noted, the real or perceived environmental demands can be appraised as threatening or benign, and the ensuing biological, behavioral, and social coping responses can be labeled as "good," "tolerable," and "toxic." Both the appraisal of stressor and the following stress response are heavily influenced by the degree to which an individual has control over a given stressor and has support systems and resources for handling a given stressor.[10] Moreover, these physiological responses are not static and change dynamically in response to the duration and severity of the stressor.

Sterling and Eyer introduced a concept of allostasis in 1980s to describe a regulatory theory of "stability through change." In order to be fit, an organism must anticipate changing conditions and employ feed-forward signals to adjust all parameters to meet predicted needs.[11] In a recent review, Sterling and Schulkin clarify that allostasis and homeostasis are not mutually exclusive, but rather complementary: where predictions fail, there are errors to correct, therefore requiring both types of regulation.[12] They define the concept of allostasis as a brain-centered, predictive mode of physiological regulation. "The brain, sensing the internal and external milieu, and consulting its database, predicts what is likely to be needed; then, it computes the best response. The brain rewards a better-than-predicted result with a pulse of dopamine, thereby encouraging the organism to learn effective regulatory behaviors. The brain, by prioritizing behaviors and dynamically adjusting the flows of energy and nutrients, reduces costly errors and exploits more opportunities."[12]

McEwen and colleagues later introduced the term "allostatic load or overload" to refer to the consequence of allodynamic regulatory wear and tear on the body and brain promoting ill health.[13] Allostatic load can derive from either too much stress or inefficient management of allostasis. Examples of the latter include failure of turning off the response when no longer needed, inability of turning on an adequate response in the first place, or dampening the allostatic response when the same stressor recurs.[13] According to the theory of allostasis and allostatic load/overload, multiple interacting mediators operate in a nonlinear network to influence functions of multiple systems, such as brain function, metabolism, cardiovascular function, neuroendocrine function, and immune function.[10]

However, allostasis and allostatic load have yet been widely accepted whereas the term "stress" remains ubiquitous. In our publications, we adopt the classic stress literature terms "eustress" (positive stress) and "distress" (negative stress) to describe the relevant environmental milieu, health outcomes, and disparate underlying mechanisms.[1,14] Hans Selye, the pioneer importing the concept of stress into experimental medicine, noted that departures from homeostasis could be either "eustressful" or "distressful," and that health effects would vary accordingly.[15,16] Eustress is related to adaptive responses to benign environments leading to beneficial effects on health, whereas maladaptive distress is associated with exposure to more severe aversive or hostile environments resulting in allostatic load and ill health.[15,16] Eustress is a seldomly used term but we consider it a viable concept as research has revealed distinct activation patterns of neuroendocrine axes upon exposure to perceived "positive stress" versus "negative stress."

Psychosocial Factors and Cancer

The notion that psychosocial factors can affect cancer progression has long been suspected.[17] Numerous clinical and epidemiological studies have recognized that certain psychosocial factors are risk factors for the development and progression of cancer, such as stress, chronic depression, and lack of social support.[17,18] Stress-related psychosocial factors are associated with a higher cancer incidence in premorbid healthy people, poorer survival in cancer patients, and higher cancer mortality[19] although the positive link between stressful life events and cancer initiation is less consistent.[20–23] In contrast, psychosocial factors such as hopelessness, denial, suppression of negative emotions, and lack of social support are found more reliable to predict progression of already-diagnosed cancers.[18] Of note, "stress" in these literatures should be more precisely referred as "distress."

Animal studies parallel these clinical and epidemiological data demonstrating that experimentally imposed distress can modulate cancer progression.[24] According to classical literature of stress, the brain perceives a threat and activates the sympathetic-adrenal-medullary (SAM) axis and/or the HPA axis, resulting in the release of catecholamines (mainly epinephrine and norepinephrine), glucocorticoids (cortisol in humans and corticosterone in rodents), and other stress hormones from the adrenal gland, brain, and sympathetic nerve terminals within innervated tissues. These factors can modulate the activity of various components of the tumor microenvironment, which are the focus of an emerging field of neural regulation of cancer.

Mechanistic studies have identified specific pathways that can mediate the pro-cancer effects of experimentally imposed distress. The majority of studies on stress–cancer relationship support the notion that psychosocial and behavioral risk factors initiate a cascade of information-processing pathways in the brain triggering fight-or-flight stress response by activating the SAM axis, and/or defeat/withdraw responses through the HPA axis, thereby affecting multiple aspects of tumorigenesis and progression.[25,26] In an integrated model of bio-behavioral influences on cancer pathogenesis,[26] psychosocial/behavioral factors affect cancer-related processes by regulating neuroendocrine hormones, such as glucocorticoids and catecholamines that directly and indirectly act on tumor microenvironment. Direct effects include promoting tumor cell proliferation, tumor-related angiogenesis, invasion, metastasis, immune evasion, and drug resistance. Indirect effects of stress hormones include activating oncogenic viruses and altering immune function such as antibody production, cytokine profiling, and immune cell trafficking. These pleiotropic effects of stress hormones resulting from activation of the SAM and HPA axes collectively support tumor initiation and progression.[27–29] In addition, stress hormones can compromise cancer immunotherapy.[30,31]

It is important to note that the vast majority of mechanistic research on the stress–cancer relationship subject animals to experimental stressors associated with negative aspects of severe stress, better referred to distress, such as restraint stress,[32–34] social isolation (SI),[35–37] and social confrontation/defeat.[30,38] In contrast, the positive functions of a milder stress or challenging but manageable environment (eustress/hormesis) have been neglected. Failure to appreciate the distinction between eustress and distress may misunderstand the nature of pathways linking environmental milieu to cancer and hinder the development of interventions for cancer prevention and treatment.

Environmental Enrichment as a Eustress Model

Our research has characterized various health benefits of EE, including anti-obesity, anticancer, antiaging, and fine-tuning immunity. Hypothalamic brain-derived neurotrophic factor (BDNF) plays a major role in orchestrating many of these adaptive responses to the social, physical, and cognitive stimuli provided by EE (Chapters 2–7).[14,39–44] A wealth of experimental animal studies has almost invariably shown that EE has beneficial effects on an animal's health and well-being. However, EE also moderately, but significantly, increases corticosterone level in serum and norepinephrine level in white adipose tissue (WAT).[14,39] Both glucocorticoid and norepinephrine are signature stress hormones. It may appear paradoxical that chronic increase of stress hormones can be associated with an anticancer phenotype and other health benefits. It is worth noting that both corticosterone and norepinephrine are metabolic regulators catabolizing energy stores to meet immediate metabolic demands. EE raises energy expenditure, thus it is not surprising that both the HPA axis and SNS are activated and WAT is mobilized to meet this energy demand.[1] As EE elicits a mild increase of classical stress hormones but is associated with overall beneficial effects on health and well-being, we believe EE can be used as a valuable model of eustress.

Our recent investigations on immune functions support this notion. As discussed in Chapter 6, EE boosts the anticancer immunity of T cells and natural killer (NK) cells in the spleen and lymph nodes while protects against autoimmunity by regulating T cell development in the thymus. Importantly, these immunomodulatory effects of EE are mediated either by the SNS or by the HPA axis, and sometimes by both, depending on the immune cell populations, the lymphoid organs, and the state of disease[42-44] (**Fig. 8.1**).

How to reconcile this EE-induced beneficial immune modulation with the large body of work on the immunocompromising effects of stress? Appreciation of the context of a stressor offers an explanation. Eustress-associated environmental challenges (e.g. EE) may be appraised by the brain differently than those stressors associated with distress (e.g. social defeat), thereby resulting in distinct brain responses, and the ensuing specific or coordinated activation of the SNS and HPA axis. These regulatory pathways are

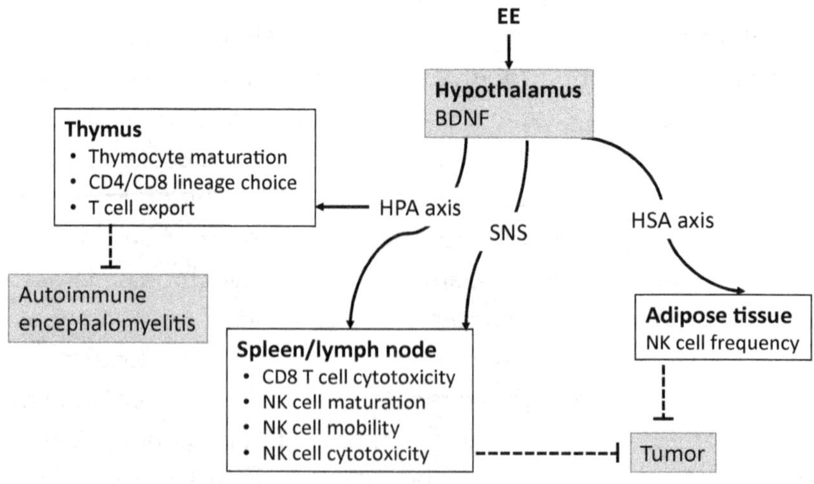

Fig. 8.1.   EE immunomodulatory effects driven by hypothalamic BDNF.

not linear but rather are connected within a complex network. The overall immune outcomes are influenced by the type of neural and neuroendocrine activity, the immune cell populations, the levels of stress mediators, and the temporal and spatial regulation of stress hormones. Whether there is an immune demand matters as well. For example, we observed that EE induced thymus involution in naïve mice, but prevented the autoimmunity-induced thymus involution in a mouse model of multiple sclerosis.[43] Experiencing eustress may train the immune system to be more adaptive and agile, and therefore can launch a proper immune response when such a demand occurs. In this sense, EE might be viewed as a behavioral "vaccine."

Social Isolation as a Distress Model

Loneliness is increasingly becoming the sad reality of modern life. For example, Britain alone has 9 million people often or always feeling lonely according to a 2017 report by the Jo Cox Commission on Loneliness. This crisis promotes United Kingdom to appoint a minister for loneliness. In the United States, more than 50% seniors experience loneliness.[45] Covid-19 pandemic has drastically disrupted social life worldwide and its debilitating effects could be disastrous and long lasting across age and sex groups. Numerous studies have identified social isolation (SI) as one of the most important risk factors for all-cause mortality,[46,47] and key risk factor for a variety of chronic diseases including cancer. Social support strongly predicts mental well-being and is linked to improved health outcomes among cancer patients[25] whereas SI predicts risk for mortality.[3,48] Several endogenous mechanisms are proposed such as inflammatory signals, glucocorticoids, and oxytocin. However, the underlying mechanisms are poorly defined. Animal research is undoubtedly necessary to identify the mechanisms mediating the detrimental effects of SI on both mental and physical well-being, particularly in states of compromised health.[46,47,49]

In humans, the detrimental effects of long-term SI and psychosocial stress on mental and physical health are well established.[50]

Rodent models of SI have proven highly effective at recapitulating human health outcomes that are strongly influenced by social milieu, including cardiovascular diseases, stroke, anxiety, depression, neuropathic pain,[46] neophobia, aggression, and cognitive rigidity.[47,51,52] SI is associated with increased tumor progression in animal models of breast cancer[47,53–55] and Ehrlich tumor.[56] SI may be the best model available, although not ideal, to study loneliness/social deprivation and its detrimental influence on cancer.

What Are the Mechanisms Driving Opposite Effects of Eustressful Environmental Enrichment versus Distressful Social Isolation on Cancer?

With regard to psychosocial environments, EE can represent social integration whereas SI can recapitulate social deprivation. Metabolic and immune mechanisms have been identified to mediate the anticancer effects of EE (Chapters 2 and 6). As to distress paradigms, animal studies suggest that prolonged activation of the HPA axis and the SAM axis by chronic stress may promote cancer progression and metastasis.[26] Dysfunction of immune system has also been implicated in distressed animals. A caveat of these studies is that the experimentally imposed stressors are often more severe than SI. For example, social defeat might model bullying while chronic unpredictable stress could model severe physical and psychological harassment. Hence, SI might not share similarity with these severe stressors in terms of impacts on cancer and the underlying mechanisms.

Hasegawa and Saiki report that SI promotes B16 melanoma growth in male C57BL/6 mice,[36] and oral administration of β blocker propranolol can abrogate the stress-accelerated B16 melanoma growth.[36] In contrast, our study using the same B16 melanoma transplant to the same strain C57BL/6 mice demonstrates that EE induces a remarkable tumor suppression. And oral propranolol can completely block the EE-induced leptin drop and inhibition of tumor growth.[14] It

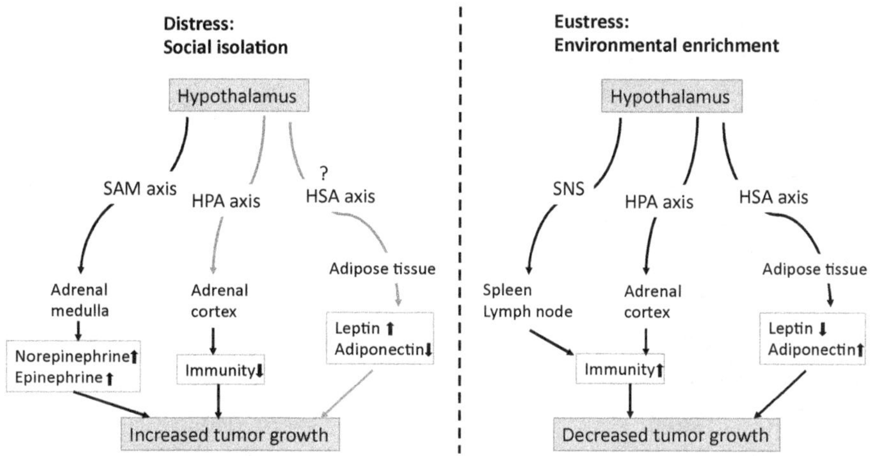

Fig. 8.2.   Mechanisms underlying the opposite effects of eustress versus distress on tumor growth.

appears that β blocker can abolish both the cancer-promoting effect of SI and the cancer-inhibiting effect of EE. How to reconcile the contradiction? We proposed a hypothesis in a review article in 2012,[1] and have revised the hypothesis according to recent research findings (**Fig. 8.2**). This seemingly paradoxical phenomenon reflects the distinct physiological responses to eustressful EE versus distressful SI that may involve three axes: the well-known HPA and SAM as well as the lesser-known hypothalamic-sympathoneural-adipocyte (HSA) axis.

The HPA axis is activated in response to both EE and SI, but the extent and duration may vary dependent of respective stress appraisal, leading to opposing modulation of immune function. EE enhances CD8 T cell immunity and NK cell immunity via activation of both the SNS and the HPA axis. Lesser is known how SI hampers anticancer immunity.

SI may activate the SAM axis thereby resulting in elevated norepinephrine levels in the circulation and possibly a local increase in the solid tumor itself. The increase of norepinephrine in tumor microenvironment can facilitate melanoma growth by stimulating proangiogenic factors including VEGF, and other direct and indirect actions similar to the observations reported in other cancer models.[37] In contrast, EE results in a significant increase of norepinephrine specifically in adipose tissues but not in muscle, and causes no significant change of circulating norepinephrine or epinephrine, suggesting minimal activation of the SAM[39] (**Fig. 8.2**).

A robust activation of the HSA axis is associated with and responsible in part for the EE-induced melanoma inhibition. The HSA axis response in SI remains to be investigated. We speculate that SI may suppress the HSA axis.

Our working hypothesis is that EE inhibits melanoma growth mainly through activating the HSA axis in combination with enhanced T cell and NK cell immunity through the SNS and/or the HPA axis, while SI promotes melanoma growth mainly through activating the SAM axis (possibly also suppressing the HSA axis, **Fig. 8.2**). Elucidating these regulatory mechanisms will have significant implications in individualized treatment. For example, several preclinical studies have shown that β blockers abrogate the deleterious effect of distress on cancer growth.[34,37] Some epidemiological and clinical studies support the link between the use of β blockers and reduced cancer risk,[57,58] and have led to the proposal of using β blocker as a therapeutic intervention for cancer.[59–61] However, recent clinical- and population-based studies on β blocker use and cancer mortality reveal inconsistent outcomes ranging from improved survival,[62,63] no effect,[64–66] to reduced survival.[67,68]

It is important to note that mediators of stress operate in a nonlinear network and the interactions are very complex. When any one mediator is altered, there are compensatory changes in the other mediators that depend on the time course and the magnitude of changes of each of the mediators.[10] As a result, we must analyze how environmental and psychosocial factors influence cancer in the context of the relevant environmental circumstance, individual coping strategy and adaptation, as well as impact on the specific cancer microenvironment biology. For individuals who are experiencing distress and inability to cope when their SAM axis is overactive, β blockers may be considered as an adjuvant therapy for cancer. On the other hand, when the HSA axis activation is the dominant force, for example, promoting eustress (active and engaging lifestyle) as a preventive strategy or supplementary treatment, the use of β blockers might attenuate eustress-induced tumor-inhibitory effects.

The complex interplay between the CNS and cancer often complicates the interpretation of human studies because it is immensely difficult to tease apart pathways in a clinical setting.[1] Laboratory animal studies in which environmental and psychosocial conditions can be properly controlled make it possible to dissect out the pathways and elucidate mechanisms, and to identify cellular and molecular mediators in the brain that may reveal potential therapeutic targets for cancer treatment. In this respect, animal models, even though far from representing human conditions faithfully, are indispensable and deserve attention.

References

1. Cao L, During MJ. (2012) What is the brain-cancer connection? *Ann Rev Neurosci* **35**:331–345.
2. House JS, Landis KR, Umberson D. (1988) Social relationships and health. *Science* **241**:540–545.
3. Holt-Lunstad J, Smith TB, Layton JB. (2010) Social relationships and mortality risk: A meta-analytic review. *PLoS Med* **7**:e1000316.
4. Cacioppo JT, Norris CJ, Decety J, *et al.* (2009) In the eye of the beholder: Individual differences in perceived social isolation predict regional brain activation to social stimuli. *J Cogn Neurosci* **21**:83–92.
5. Cacioppo JT, Ernst JM, Burleson MH, *et al.* (2000) Lonely traits and concomitant physiological processes: The MacArthur social neuroscience studies. *Int J Psychophysiol* **35**:143–154.
6. Cole SW, Hawkley LC, Arevalo JM, Cacioppo JT. (2011) Transcript origin analysis identifies antigen-presenting cells as primary targets of

socially regulated gene expression in leukocytes. *Proc Natl Acad Sci U S A* **108**:3080–3085.

7. Holt-Lunstad J. (2018) Why social relationships are important for physical health: A systems approach to understanding and modifying risk and protection. *Annu Rev Psychol* **69**:437–458.

8. Cannon W. (1932) *The Wisdom of the Body.* W.W. Norton, New York.

9. Joels M, Baram TZ. (2009) The neuro-symphony of stress. *Nat Rev Neurosci* **10**:459–466.

10. McEwen BS, Gianaros PJ. (2010) Central role of the brain in stress and adaptation: Links to socioeconomic status, health, and disease. *Ann N Y Acad Sci* **1186**:190–222.

11. Sterling P, Eyer J. (1988) Allostasis: A new paradigm to explain arousal pathology. In: S Fisher, J Reason (eds), *Handbook of Life Stress, Cognition and Health.* John Wiley & Sons, New York.

12. Schulkin J, Sterling P. (2019) Allostasis: A brain-centered, predictive mode of physiological regulation. *Trends Neurosci* **42**:740–752.

13. McEwen BS. (1998) Protective and damaging effects of stress mediators. *N Engl J Med* **338**:171–179.

14. Cao L, Liu X, Lin E-JD, *et al.* (2010) Environmental and genetic activation of a brain-adipocyte BDNF/leptin axis causes cancer remission and inhibition. *Cell* **142**:52–64.

15. Selye H. (1974) *Stress without Distress.* McClelland and Stewart, Ltd., Toronto.

16. Milsum JH. (1985) A model of the eustress system for health/illness. *Behav Sci* **30**:179–186.

17. Reiche EM, Nunes SO, Morimoto HK. (2004) Stress, depression, the immune system, and cancer. *Lancet Oncol* **5**:617–625.

18. Armaiz-Pena GN, Lutgendorf SK, Cole SW, Sood AK. (2009) Neuroendocrine modulation of cancer progression. *Brain Behav Immun* **23**:10–15.

19. Chida Y, Hamer M, Wardle J, Steptoe A. (2008) Do stress-related psychosocial factors contribute to cancer incidence and survival? *Nat Clin Pract Oncol* **5**:466–475.

20. Duijts SF, Zeegers MP, Borne BV. (2003) The association between stressful life events and breast cancer risk: A meta-analysis. *Int J Cancer* **107**:1023–1029.

21. Lillberg K, Verkasalo PK, Kaprio J, *et al.* (2003) Stressful life events and risk of breast cancer in 10,808 women: A cohort study. *Am J Epidemiol* **157**:415–423.

22. Price MA, Tennant CC, Butow PN, *et al.* (2001) The role of psychosocial factors in the development of breast carcinoma: Part II. Life event stressors, social support, defense style, and emotional control and their interactions. *Cancer* **91**:686–697.

23. Kruk J, Aboul-Enein BH, Bernstein J, Gronostaj M. (2019) Psychological stress and cellular aging in cancer: A meta-analysis. *Oxid Med Cell Longev* **2019**:1270397.

24. Thaker PH, Sood AK. (2008) Neuroendocrine influences on cancer biology. *Semin Cancer Biol* **18**:164–170.

25. Glaser R, Kiecolt-Glaser JK. (2005) Stress-induced immune dysfunction: Implications for health. *Nat Rev Immunol* **5**:243–251.

26. Antoni MH, Lutgendorf SK, Cole SW, *et al.* (2006) The influence of bio-behavioural factors on tumour biology: Pathways and mechanisms. *Nat Rev Cancer* **6**:240–248.

27. Green McDonald P, O'Connell M, Lutgendorf SK. (2013) Psychoneuroimmunology and cancer: A decade of discovery, paradigm shifts, and methodological innovations. *Brain Behav Immun* **30 Suppl**: S1–9.

28. Armaiz-Pena GN, Cole SW, Lutgendorf SK, Sood AK. (2013) Neuroendocrine influences on cancer progression. *Brain Behav Immun* **30 Suppl**: S19–25.

29. Cole SW. (2013) Nervous system regulation of the cancer genome. *Brain Behav Immun* **30 Suppl**: S10–18.

30. Yang H, Xia L, Chen J, *et al.* (2019) Stress-glucocorticoid-TSC22D3 axis compromises therapy-induced antitumor immunity. *Nat Med* **25**:1428–1441.

31. He XY, Ng D, Van Aelst L, Egeblad M. (2019) Stressing out about cancer immunotherapy. *Cancer Cell* **36**:468–470.

32. Steplewski Z, Vogel WH, Ehya H, *et al.* (1985) Effects of restraint stress on inoculated tumor growth and immune response in rats. *Cancer Res* **45**:5128–5133.

33. Saul AN, Oberyszyn TM, Daugherty C, *et al.* (2005) Chronic stress and susceptibility to skin cancer. *J Natl Cancer Inst* **97**:1760–1767.

34. Sloan EK, Priceman SJ, Cox BF, *et al.* (2010) The sympathetic nervous system induces a metastatic switch in primary breast cancer. *Cancer Res* **70**:7042–7052.

35. Palermo-Neto J, de Oliveira Massoco C, Robespierre de Souza W. (2003) Effects of physical and psychological stressors on behavior, macrophage activity, and Ehrlich tumor growth. *Brain Behav Immun* **17**:43–54.

36. Hasegawa H, Saiki I. (2002) Psychosocial stress augments tumor development through beta-adrenergic activation in mice. *Jpn J Cancer Res* **93**:729–735.

37. Thaker PH, Han LY, Kamat AA, *et al.* (2006) Chronic stress promotes tumor growth and angiogenesis in a mouse model of ovarian carcinoma. *Nat Med* **12**:939–944.

38. Stefanski V, Ben-Eliyahu S. (1996) Social confrontation and tumor metastasis in rats: Defeat and beta-adrenergic mechanisms. *Physiol Behav* **60**:277–282.

39. Cao L, Choi EY, Liu X, *et al.* (2011) White to brown fat phenotypic switch induced by genetic and environmental activation of a hypothalamic-adipocyte axis. *Cell Metab* **14**:324–338.

40. During MJ, Liu X, Huang W, *et al.* (2015) Adipose VEGF links the white-to-brown fat switch with environmental, genetic, and pharmacological stimuli in male mice. *Endocrinology* **156**:2059–2073.

41. McMurphy T, Huang W, Liu X, *et al.* (2019) Hypothalamic gene transfer of BDNF promotes healthy aging in mice. *Aging Cell* **18**:e12846.

42. Mansour AG, Xiao R, Bergin SM, *et al.* (2020) Enriched environment enhances NK cell maturation through hypothalamic BDNF in male mice. *Eur J Immunol* **51**:557–566.

43. Xiao R, Bergin SM, Huang W, *et al.* (2019) Enriched environment regulates thymocyte development and alleviates experimental autoimmune encephalomyelitis in mice. *Brain Behav Immun* **75**:137–148.

44. Xiao R, Bergin SM, Huang W, *et al.* (2016) Environmental and genetic activation of hypothalamic BDNF modulates T-cell immunity to exert an anticancer phenotype. *Cancer Immunol Res* **4**:488–497.

45. Gerst-Emerson K, Jayawardhana J. (2015) Loneliness as a public health issue: The impact of loneliness on health care utilization among older adults. *Am J Public Health* **105**:1013–1019.

46. Karelina K, DeVries AC. (2011) Modeling social influences on human health. *Psychosom Med* **73**:67–74.

47. Hinzey A, Gaudier-Diaz MM, Lustberg MB, DeVries AC. (2016) Breast cancer and social environment: Getting by with a little help from our friends. *Breast Cancer Res* **18**:54.

48. Berkman LF, Syme SL. (1979) Social networks, host resistance, and mortality: A nine-year follow-up study of Alameda County residents. *Am J Epidemiol* **109**:186–204.

49. Zelikowsky M, Hui M, Karigo T, *et al.* (2018) The neuropeptide Tac2 controls a distributed brain state induced by chronic social isolation stress. *Cell* **173**:1265–1279.e1219.

50. Cacioppo JT, Hawkley LC, Norman GJ, Berntson GG. (2011) Social isolation. *Ann N Y Acad Sci* **1231**:17–22.

51. Lapiz MD, Fulford A, Muchimapura S, *et al.* (2003) Influence of post-weaning social isolation in the rat on brain development, conditioned behavior, and neurotransmission. *Neurosci Behav Physiol* **33**:13–29.

52. Fone KC, Porkess MV. (2008) Behavioural and neurochemical effects of post-weaning social isolation in rodents-relevance to developmental neuropsychiatric disorders. *Neurosci Biobehav Rev* **32**:1087–1102.

53. Hasen NS, O'Leary KA, Auger AP, Schuler LA. (2010) Social isolation reduces mammary development, tumor incidence, and expression of epigenetic regulators in wild-type and p53-heterozygotic mice. *Cancer Prev Res (Phila)* **3**:620–629.

54. Williams JB, Pang D, Delgado B, *et al.* (2009) A model of gene-environment interaction reveals altered mammary gland gene expression and increased tumor growth following social isolation. *Cancer Prev Res (Phila)* **2**:850–861.

55. Hermes GL, Delgado B, Tretiakova M, *et al.* (2009) Social isolation dysregulates endocrine and behavioral stress while increasing malignant burden of spontaneous mammary tumors. *Proc Natl Acad Sci U S A* **106**:22393–22398.

56. Palermo-Neto J, Fonseca ES, Quinteiro-Filho WM, *et al.* (2008) Effects of individual housing on behavior and resistance to Ehrlich tumor growth in mice. *Physiol Behav* **95**:435–440.

57. Algazi M, Plu-Bureau G, Flahault A, *et al.* (2004) [Could treatments with beta-blockers be associated with a reduction in cancer risk?]. *Rev Epidemiol Sante Publique* **52**:53–65.

58. Perron L, Bairati I, Harel F, Meyer F. (2004) Antihypertensive drug use and the risk of prostate cancer (Canada). *Cancer Causes Control* **15**:535–541.

59. Melamed R, Rosenne E, Shakhar K, *et al.* (2005) Marginating pulmo-nary-NK activity and resistance to experimental tumor metastasis: Suppression by surgery and the prophylactic use of a beta-adrener-gic antagonist and a prostaglandin synthesis inhibitor. *Brain Behav Immun* **19**:114–126.

60. De Giorgi V, Grazzini M, Gandini S, *et al.* (2011) Treatment with beta-blockers and reduced disease progression in patients with thick melanoma. *Arch Intern Med* **171**:779–781.

61. Lemeshow S, Sørensen HT, Phillips G, *et al.* (2011) beta-Blockers and survival among Danish patients with malignant melanoma: A popula-tion-based cohort study. *Cancer Epidemiol Biomarkers Prev* **20**:2273–2279.

62. Choi CH, Song T, Kim TH, *et al.* (2014) Meta-analysis of the effects of beta blocker on survival time in cancer patients. *J Cancer Res Clin Oncol* **140**:1179–1188.

63. Udumyan R, Montgomery S, Fang F, *et al.* (2017) Beta-blocker drug use and survival among patients with pancreatic adenocarcinoma. *Cancer Res* **77**:3700–3707.

64. Reda S, Ahl R, Szabo E, *et al.* (2020) Pre-operative beta-blocker ther-apy does not affect short-term mortality after esophageal resection for cancer. *BMC Surg* **20**:333.

65. Musselman RP, Bennett S, Li W, *et al.* (2018) Association between perioperative beta blocker use and cancer survival following surgical resection. *Eur J Surg Oncol* **44**:1164–1169.

66. Coelho M, Squizzato A, Cassina N, *et al.* (2020) Effect of beta-block-ers on survival of lung cancer patients: A systematic review and meta-analysis. *Eur J Cancer Prev* **29**:306–314.

67. Couttenier A, Lacroix O, Silversmit G, *et al.* (2019) Beta-blocker use and mortality following ovarian cancer diagnosis: A population-based study. *Cancer Epidemiol* **62**:101579.

68. Gonzalez R, Gockley AA, Melamed A, *et al.* (2020) Multivariable anal-ysis of association of beta-blocker use and survival in advanced ovar-ian cancer. *Gynecol Oncol* **157**:700–705.

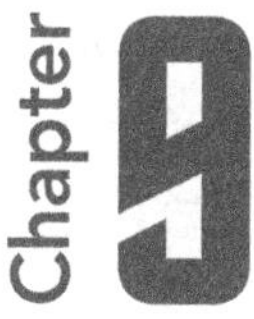

Why We Should Care about Laboratory Animal Housing: Implications of Environmental Enrichment Studies in Biomedical Research

Healthier and Happier Mice Make Better Science

Tens of millions of mice and rats are used in US labs each year. Vast majority of these laboratory rodents are housed in standard environment (SE). Numerous studies have established that environmental enrichment (EE) benefits the mental and physical health of laboratory animals including rodents. Yet the biomedical research community at large does not adequately appreciate the impact of housing environment on physiology and pathophysiology of laboratory animals essential for basic and translational research. It is understandable that advocating of housing most animals in species-appropriate EE housing has met resistance because of lack of awareness, absence of standardization of EE paradigm, and perhaps more critically the enormous cost of space, material, and labor to make such a change.[1] Why should we care about laboratory animal housing? Because healthier and happier mice make better science.

One of the most asked questions about EE research is the relevance to human health. There are several angles to look at this question. Laboratory animals are used to understand fundamental biology while vast majority of them are used for biomedical research with the ultimate goal of translating to treat human diseases and improve human health. As we call them animal models, we certainly should care deeply whether these animal models can faithfully or at least as close as possible to "model" human conditions. I was often asked when presenting our research on EE: Are we enriched? My answer is probably yes for those among the audience. We, the biomedical research community, are perhaps "over enriched" as many are experiencing hectic schedule, high pressure of performance, and intense competition of research funding and career advancement. But people who are deprived of healthy physical and social environments do exist. In this respect, mice living in SE can be seen as a model recapitulating some aspects of these unfortunate ones who are at risk of poor mental and physical health. In other words, animals living in EE may represent ordinary or normal humans more appropriately. If EE should be a default housing condition for laboratory animals, SE housing can be used to study unhealthy living conditions such as sedentary lifestyle and boredom.

It should be noted that mice in SE live a comfortable life with free access to food and water, in temperature- and humidity-controlled environment, and usually are protected from bacterial and viral infections. Laboratory mice are also free from predators. However, SE is not optimal for rodent health and well-being as EE results in better mental and physical health in normal mice and a variety of disease models as summarized in Chapters 1–8. Some researchers view SE as a so-called "impoverished" environment conferring minimal physical, social, cognitive, motor, and somatosensory stimulation.[2] Indeed, SE renders animals prone to obesity and other health risks.[3] We agree with the notion that EE is more analogous to the normal human experience than the SE.[4] Others insist that SE is appropriate for animal's well-being. Despite the debate, there should be consensus that social and physical environments can influence profoundly an individual's physiology and risk of developing a disease and its prognosis. Hence, mechanistic studies in animals should take the housing condition into consideration as a variable just like sex and age.

Many of therapeutics found to be promising in preclinical animal studies turn out to be disappointing in clinical studies. The causes of failure of translating are likely several, such as the intrinsic difference of biology between species. Could housing of laboratory animals contribute? Most preclinical studies are conducted in SE and sometimes in singly housing for convenience of collecting individual data, environments putting animals in a vulnerable situation. Interventions that have been proved to be highly effective in the vulnerable animals might become less successful in patients who are not suffering from those deprivations. Hence, preclinical studies may be performed in both SE and EE in order to better evaluate the translational potentials. This practice certainly increases expenses of animal studies, but it can be cost-effective or even cost-saving given the huge waste due to the dismal success rate of translating to the clinic.

Another pushback to widely adopting EE is that EE introduces unnecessary variability to experimental research.[1] Admittedly, EE protocols vary among laboratories, but this protocol-derived variability contributes relatively little to total variance observed in EE experiments.[5] In our opinion, the main goal of EE is to discover conserved biological mechanisms that are therapeutically or preventively relevant, and can be implicated in human health and disease. Thus, the fact that EE paradigms with technical variability among laboratories largely result in similar phenotypes should be seen as a strength of the EE model system rather than a weakness.

Taking animal housing as a variable might facilitate research of precision medicine. Current focus of the field is the genetic makeup of each individual. For any given disease, considerable variance exists in patients with regard to the risk and prognosis, for which genetic factors cannot fully account. Should each individual's broad living environment be treated as an important element for precision medicine? Animal studies support this notion. From this perspective, we argue that EE might be a more apt model for understanding disease development and progression than SE alone, providing a modeling system for interindividual differences in exposure to complex stimuli that more closely mirrors the complexity of the human experience.[6,7]

Although many of the biomedical research community adopt a deductive view by emphasizing discrete disease processes, a holistic or integrative view is increasingly gaining traction. EE can enable interrogation of systemic processes, mind-and-body connection, and interaction between internal and external cues, and therefore facilitate integrative biology research.

In addition, EE may reveal effects of a therapeutic otherwise are not found in SE. For instance, we observed additive metabolic benefits of combining CSF1R inhibitor PLX5622 and EE in middle-aged mice. Some of the effects of CSF1R inhibitor were not found in middle-aged mice living in SE.[8] Thus, investigating testing agents in laboratory animals living in EE may offer insight into biological pathways that are likely at play in patient populations, but are hidden in animals housed in SE. To that end, identifying drugs that have additive effects on top of or in combination with EE pathways becomes highly relevant for translatability. Attention to pathway-overlapping interactions between therapeutics has been raised in order to improve therapeutic efficacy. However, simply putting together two individually effective interventions is not necessarily successful. For example, metformin is widely considered as the best initial pharmacological option for managing type 2 diabetes (T2D).[9] Meanwhile, increased physical exercise is beneficial to patients with metabolic syndrome.[10] Naturally, the combination of these first-line treatment modalities of metformin and exercise has been widely recommended for managing diabetes. However, recent studies have casted doubt on this combinational treatment as antagonistic, rather than synergistic, effects have been found.[11–13] Hence, it is imperative for researchers to carefully assess combining prescriptions in preclinical animal models that are amenable to implementation in real patient populations.

Besides EE, ambient temperature has been shown to exert significant influence. For example, the confusion over the role of uncoupling protein 1 (UCP1) in bioenergetics is ascribed to housing temperature for the laboratory animals.[14] As mentioned in Chapter 3, UCP1 is a classic uncoupler that mediates adaptive thermogenesis in response to β-adrenergic receptor activation. Overexpressing UCP1 in adipose tissue or skeletal muscle protects against obesity,[15,16] but surprisingly obesity does not develop in UCP1 knockout mice under regular laboratory conditions.[17] Feldmann and colleagues later solved this controversy by housing mice at thermoneutrality.[18] Thermoneutrality refers to the temperature at which an animal needs to expend the lowest energy for maintaining body temperature. The thermoneutral zone is from 28°C to 30°C for naked humans, and from 22°C to 25°C for people wearing clothes indoors. Thermoneutrality for mice is around 30°C. However, laboratory mice are usually housed at approximately 22°C, a "room temperature" comfortable to us, but cold to them. As a result, mice under chronic cold stress must increase their energy metabolism and food consumption by ~50%.[19] This altered metabolism induced by chronic thermal stress masks the obesogenic phenotype in UCP1 knockout mice. Indeed, when being maintained at thermoneutral temperature, UCP1 knockout mice become obese even on normal chow diet, and exhibit more dramatic obesity when fed a high-fat diet.[18] By simply changing housing temperature, the investigators reveal a profound phenotypic impact of UCP1 that is obscured by UCP1-independent processes activated to maintain body temperature at "room temperature."

In addition to metabolism, studies indicate significant impact of ambient housing temperature on immunity and cancer in mice.[20,21] Kokolus and colleagues report a striking reduction in tumor formation, growth rate, and metastasis in mice living at thermoneutral temperature free from mild chronic cold stress. This improved control of tumor growth is dependent on the adaptive immune system, associated with increased numbers of tumor infiltrating antigen-specific CD8

T cells and activated CD8 T cells whereas decreased numbers of immunosuppressive myeloid-derived suppressor cells (MDSCs) and regulatory T cells at thermoneutrality. Notably, tumor-bearing mice prefer a higher ambient temperature than non-tumor-bearing mice, indicating tumor-bearing mice experiencing a greater cold stress.[22] A recent study describes several physiologically relevant thermal treatments to influence MDSC accumulation in tumor-bearing mice. These temperature-based protocols, such as weekly whole-body hyperthermia, housing at thermoneutrality, and providing a localized heat source to mice housed at sub-thermoneutral temperature, all result in decreased MDSC accumulation and reduced tumor growth compared to mice housed at standard temperature. Treatment of low-dose β-blocker propranolol mimics the effects of the thermal treatments on MDSC and tumor growth.[23] These findings suggest that cold stress–induced thermogenesis may suppress antitumor immunity. Therefore, preclinical studies in mice housed at standard room temperature may underestimate the efficacy of a cancer immune therapeutic.[24]

Accumulating evidence indicates negative impacts on physiology of mice housed under standard vivarium conditions regarding various housing parameters such as temperature, density, bedding, cage environment, cage tops, cage color, noise, light intensity, and husbandry.[3,14,25–29] The resulting concern is prompting biomedical researchers to consider how these factors influence experimental outcomes in animal studies. Acknowledgment of environmental impact and keen appreciation of the nuances of physiological systems may lead to better strategies to "humanize" animal models that are critical for basic and translational research.

The Search for EE Translation

If SE is considered an impoverishment, EE can mitigate these detrimental effects. Reversely, if SE is seen as an appropriate living condition, EE appears to improve health and resilience to disease. The latter is the mostly accepted view. How to translate findings from EE research in laboratory animals to humans has been a topic of debate.[4] It is difficult to match animal toys, shelters, bedding, etc., to the human conditions, but such attempts might not be necessary since EE must be species appropriate. The fundamental premise of EE research is that the underneath pathways are conserved among species including humans. Therefore, the goal of translational research is to seek human interventions that regulate the shared pathways discovered by EE studies in animals, either through lifestyle modifications or targeted pharmacotherapies.[30] In several reviews and book chapters,[6,7,31,32] my colleagues and I have discussed the implication of EE for human health and the challenge of translatability. Talented graduate students and postdoc researchers of our lab, Nicholas Queen, Seemaab Ali, Quais Hassan, II, and Run Xiao, have excellently articulated our thoughts on how to harness knowledge garnered from laboratory EE model to guide the design and development of human interventions. Although these recent articles are focused on aging and cancer, the concepts may generalize to overall health and a wide range of diseases. This chapter will reiterate these ideas with the desire of stimulating research to bridge the bench-to-bedside gap toward maximizing human health.

Lifestyle Interventions

EE is a laboratory condition that recapitulates some aspects of an active lifestyle, and therefore can facilitate mechanistic studies, which are vital to understand conserved mechanisms that contribute to human health and disease. For example, numerous clinical data have shown that lifestyle factors (education level, work position, cognitive and social activities) and behavioral interventions (physical exercise and cognitive stimulation) make important impacts on health and disease.[33–37] It is perhaps futile to pinpoint each component of EE setting to a correspondent human analog, and it is impossible to match every human lifestyle factor to EE of animals. However, it is not difficult to see the links between animal EE and human lifestyle/behavioral interventions, anchored on the three key components — increased physical activity, cognitive stimulation, and social engagement. All of the three are influenced by intrinsic drive but can also be nudged by physical and social environments.

Physical Activity

Increasing physical activity is one of the most effective measures to improve well-being and prevent a variety of disease processes, including T2D,[38–40] cardiovascular disease (CVD),[41,42] obesity,[43] ischemic stroke,[44,45] cancer,[46,47] and affective disorders,[48,49] among others. These benefits of physical exercise have been replicated in animal studies. Voluntary exercise is thought to modulate hypothalamic-pituitary-adrenal (HPA) axis signaling,[50] immune function,[51,52] muscle maintenance,[53] adipose remodeling,[51,54] neurogenesis,[55,56] and health span.[57,58]

Animal studies across healthy, obese, and aging models have shown a positive correlation between physical activity and brain-derived neurotrophic factor (*Bdnf*) levels within brain and peripheral tissues.[59–63] Providing opportunities to exercise is no doubt a critical component of EE. It is worthy of noting that a great deal of research has sought to define the magnitude that voluntary physical activity contributes to the EE phenotype in animal models. Some evidence indicates that voluntary physical activity and EE act on dissociable pathways even both share phenotypic similarities.[64] Other work suggests that voluntary physical activity may "prime" physiological change induced within EE.[65,66] Several reviews comprehensively cover these topics.[67–69]

Based on our own research,[70–72] we take the stand that the full EE phenotype often surpasses what is accomplished with exercise alone, suggesting the confluence of EE stimuli are vital for the observed improvements in health.[6] This brings about the following questions: What element within EE can add on top of the well-characterized physical exercise? What social or psychological elements might positively or negatively influence exercise benefits? How can we design exercise interventions to maximize its benefits? It is natural to understand that exercising with buddies or playing team sports are great ways to motivate physical activities. But EE studies in animals suggest it is possible to enhance the benefits of exercise by enriching the macroenvironment through shared or distinct mechanisms. Raising the awareness of social and psychological influence on exercise may not only improve research on exercise biology and sports medicine, but also guide the design and implementation of exercise intervention tailoring to individuals or community.

Socialization and Mental Stimulation

Enrichment of an animal's environment provides opportunities to exercise, socialize, and play. Additional peers may improve social life. As we noted in Chapter 1, even without changing the number of peers sharing the living environment, the presence of objects (running wheel, toys, etc.) may incentivize social engagement and in some cases necessitate such social connection. EE of animals provides cognitive stimulations by regular rearrangement of objects within EE environment.

Obviously, rodent models are no match for human intelligence and social structure. However, lifestyle factors, in their broad sense, are increasingly included in the health history questionnaire of a patient following the rising awareness of their critical impacts on health. Measures to encourage healthy lifestyles are being taken in addition to exercise, smoking cessation, and eating a balanced diet. For instance, art is recognized as a vital, rather than optional, human experience important for well-being, which results in offering free or reduced admission to museums to those receiving social assistance. People who actively seek out inherently complicated careers or hobbies, engage in spiritual or religious activities, or appreciate auditory and visual aesthetics tend to enjoy better health and quality of life, all are difficult if not impossible to recapitulate in animal models.[6] What a human may perceive as beauty and enjoyable, another animal may ignore or avoid.

We actually did a pet project several years ago to examine the metabolic outcomes in SE mice upon exposure to music several hours a day. Then we realized that music to our ears is likely white noise to mice, and such experiment must be properly controlled. Furthermore, the effects of a particular stimulus can differ among individual people. I chose to play new-age music to the mice because of my own taste. In hindsight, this was not a proper study design due to lacking consideration of not only species-specific effects but also individual perception. Perhaps, sounds in the nature are better options to study auditory effects on mice, but definitely not cat meow sound. Adding more complexity, perception of a given stimulus is not static but may change within a particular person as time goes by. For humans, it is difficult to tell where instinct ends and personality begins.[6]

One element of EE that is not often mentioned is sense of safety and self-control by retreats, more hiding places, extra bedding within an EE. In our opinion, this component is important to avoid unwanted conflicts with peers and to elicit eustressful or allostatic adaptions. Human social life can be incredibly complicated, and there is no one-size-fits-all solution. Some prefer open floor design of office space, whereas others enjoy segregated cubicles. Extroverts can gain strengths from larger audience in person, whereas introverts may feel much more comfortable to speak up in small group and in situations they can control. In the time of zoom meeting everywhere, it is not surprising to see reactions varying from exhaustion to joy. Whether animal model of EE can mirror some human psychology, at least to some extent, require further investigations. Nevertheless, the importance of safety and self-control is no doubt conserved between mice and humans, and the regulatory mechanisms are likely shared.

These difficulties don't make EE studies in animals useless. Many EE mechanisms such as BDNF, leptin, adiponectin, and the HPA axis–mediated stress response are known to be conserved between mice and humans. These are potential biomarkers for bio-behavioral interventions in humans. For example, clinical researchers at the Ohio State University have been conducting "gardening" projects to diabetes patients or cancer survivors. Many of the participants are from underprivileged communities. The program offers nutritional counseling and organizes gardening activities in groups. Participants take home harvest of vegetables and fruits. The program is successful at promoting healthy lifestyle and improving quality of life. Such a program consists physical, social, and mental stimuli of an EE. It will be interesting to examine the biomarkers of EE identified from animal studies in this kind of human interventions.

On the other hand, there may exist additional mechanisms unique to human-centric stimuli. The biomarkers or pathways that are identified in humans can be tested in laboratory EE models, even different environmental cues are employed, representing a bedside-to-bench approach. If these biomarkers are wholly conserved, laboratory EE models will allow in-depth mechanistic interrogations that will ultimately benefit humans.

Therapeutic Value of EE and Lifestyle Interventions

In a review article, Nicholas Queen and Quais Hassan, II, both are graduate students, put forward excellent writing of our views on potential therapeutic values of EE and lifestyle interventions to improve health span and how EE model may inform future public health and medical considerations as researchers and clinicians connect the bench and bedside.[6] These ideas can be applied to people across the life span, and therefore are reiterated here. The following section "Optimization of Environment in Medicine" is excerpt from our recent review article.[6]

Optimization of Environment in Medicine

Anecdotally, most people would agree that physical environment and psychological stress can affect recovery from disease or injury. However, it wasn't until an article published in *Science* in 1984 by Roger Ulrich[73] that rigorous scientific study of the effects of design in the healthcare environment was truly considered. In 2008, an extensive literature review by Ulrich *et al.* deeply examined how exposure to factors such as natural and artificial light, noise, plants, art, air quality, color, simulated and actual views of nature, and support groups or other social opportunities could greatly affect the healing process.[74] Exploration, categorization, and evaluation of these factors over the last 35 years has led to the development and iterative refinement of frameworks for "evidence-based design" and best practices in which to create "optimal healing environments," both inside and out of clinical encounters.[75–78]

Early classifications of features required for healing predominantly focused on the perspective of a patient's external environment including a sense of control of surroundings, access to social support, and access to positive distractions.[77] Over time, others expanded and refined these classifications to evaluate the internal, interpersonal, and behavioral environments, in addition to external experiences of patients.[76] A recent review of the emotional, psychological, social, behavioral, and functional antecedents of healing has specifically indicated that creation of a homelike environment, with access to views and nature, appropriate light exposure, noise control, and a room layout that minimizes barriers not only improves patient safety and satisfaction, but also improves recovery, representing the emphasis that evidence-based design places on environmental factors.[75] More specific explorations of these factors include studying patient exposure to natural and artificial light on sleep quality and subsequent recovery,[79] how the design of mental health facilities affects stress and behavior,[80,81] and how perceptions of loneliness diminish recovery from stroke.[82] Studies evaluating the effects of acoustics and sound on medical outcomes[83–85] have also concluded that sound can both help and hinder recovery. Although ambient noise from poor building design, conversations heard from hallways or shared patient rooms, and various machines and medical devices negatively impact patients through impaired sleep and increased stress, relaxing music and music of a patient's choice have been demonstrated to aid healing and decrease stress.

One underlying factor acknowledged in all of these studies and reviews is the significance of a patient's perception of control, a factor considered important early on in this field.[77] Even when both patients and healthcare providers ultimately have little to no control over outcomes, patients benefit from feeling like they can exert some influence over their situation. In a study exploring how perceptions of the treatment environment in a palliative care setting affected patient perceptions of positive emotion during treatment,[86] patients reported that personalized decorations, maintaining a familiar daily rhythm with familiar tasks, and creation of a sense of "coziness" or "homeliness" was important for their sense of well-being and experience of positive emotions. It is clear that these factors do not only impact terminally ill patients and that the contribution of environmental factors on psychological and physical health extend to people in all states of health.

Another well-explored aspect of improving health and the healing process is exposure to nature. Instead of incidentally viewing nature through a window, patients and their families are now receiving in-depth real and simulated exposure in and out of the healthcare setting surpassing just a therapeutic adjunct. Recent work in this area has included studying psychological benefits from exposure to nature through indoor and outdoor spaces in general,[87,88] as well as during childbirth,[89] before colonoscopy,[90] for those visiting someone in an intensive care unit,[91] and exposure to sights, sounds, and scents from a traditional Japanese garden for those with cognitive impairment.[92] These studies and reviews emphasize that exposure to nature decreases stress, increases happiness and satisfaction with treatment, improves sleep, and leads to measurable improvements in recovery: additionally, these exposures provide socialization and an improved perception of control of one's environment. It is important to consider the complexity of healthcare environments in such studies; care must be taken to evaluate whether these nature-related stress reductions are correlative or causative, controlling for relevant variables. The development and use of biomarkers will push this field forward, alongside clinical outcome metrics.

It is important to iterate that the therapeutic benefits of factors useful in creating optimal healing environments are not limited to healthcare settings or even in unhealthy individuals. More recent work has explored the use of nature-based stimuli as a therapeutic driver for well-being in healthy aged individuals.[93–95] Horticultural therapy within community or home gardens and the inclusion of green spaces within neighborhoods, hospitals, and nursing homes shows incredible promise to benefit people across a wide spectrum of health. Experiencing complex stimuli such as nature shows immense benefits to one's well-being, in sickness and in health, and even when simulated through pictures or video or through temporary exposure.

Therapeutic Translation Originating from Laboratory EE Studies

Attempts to translate EE-mediated therapy originated from animal models remain in their infancy. Three clinical trials by Woo and Leon are among the first examples of direct translation of EE in animal models of autism spectrum disorder (ASD) to clinical studies.[96–98] These randomized clinical trials have shown that EE in the form of Sensory Enrichment Therapy is capable of ameliorating symptoms of ASD. The most recent trial enrolled 1002 children (United States and international) across a wide age range (1–15 years old) and the EE therapy was delivered via an online system. This EE therapy appears to be an effective, low-cost treatment of ASD symptoms across different ages, geographic location, gender, and symptom severity under real-world conditions.[98] Additionally, EE has been shown to improve the symptoms of children with Rett syndrome.[99] These studies provide a clear example of how preclinical studies in animal models of brain disorders can directly inform clinical investigations and trials.

Chapter 4 describes our efforts to develop gene therapies targeting genes that are critical players among the regulatory network driving the beneficial effects of EE on health and disease. Such research has yielded technical advances and promising preclinical data leading to licensing of autoregulatory BDNF gene therapy to a biotech company that intends to bring this gene therapy to clinic. Moreover, our research on EE has drawn attention to adipose tissue, which has been under the radar in the field. To meet the basic research need, we have developed rAAV vector systems enabling selective and efficient genetic manipulation of adipose tissue. As a result, these technological advances may tread a new path to adipose-oriented molecular therapies for metabolic disorders and beyond (either genetic or acquired diseases).

Gene therapy is unlikely a possibility for prevention and treatment of many common diseases. Nevertheless, EE research in animal models has provided insights for researchers to develop novel environmimetics and epimimetics for pharmacological use — concepts proposed by Hannan and colleagues. These goals are exceptionally important since lifestyle interventions are difficult to implement in the long-term and are rarely a panacea.[30,100]

In summary, I hope the book help to convince biomedical research community and the public that we should care about laboratory animal housing. Improving laboratory animal housing conditions can benefit not only animal welfare but also basic and translational research with the ultimate goal to improve human health, well-being, and disease prevention and treatment.

References

1. Hutchinson E, Avery A, VandeWoude S. (2005) Environmental enrichment for laboratory rodents. *ILAR J* **46**:148–161.
2. Kempermann G. (2019) Environmental enrichment, new neurons and the neurobiology of individuality. *Nat Rev Neurosci* **20**:235–245.
3. Martin B, Ji S, Maudsley S, Mattson MP. (2010) "Control" laboratory rodents are metabolically morbid: Why it matters. *Proc Natl Acad Sci U S A* **107**:6127–6133.
4. Burrows EL, McOmish CE, Hannan AJ. (2011) Gene–environment interactions and construct validity in preclinical models of psychiatric disorders. *Prog Neuro-Psychopharmacol Biol Psychiatry* **35**:1376–1382.
5. Wolfer DP, Litvin O, Morf S, *et al.* (2004) Laboratory animal welfare: Cage enrichment and mouse behaviour. *Nature* **432**:821.
6. Queen NJ, Hassan QN, 2nd, Cao L. (2020) Improvements to healthspan through environmental enrichment and lifestyle interventions: Where are we now? *Front Neurosci* **14**:605.
7. Hassan QN, 2nd, Queen NJ, Cao L. (2020) Regulation of aging and cancer by enhanced environmental activation of a hypothalamic-sympathoneural-adipocyte axis. *Transl Cancer Res* **9**: 5687–5699.
8. Ali S, Mansour AG, Huang W, *et al.* (2020) CSF1R inhibitor PLX5622 and environmental enrichment additively improve metabolic outcomes in middle-aged female mice. *Aging (Albany NY)* **12**:2101–2122.
9. Inzucchi SE, Lipska KJ, Mayo H, *et al.* (2014) Metformin in patients with type 2 diabetes and kidney disease: A systematic review. *JAMA* **312**:2668–2675.

10. Sampath Kumar A, Maiya AG, Shastry BA, *et al.* (2019) Exercise and insulin resistance in type 2 diabetes mellitus: A systematic review and meta-analysis. *Ann Phys Rehabil Med* **62**:98–103.

11. Boulé NG, Robert C, Bell GJ, *et al.* (2011) Metformin and exercise in type 2 diabetes: Examining treatment modality interactions. *Diabetes Care* **34**:1469–1474.

12. Boulé NG. (2012) Complex relationship between metformin and exercise in diabetes treatment: Should we reconsider our recommendations? *Diabetes Manage* **2**:5–8.

13. Konopka AR, Laurin JL, Schoenberg HM, *et al.* (2019) Metformin inhibits mitochondrial adaptations to aerobic exercise training in older adults. *Aging Cell* **18**:e12880.

14. Lodhi IJ, Semenkovich CF. (2009) Why we should put clothes on mice. *Cell Metab* **9**:111–112.

15. Kopecky J, Rossmeisl M, Hodný Z, *et al.* (1996) Reduction of dietary obesity in aP2-Ucp transgenic mice: Mechanism and adipose tissue morphology. *Am J Physiol* **270**:E776–786.

16. Li B, Nolte LA, Ju J-S, *et al.* (2000) Skeletal muscle respiratory uncoupling prevents diet-induced obesity and insulin resistance in mice. *Nat Med* **6**:1115–1120.

17. Enerback S, Jacobsson A, Simpson EM, *et al.* (1997) Mice lacking mitochondrial uncoupling protein are cold-sensitive but not obese. *Nature* **387**:90–94.

18. Feldmann HM, Golozoubova V, Cannon B, Nedergaard J. (2009) UCP1 ablation induces obesity and abolishes diet-induced thermogenesis in mice exempt from thermal stress by living at thermoneutrality. *Cell Metab* **9**:203–209.

19. Golozoubova V, Gullberg H, Matthias A, *et al.* (2004) Depressed thermogenesis but competent brown adipose tissue recruitment in mice devoid of all hormone-binding thyroid hormone receptors. *Mol Endocrinol* **18**:384–401.

20. Hylander BL, Repasky EA. (2016) Thermoneutrality, mice, and cancer: A heated opinion. *Trends Cancer* **2**:166–175.

21. Gandhi S, Oshi M, Murthy V, *et al.* (2021) Enhanced thermogenesis in triple-negative breast cancer is associated with pro-tumor immune microenvironment. *Cancers* **13**:2559.

22. Kokolus KM, Capitano ML, Lee C-T, *et al.* (2013) Baseline tumor growth and immune control in laboratory mice are significantly influenced by subthermoneutral housing temperature. *Proc Natl Acad Sci U S A* **110**:20176–20181.

23. MacDonald C, Ministero S, Pandey M, *et al.* (2021) Comparing thermal stress reduction strategies that influence MDSC accumulation in tumor bearing mice. *Cell Immunol* **361**:104285.

24. Eng JWL, Reed CB, Kokolus KM, *et al.* (2015) Housing temperature-induced stress drives therapeutic resistance in murine tumour models through beta(2)-adrenergic receptor activation. *Nat Commun* **6**:6426.

25. Karp CL. (2012) Unstressing intemperate models: How cold stress undermines mouse modeling. *J Exp Med* **209**:1069–1074.

26. Toth LA. (2015) The influence of the cage environment on rodent physiology and behavior: Implications for reproducibility of pre-clinical rodent research. *Exp Neurol* **270**:72–77.

27. Toth LA, Trammell RA, Ilsley-Woods M. (2015) Interactions between housing density and ambient temperature in the cage environment: Effects on mouse physiology and behavior. *J Am Assoc Lab Anim Sci* **54**:708–717.

28. Stemmer K, Kotzbeck P, Zani F, *et al.* (2015) Thermoneutral housing is a critical factor for immune function and diet-induced obesity in C57BL/6 nude mice. *Int J Obes (Lond)* **39**:791–797.

29. Tian XY, Ganeshan K, Hong C, *et al.* (2016) Thermoneutral housing accelerates metabolic inflammation to potentiate atherosclerosis but not insulin resistance. *Cell Metab* **23**:165–178.

30. Hannan AJ. (2020) Epimimetics: Novel therapeutics targeting epigenetic mediators and modulators. *Trends Pharmacol Sci* **41**:232–235.

31. Cao L, Ali S, Queen NJ. (2021) Hypothalamic gene transfer of BDNF promotes healthy aging. *Vitam Horm* **115**:39–66.

32. Xiao R, Ali S, Caligiuri MA, Cao L. (2021) Enhancing effects of environmental enrichment on the functions of natural killer cells in mice. *Front Immunol* **12**:695859.

33. Sampedro-Piquero P, Begega A. (2017) Environmental enrichment as a positive behavioral intervention across the lifespan. *Curr Neuropharmacol* **15**:459–470.

34. Webb VL, Wadden TA. (2017) Intensive lifestyle intervention for obesity: Principles, practices, and results. *Gastroenterology* **152**:1752–1764.

35. Bluher M. (2019) Obesity: Global epidemiology and pathogenesis. *Nat Rev Endocrinol* **15**:288–298.

36. Peisch SF, Van Blarigan EL, Chan JM, *et al.* (2017) Prostate cancer progression and mortality: A review of diet and lifestyle factors. *World J Urol* **35**:867–874.

37. Walsh R. (2011) Lifestyle and mental health. *Am Psychol* **66**:579–592.

38. Anonymous. (2004) Physical activity/exercise and diabetes. *Diabetes Care* **27**:s58–s62.

39. Colberg SR, Sigal RJ, Fernhall B, *et al.* (2010) Exercise and type 2 diabetes: The American College of Sports Medicine and the American Diabetes Association: Joint position statement. *Diabetes Care* **33**:e147–167.

40. Aune D, Norat T, Leitzmann M, *et al.* (2015) Physical activity and the risk of type 2 diabetes: A systematic review and dose–response meta-analysis. *Eur J Epidemiol* **30**:529–542.

41. Mora S, Cook N, Buring JE, *et al.* (2007) Physical activity and reduced risk of cardiovascular events: Potential mediating mechanisms. *Circulation* **116**:2110.

42. Wannamethee SG, Shaper AG. (2001) Physical activity in the prevention of cardiovascular disease. *Sports Med* **31**:101–114.

43. Wadden TA, Bray GA. (2018) *Handbook of Obesity Treatment*. Guilford Publications, New York.

44. Kiely DK, Wolf PA, Cupples LA, *et al.* (1994) Physical activity and stroke risk: The Framingham study. *Am J Epidemiol* **140**:608–620.

45. Lee CD, Folsom AR, Blair SN. (2003) Physical activity and stroke risk: A meta-analysis. *Stroke* **34**:2475–2481.

46. Ruiz-Casado A, Martín-Ruiz A, Pérez LM, *et al.* (2017) Exercise and the hallmarks of cancer. *Trends Cancer* **3**:423–441.

47. Brown JC, Winters-Stone K, Lee A, Schmitz KH. (2012) Cancer, physical activity, and exercise. *Compr Physiol* **2**:2775–2809.

48. Kandola A, Vancampfort D, Herring M, *et al.* (2018) Moving to beat anxiety: Epidemiology and therapeutic issues with physical activity for anxiety. *Curr Psychiatry Rep* **20**:63.

49. Schuch FB, Stubbs B. (2019) The role of exercise in preventing and treating depression. *Curr Sports Med Rep* **18**:299–304.

50. Droste SK, Gesing A, Ulbricht S, *et al.* (2003) Effects of long-term voluntary exercise on the mouse hypothalamic-pituitary-adrenocortical axis. *Endocrinology* **144**:3012–3023.

51. Vieira VJ, Valentine RJ, Wilund KR, *et al.* (2009) Effects of exercise and low-fat diet on adipose tissue inflammation and metabolic complications in obese mice. *Am J Physiol-Endocrinol Metab* **296**:E1164–E1171.

52. Pedersen L, Idorn M, Olofsson GH, *et al.* (2016) Voluntary running suppresses tumor growth through epinephrine-and IL-6-dependent NK cell mobilization and redistribution. *Cell Metab* **23**:554–562.

53. White Z, Terrill J, White RB, *et al.* (2016) Voluntary resistance wheel exercise from mid-life prevents sarcopenia and increases markers of mitochondrial function and autophagy in muscles of old male and female C57BL/6J mice. *Skeletal Muscle* **6**:45.

54. Stanford KI, Middelbeek RJW, Goodyear LJ. (2015) Exercise effects on white adipose tissue: Beiging and metabolic adaptations. *Diabetes* **64**:2361–2368.

55. van Praag H, Kempermann G, Gage FH. (1999) Running increases cell proliferation and neurogenesis in the adult mouse dentate gyrus. *Nat Neurosci* **2**:266–270.

56. Cooper C, Moon HY, van Praag H. (2018) On the run for hippocampal plasticity. *Cold Spring Harb Perspect Med* **8**:a029736.

57. Kujala UM. (2018) Is physical activity a cause of longevity? It is not as straightforward as some would believe. A critical analysis. *British J Sports Med* **52**:914–918.

58. Holloszy JO, Smith EK, Vining M, Adams S. (1985) Effect of voluntary exercise on longevity of rats. *J Appl Physiol* **59**:826–831.

59. Gómez-Pinilla F, Ying Z, Roy RR, *et al.* (2002) Voluntary exercise induces a BDNF-mediated mechanism that promotes neuroplasticity. *J Neurophysiol* **88**:2187–2195.

60. Stranahan AM, Lee K, Martin B, *et al.* (2009) Voluntary exercise and caloric restriction enhance hippocampal dendritic spine density and BDNF levels in diabetic mice. *Hippocampus* **19**:951–961.

61. Molteni R, Wu A, Vaynman S, *et al.* (2004) Exercise reverses the harmful effects of consumption of a high-fat diet on synaptic and behavioral plasticity associated to the action of brain-derived neurotrophic factor. *Neuroscience* **123**:429–440.

62. Erickson KI, Miller DL, Roecklein KA. (2012) The aging hippocampus: Interactions between exercise, depression, and BDNF. *Neuroscientist* **18**:82–97.

63. Adlard P, Cotman C. (2004) Voluntary exercise protects against stress-induced decreases in brain-derived neurotrophic factor protein expression. *Neuroscience* **124**:985–992.

64. Olson AK, Eadie BD, Ernst C, Christie BR. (2006) Environmental enrichment and voluntary exercise massively increase neurogenesis in the adult hippocampus via dissociable pathways. *Hippocampus* **16**:250–260.

65. Fabel K, Wolf SA, Ehninger D, *et al.* (2009) Additive effects of physical exercise and environmental enrichment on adult hippocampal neurogenesis in mice. *Front Neurosci* **3**:50.

66. Kronenberg G, Bick-Sander A, Bunk E, *et al.* (2006) Physical exercise prevents age-related decline in precursor cell activity in the mouse dentate gyrus. *Neurobiol Aging* **27**:1505–1513.

67. Rogers J, Renoir T, Hannan AJ. (2019) Gene-environment interactions informing therapeutic approaches to cognitive and affective disorders. *Neuropharmacology* **145**:37–48.

68. Bekinschtein P, Oomen CA, Saksida LM, Bussey TJ. (2011) Effects of environmental enrichment and voluntary exercise on neurogenesis, learning and memory, and pattern separation: BDNF as a critical variable? *Semin Cell Dev Biol* **22**:536–542.

69. Pang TYC, Hannan AJ. (2013) Enhancement of cognitive function in models of brain disease through environmental enrichment and physical activity. *Neuropharmacology* **64**:515–528.

70. Cao L, Choi EY, Liu X, *et al.* (2011) White to brown fat phenotypic switch induced by genetic and environmental activation of a hypothalamic-adipocyte axis. *Cell Metab* **14**:324–338.

71. McMurphy T, Huang W, Queen NJ, *et al.* (2018) Implementation of environmental enrichment after middle age promotes healthy aging. *Aging* **10**:1698–1721.

72. Cao L, Liu X, Lin E-JD, *et al.* (2010) Environmental and genetic activation of a brain-adipocyte BDNF/leptin axis causes cancer remission and inhibition. *Cell* **142**:52–64.

73. Ulrich RS. (1984) View through a window may influence recovery from surgery. *Science* **224**:420.

74. Ulrich RS, Zimring C, Zhu X, *et al.* (2008) A review of the research literature on evidence-based healthcare design. *HERD* **1**:61–125.

75. DuBose J, MacAllister L, Hadi K, Sakallaris B. (2018) Exploring the concept of healing spaces. *HERD* **11**:43–56.

76. Sakallaris BR, MacAllister L, Voss M, *et al.* (2015) Optimal healing environments. *Glob Adv Health Med* **4**:40–45.

77. Ulrich RS. (1991) Effects of interior design on wellness: Theory and recent scientific research. *J Health Care Inter Design* **3**:97–109.

78. Ulrich R. (1997) A theory of supportive design for healthcare facilities. *J Health Care Inter Design* **9**:3–7; discussion 21.

79. Hadi K, Du Bose JR, Choi Y-S. (2019) The effect of light on sleep and sleep-related physiological factors among patients in healthcare facilities: A systematic review. *HERD* **12**:116–141.

80. Connellan K, Gaardboe M, Riggs D, *et al.* (2013) Stressed spaces: Mental health and architecture. *HERD* **6**:127–168.

81. Ulrich RS, Bogren L, Gardiner SK, Lundin S. (2018) Psychiatric ward design can reduce aggressive behavior. *J Environ Psychol* **57**:53–66.

82. Anåker A, von Koch L, Heylighen A, Elf M. (2019) "It's lonely": Patients' experiences of the physical environment at a newly built stroke unit. *HERD* **12**:141–152.

83. Ulrich R. (2008) Effects of healthcare acoustics on medical outcomes. *J Acoust Soc Am* **123**:3094.

84. Joseph A, Ulrich R. (2007) Sound control for improved outcomes in healthcare settings. *Center Health Design* **4**:1–17.

85. Blomkvist V, Eriksen C, Theorell T, *et al.* (2005) Acoustics and psychosocial environment in intensive coronary care. *Occup Environ Med* **62**:e1.

86. Timmermann C, Uhrenfeldt L, Hoybye M, Birkelund R. (2014) A palliative environment: Caring for seriously ill hospitalized patients. *Palliat Support Care* **13**:1–9.

87. Lacanna G, Wagenaar C, Avermaete T, Swami V. (2019) Evaluating the psychosocial impact of indoor public spaces in complex healthcare settings. *HERD* **12**:11–30.

88. Sachs NA. (2019) A breath of fresh air: Outdoor spaces in healthcare facilities can provide clean air and respite. *HERD* **12**:226–230.

89. Aburas R, Pati D, Casanova R, Adams NG. (2017) The influence of nature stimulus in enhancing the birth experience. *HERD* **10**:81–100.

90. Sjölander A, Jakobsson Ung E, Theorell T, *et al.* (2019) Hospital design with nature films reduces stress-related variables in patients undergoing colonoscopy. *HERD* **12**:186–196.

91. Ulrich RS, Cordoza M, Gardiner SK, *et al.* (2019) ICU patient family stress recovery during breaks in a hospital garden and indoor environments. *HERD* **13**:83–102.

92. Goto S, Gianfagia TJ, Munafo JP, *et al.* (2017) The power of traditional design techniques: The effects of viewing a Japanese garden on individuals with cognitive impairment. *HERD* **10**:74–86.

93. Gagliardi C, Piccinini F. (2019) The use of nature – based activities for the well-being of older people: An integrative literature review. *Arch Gerontol Geriatr* **83**:315–327.

94. Gagliardi C, Santini S, Piccinini F, *et al.* (2019) A pilot programme evaluation of social farming horticultural and occupational activities for older people in Italy. *Health Soc Care Community* **27**:207–214.

95. Santini S, Piccinini F, Gagliardi C. (2019) Can a green care informal learning program foster active aging in older adults? Results from a qualitative pilot study in Central Italy. *J Appl Gerontol* **27**:207–214.

96. Woo CC, Leon M. (2013) Environmental enrichment as an effective treatment for autism: A randomized controlled trial. *Behav Neurosci* **127**:487–497.

97. Woo CC, Donnelly JH, Steinberg-Epstein R, Leon M. (2015) Environmental enrichment as a therapy for autism: A clinical trial replication and extension. *Behav Neurosci* **129**:412–422.

98. Aronoff E, Hillyer R, Leon M. (2016) Environmental enrichment therapy for autism: Outcomes with increased access. *Neural Plast* **2016**:2734915.

99. Downs J, Rodger J, Li C, *et al.* (2018) Environmental enrichment intervention for Rett syndrome: An individually randomised stepped wedge trial. *Orphanet J Rare Dis* **13**:3.
100. Kelly A, Hannan AJ. (2019) Therapeutic impacts of environmental enrichment: Neurobiological mechanisms informing molecular targets for enviromimetics. *Neuropharmacology* **145**:1–2.

Index

CPSIA information can be obtained
at www.ICGtesting.com
Printed in the USA
JSHW052314030522
25141JS00004B/7